Textbook
of
Performing Arts Medicine

Textbook
of
Performing Arts Medicine

Editors

Robert Thayer Sataloff, MD, DMA
Professor of Otolaryngology
Thomas Jefferson University
Director, Jefferson Arts—Medicine Center
Faculty, The Curtis Institute of Music and
The Academy of Vocal Arts
Philadelphia, Pennsylvania

Alice G. Brandfonbrener, MD
Assistant Professor of Clinical Medicine
Northwestern University Medical School
Director, Medical Program for
Performing Artists
Chicago, Illinois

Richard J. Lederman, MD, PhD
Department of Neurology
Director, Medical Center for Performing Artists
Cleveland Clinic Foundation
Cleveland, Ohio

Raven Press New York

Raven Press, Ltd., 1185 Avenue of the Americas, New York, New York 10036

Made in the United States of America

Library of Congress Cataloging-in-Publication Data

Textbook of performing arts medicine / [edited by] Robert Thayer Sataloff, Alice Brandfonbrener, Richard J. Lederman.
    p.   cm.
    Includes bibliographical references.
    Includes index.
    ISBN 0-88167-698-5
    1. Performing arts medicine. I. Sataloff, Robert Thayer. II. Brandfonbrener, Alice. III. Lederman, Richard J.
    [DNLM: 1. Dancing. 2. Music. 3. Occupational Diseases. WA 400 T3558]
RC965.P46T48   1990
616.9'802—dc20
DNLM/DLC
for Library of Congress   90-9001
                                                        CIP

9 8 7 6 5 4 3 2 1

To our patient and devoted spouses:
Dahlia M. Sataloff, M. D., Martin Brandfonbrener, M. D.,
and Barbara Lederman, J. D.

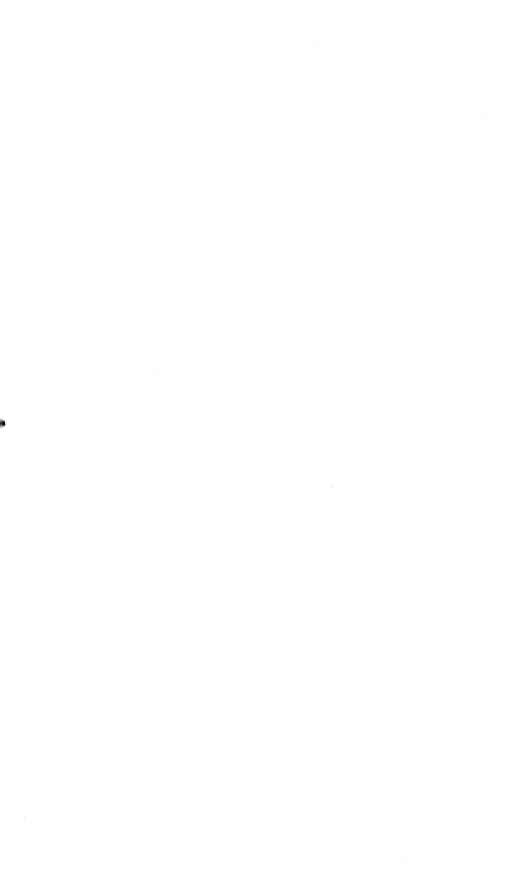

Foreword

It is with the greatest pleasure (enhanced, I admit, by the tiniest glimmer of smugness) that I write the foreword to this timely volume. As one pianist victim of performance-related dysfunction, I am constantly reminded of how far the medical profession has come over the last few years toward recognition of specific physical problems incurred by performing artists in the line of duty. Today, the idea of a book devoted to arts medicine is, while perhaps not exactly routine, nevertheless perfectly comprehensible. A decade ago, the very subject did not exist.

A decade ago, medical assistance—and, to a great extent, even medical sympathy—for an affliction such as mine was unavailable. In 1979, when I first sought help for a hand problem, my symptoms were described by the physicians I consulted as "bizarre" and "exotic." Today, similar symptoms in pianists are known to be not uncommon. Ten years ago, when I first sought help, I was considered to be either slightly crazy or terminally ill. Today, an instrumentalist similarly afflicted stands a good chance of obtaining at least an intelligent diagnosis. Ten years ago, I was bounced back and forth among a dozen orthopedists and neurologists, none of whom really wanted to have anything to do with me. Recently, I had the deliciously evil pleasure of lecturing a ballroom full of orthopedists and neurologists about the error of their ways.

Ten years ago, mine was a voice in the wilderness. Today, much of the undergrowth in that wilderness has been cleared away, and a pianist with symptoms similar to mine may visit performing arts clinics in Boston, Chicago, Cleveland, New York, Philadelphia, San Francisco, and in many other cities throughout the United States. Practically every week I receive information about new medical clinics for treating ailments of performing artists. For this I am grateful. I am also grateful to have been instrumental—albeit inadvertently—in the development of this new medical subspecialty, and also in alerting musicians—performers, teachers, and students alike—to the physical hazards they face. Simple awareness of these dangers on the part of the musician, as well as the musical and medical advisors, may go a long way toward prevention. If I had only known 12 or 15 years ago what almost every pianist now knows about these physical perils, I probably could have arrested the development of my problem before it became incapacitating.

At the time I first became conscious that something was very wrong with the way my right hand was functioning at the piano, there was literally no place for me to go, and no doctor who would really listen to what I was saying. My symptoms were so specialized that I needed a keyboard to demonstrate convincingly what was wrong. I had no pain, no numbness, no tingling. Only in certain very specific, extended positions of my right hand at the keyboard—playing a series of octaves, for example—did my trouble surface. I was able to play the first octave normally, but the act of striking each subsequent one caused my fourth finger to draw in more and more, dragging the fifth along with it as my hand contracted and, of course, I hit wrong notes. It was never any different. My hand could always normally negotiate certain patterns at the keyboard and, just as predictably, could never negotiate certain other patterns without contracting. I tried to articulate these symptoms verbally; I demonstrated physically as well as I could on examining-room tabletops. I was tested for all sorts of neurological blockages, tangles, injuries, and diseases, but when no abnormality could be found, I was regarded with exasperation as one of those mentally unbalanced artists—"aren't they all?"—and sent away.

Hard as it is to believe as I write this, not quite 10 years later, when occurrence of performance-induced dysfunction is so widely accepted, none of the 18 doctors I consulted during the fall and winter of 1979 would even consider the possibility that my disability might have been caused, or at least triggered, by playing the piano. Either I was nuts or, as some of the specialists decided, I must be suffering from one of several disorders of the central nervous system. "See? Those two fingers are curling, the earliest symptoms of Parkinson's disease," I was informed by one world-famed neurologist. "But," I reminded him, "only on my right hand" (the hand that gets most of the slamming). "Don't worry," he soothed me. "Your left hand will start to curl soon, too."

Ultimately, the nature of my performance-induced injury was finally recognized early in 1980. My experience led my friend and colleague, Leon Fleisher, whose right hand had been disabled for many years, to seek consultation as well. After a *New York Times* article appeared about our plight, instrumentalists from all over North America began to solicit help regarding physical disabilities possibly related to their work. By the summer of 1982, musicians with physical dysfunctions had begun to discover that what they had previously considered to be their unique miseries were, in fact, widely shared. Soon, doctors began to realize that most of the physical complaints of the musicians they examined were attributable, at least in part, to the mechanics of playing or in some cases simply holding their instruments.

And now, thanks to the extraordinary and continuing publicity that the field of arts medicine receives, such information is virtually common knowledge. Now we know that inflamed tendons and nerve compression, if not motor control disorders, are fairly typical afflictions of instrumentalists. We know that violinists can suffer neck, shoulder, and arm pain simply because of the way they grip the instrument. We know that trumpet players are prone to develop outpouching of the upper airway from the strain of hitting high notes. We know about harpist's cramp and flutist's skin eruption and bassoonist's thumb, and even that the height of a cellist's chair can cause formerly unsuspected difficulties. Performers have become infinitely more aware of the dangers that await in the pursuit of their daily routines.

I know that my piano students today are far more conscious of what they are doing physically at the instrument than my contemporaries and I were when we were students. Certainly I am more aware of my students' physical behavior at the instrument. If they complain of any strain or if they sustain any kind of injury that interferes even slightly with their playing, I advise them not to play at all until they can use the injured part of the body normally. By "normally," I mean what is normal for them, because there is no absolute right or wrong way to hold the hand, arm, wrists, etc., or to sit at the instrument. It has to be done in the way that is most natural for the individual—and there are almost as many different ways of playing naturally as there are individuals who play.

I think the most I can do as a teacher is to make sure that my students learn to be aware of what they are doing. They should learn to be conscious early on if they are sliding into physical habits that distort their natural position. This new awareness brings with it, unfortunately, the side effect of sometimes being too self-conscious, but I guess that is a lesser evil than permitting potentially devastating habits to take over, as happened with me.

For it is really only through education—and thus prevention—that we can keep these physical problems at bay. Treatment for many such dysfunctions is still in the experimental stage and so far some of them cannot be reversed. So it is up to those at risk to inform themselves about these dangers, how to avoid them, and what kind of medical help is available when necessary.

I think, therefore, that this book should be of immeasurable usefulness to performing artists of all kinds. I hope that it will prove similarly invaluable to members of the medical profession as well, particularly when presented with hand symptoms by a pianist, or foot symptoms by a dancer, or throat symptoms by a singer, or lower back symptoms by a cellist. To be sure, it is necessary for physicians to investigate all possibilities of disease. By all means, scan the brain and probe the psyche. But it is also crucial to remember that the very act of performing can also be injurious to a performer's health.

Gary Graffman

Preface

Textbook of Performing Arts Medicine is the first modern textbook in a new and exciting field of medicine. It was written because of a compelling need for information among physicians, performers, teachers, and therapists. Educational information has been difficult for most people to acquire because of the interdisciplinary nature of arts medicine. In recent years, the development of arts medicine has become possible because of collaboration among physicians, performers, music teachers, acting teachers, physical therapists, speech–language pathologists, nurses, dance instructors, and others who have not traditionally worked closely together. Teamwork has resulted in a new understanding among all the professions, and in the bridging of language barriers that have traditionally hindered musicians' access to treatment.

Interested physicians have risen to the special challenge of arts medicine. In most other areas of medicine, we are given wide latitude in our definition of "normal." Arts medicine does not permit such imprecision. The performing artist depends on the last small percentage of optimal human performance. The difference between 95% recovery of an injured finger and 100% recovery may mean the difference between a world-class performing career as a violinist and obscurity. Arts medicine physicians are learning to recognize the subtle differences between normal, supernormal, and perfection by performers' standards.

In addition to interdisciplinary teamwork, the development of performing arts medicine has been assisted through basic science research and new technology. While an enourmous amount of clinical and basic information remains to be discovered, and although performance applications of many of our new insights remain unexplored, it is clear that the field of arts medicine is firmly established. Its development is a proud saga of creative professional response to a neglected public health need. We are hopeful that this book will catalyze its further development by making information on the current state of the art in this new field readily accessible to physicians, performers, and all other professionals concerned with the care of performing artists. We look forward to continued, rapid advancement of all the subspecialties of arts medicine, and we anticipate including not only new information, but also additional subspecialties in future editions.

Robert Thayer Sataloff
Alice G. Brandfonbrener
Richard J. Lederman

Contents

Contributors

Marc Avery, M.D. *Assistant Adjunct Professor of Psychiatry, Psychiatric Consultant, Health Program for Performing Artists, University of California, San Francisco, California 94143*

Alice G. Brandfonbrener, M.D. *Assistant Clinical Professor of Medicine, Northwestern University Medical School, Director, Medical Program for Performing Artists of the Rehabilitation Institute of Chicago, Chicago, Illinois 60611*

Richard G. Eaton, M.D. *Professor of Clinical Surgery, College of Physicians and Surgeons of Columbia University, Division of Hand Surgery, Hand Center, Roosevelt Hospital, New York, New York 10019*

Susan E. Harman *Music Medicine Clearinghouse, Library, Medical and Chirurgical Faculty of the State of Maryland, Baltimore, Maryland 21201*

Richard A. Hoppmann, M.D. *Assistant Professor, University of South Carolina School of Medicine, Chief of Rheumatology, Dorns Veterans Hospital, Columbia, South Carolina 29201*

James A. Howard, D.D.S. *Clinical Assistant Professor, The University of Washington Dental Division, Children's Hospital, Seattle, Washington 98105*

Richard J. Lederman, M.D., Ph.D. *Department of Neurology, Director, Medical Center for Performing Artists, Cleveland Clinic Foundation, Cleveland, Ohio 44195*

Michael F. Marmor, M.D. *Stanford University Medical Center, Stanford, California 94305-5308*

William B. Nolan III, M.D. *Attending in Hand Surgery, Roosevelt Hospital Hand Center, New York, New York 10019*

Peter Ostwald, M.D. *Medical Director, Health Program for Performing Artists, University of California, San Francisco, California 94143*

Nicholas A. Patrone, M.D., F.A.C.P. *Clinical Associate Professor of Medicine and Pediatrics, East Carolina University School of Medicine, Greenville, North Carolina 27858*

Kyle D. Pruett, M.D. *Clinical Professor of Psychiatry, Yale Child Study Center, Coordinator of Training, Child Development Unit, Yale University, New Haven, Connecticut 06510*

Textbook of Performing Arts Medicine, edited
by R. T. Sataloff, A. Brandfonbrener, and
R. Lederman. Raven Press, Ltd.,
New York © 1991.

1

The Evolution of Performing Arts Medicine as Seen Through the Literature

Susan E. Harman

*Coordinator, Music Medicine Clearinghouse, Medical and Chirurgical Faculty Library,
Baltimore, Maryland 21201*

Over 100 years ago, an early researcher in the physiology of music making wrote, "It was always on the borderground between two great subjects of study that new phenomena were often to be looked for" (1). As today's researchers watch the field of arts medicine unfold, this quote seems prophetic. Practitioners from two disciplines which initially appeared so discordant are uniting to work toward common goals. In the last 10 or 15 years, the terrain of this borderground has become gradually more discernable, but the first tentative steps into the uncharted territory of arts medicine were taken by a great Italian physician in the early 1700s.

In his 1713 treatise, *Diseases of Tradesmen*, Bernardino Ramazzini gave what many consider the first summary of the occupational diseases of musicians. His list of possible problems included "rupture of the groin . . . distentions of the head, palpations [sic] of the temples, pulsations of the brain, inflations or swellings of the eyes and tingling in the ears . . . ruptures of the vessels of the breast," as well as fatigue of the lungs. Ramazzini's general opinion was, "There is no exercise, though never so healthful and innocent, but what may produce great disorders, if it [is] used with intemperance" (2).

For the rest of the eighteenth century and the beginning of the nineteenth, interest in the medical problems of musicians was sporadic at best. Few published reports in the medical literature alluded to any real study in this area. However, there were a number of unsubstantiated beliefs regarding the health of musicians. In 1874 Dr. W. H. Stone studied the wind pressure generated while playing musical instruments, concluding that such pressure was very unlikely to cause emphysema or other lung diseases (1). Despite a number of similar studies over the years that disproved it, this myth continued (3).

During the late 1800s a number of physicians turned their interest to musician's cramp. Writer's cramp had been recognized for some time, and telegrapher's cramp was becoming another significant problem in the occupational cramp lexicon.

1

While the majority of musician's cramp or palsy cases seemed to occur among pianists, there were also reports of cases among violinists (4), cornetists (5), and others.

George Vivian Poore, a British physician, did extensive research on pianist's cramp. He felt that the discomfort, fatigue, and loss of control could be brought on by overuse or injury. In his opinion, no two cases were exactly the same and quite often a positive diagnosis could not be made. While Poore used arsenic, counterirritation, and massage, his principal treatment was rest (6). It is ironic that today's physicians are just as mystified by "pianist's breakdown" (7).

During this same period, another problem of pianists was tackled by a number of surgeons, though not actually a disease, but many pianists complained that the ring finger was less independent and powerful than the other fingers. A Philadelphia surgeon, William S. Forbes, devised an operation he called "liberating of the ring finger." Between 1857 and 1885 he performed 14 of these tenotomies by dividing the accessory tendons of the extensor digitorum communis. Patients marveled at their increased agility and extension, and Forbes insisted there were very few complications from this minor procedure (8).

For the rest of the century, tenotomies remained the vogue for pianists, especially in the United States (9). A number of surgeons in urban centers seem to have specialized in this "corrective" procedure, some traveling to other cities at the behest of pianists and teachers (10,11). The visit of Professor E. S. Bonelli of San Francisco was enthusiastically reported in the *New York Times* of June 7, 1890 (12). While tenotomies fell from favor around 1900, there is some evidence the practice continued into this century (9).

PIANO TECHNIQUE

While physicians concentrated on what happened to the musician's playing when injured, there was a group of teachers and researchers who approached musicians from another angle. Especially among pianists, there was tremendous interest in proper technique, in all its varied definitions. Around the turn of the nineteenth century, many teachers still advocated what had become known as the "finger school" of playing, emphasizing use of the fingers only and extensive technical practice. This method worked well enough with the smaller, lighter harpsichords and pianofortes (13) but less well with the modern piano, which emerged between 1825 and 1900. Composers began to exploit the modern piano's increased power, speed, and brilliance with virtuoso pieces that pushed pianists to the limit (14). Not surprisingly, the best pianists intuitively changed their techniques to execute these difficult compositions. Those who could not or would not do so may have ended up among the breakdown casualties that Dr. Poore described (13).

Perhaps the most famous musician to suffer from a hand injury was the pianist and composer Robert Schumann. For most of his adult life, Schumann grappled with a disability of the fingers of the right hand. Over the years there have been various explanations advanced for this: use of a mechanical finger-strengthening device, excessive practice, toxic neuropathy due to mercury, or some sort of neurological lesion. The real etiology may never be known, but Schumann stands as a dramatic example of a virtuoso performing career cut short by hand disability (15).

Due to the new technical demands required of Schumann and others, piano teachers became more interested in anatomy and physiology. Teachers such as Rudolf Breithaupt and Tobias Matthay produced systematic texts that were filled with medical illustrations and discussions, advocating the use of arm weight while stressing relaxation. However, they often misunderstood scientific data and frequently disagreed with one another (13).

Out of the confusion surrounding piano technique emerged Otto Ortmann, director of the Peabody Conservatory in Baltimore. He organized a research department there and produced objective, thoroughly detailed work. In 1925 Ortmann published *The Physical Basis of Piano Touch and Tone*. This was followed in 1929 by what many consider the single most important book on piano technique ever published, *The Physiological Mechanisms of Piano Technique* (16). A proposed third volume in this series, discussing psychological aspects of technique, was incomplete when Ortmann died (13).

Unlike other pianists, Ortmann analyzed individual differences in the hand and arm and their impact on technique. He stressed coordination, basing his work on scientific procedures and laboratory experimentation. Ortmann used the most modern technology available, such as photography, dynamography, and pantography, to explore virtually every aspect of pianistic movement (17).

EARLY TWENTIETH CENTURY

In 1932 the English translation of another landmark publication appeared. Dr. Kurt Singer, a German neurologist with an extensive musical education, published *Diseases of the Musical Profession: A Systematic Presentation of Their Causes, Symptoms and Methods of Treatment*. In his preface, the translator remarked, "This volume will present a tremendous surprise," and indeed, it was virtually the first book devoted to the subject (18).

Singer discussed both the psychological and physical ailments of musicians. For "nervousness"—what today's physician might consider performance anxiety—he recommended a drastic reduction in practice time. Singer devoted a long section of his work to "psychopathic musicians," feeling that many performers' physical problems were psychologically determined (19).

Singer also discussed occupational cramps at length, listing causes, symptoms, and possible treatments. In a brief chapter he described rarer conditions, such as embouchure failure, vision problems, laryngitis, dental disorders, etc. (20). Emphysema was discussed: "An especially disagreeable disease among wind players, occasionally compelling the abandonment of the profession, is the enlargement of the lungs—emphysema" (18).

By today's standards, Singer's book is somewhat dated, and some of his opinions could be viewed as quaint or infuriating. For example: "The mother-complex is stronger in woman than the artist-complex. She inclines—predisposition assumed—more easily to peculiar hysterical states, to gloomy thoughts, to a collapse in the first conflict with life. . . . Biologically, woman's inferior creative power in music can be explained by her highest calling, that of motherhood" (18). However, Singer also provided some maxims which today's physicians would embrace: " 'Any exertion, according to its intensity, must be followed by adequate recovery' " (19).

Between 1930 and 1934 the International Labour Office (ILO), headquartered in Geneva, put out a two-volume encyclopedia entitled *Occupation and Health: Encyclopedia of Hygiene, Pathology and Social Welfare*. Two articles discussing occupational diseases of musicians, taking their cue from Singer, detailed an even longer list of problems than Ramazzini, including hand pain, myopia, cramps, dental problems, neuritis, tenosynovitis, and chronic laryngitis. Emphysema was noted and named as the most frequent problem among those occupations requiring continual respiratory effort, but it was acknowledged that no emphysema had been found in two extensive studies among musicians.

As a Labour Office publication, the encyclopedia reviewed legislation in regard to occupational diseases in various countries. In 1925, German musicians were negotiating for a contract which included pensions and death benefits. In the Netherlands, reporting of musician's cramp was required, and in the U.S.S.R., loss of the voice in singers was compensated. However, the editors stressed that "data are few and scattered throughout medical literature. Only of late years (1925–1926) have new studies commenced to appear . . . it is to be hoped that the specialists will direct their attention to the different branches of this art in order to make a more intensive study of its pathology" (21). The ILO publication's bibliography, perhaps understandably, appears to be almost entirely foreign literature. Many references refer the reader to other ILO bibliographies (21). Such vague citations would likely have discouraged many interested readers.

Indeed, various music medicine bibliographies which have attempted to reach back into the era before computerized or otherwise systematic periodical indexing, do not afford very many citations for the first half or even two-thirds of this century. One respected 1948 textbook, *Music and Medicine*, edited by Dorothy M. Schullian and Max Schoen, listed nearly 200 citations related to occupational diseases of musicians from both the music and medical literature. The vast majority of these are European and involve mostly vocal or dental problems (28). Two national clearinghouse bibliographies, concentrating mainly on English language items from both literatures, now contain some 600 citations. These include 17 from the 1800s, 1 from the 1920s, 5 from the 1930s, 4 from the 1940s, and 16 from the 1950s (23,24). *Index Medicus* itself, an indispensable aid to the early-twentieth-century physician, listed very few citations, English or foreign, between 1879 and 1966, when the National Library of Medicine began computerized indexing (25–28).

DENTAL AND VOCAL PROBLEMS

In the post–World War II era there continued to be some physicians, musicians, and others interested in music medicine. However, the various groups did not seem to communicate with each other very often or very effectively. From the earliest issues of *Music Index*, which began in 1949, the concerns of musicians can be seen. Most articles related to dental and vocal problems (29).

In 1967, M. M. Porter published a 12-part series in the *British Dental Journal* detailing practically all the dental problems that could occur in wind instrumentalists (30–41). Periodontal disease and tooth movement were primary concerns. Until recently, the total loss of teeth meant the end of a career, so this was a major threat for any wind instrumentalist (42). Music educators and orthodontists debated the interplay between orthodontia and the playing of wind instruments, with study results and opinions remaining mixed (43). Lip shields to protect soft tissue from irregular teeth were improvised from paper, foil, wax, and numerous other materials, becoming more "high tech" along with the rest of the scientific community (44).

Physician interest and involvement in the voice dates back at least to the time of Hippocrates in the fifth century B. C. His *Corpus Hippocraticum* provides some of the earliest medical speculation on the workings of the voice, recognizing the importance of the lungs, trachea, lips, and tongue in phonation. Aristotle noted the role of the voice in emotional expression. Claudius Galen, who practiced from 131 to 201 A. D., is hailed as the founder of laryngology and voice science, as noted in Von Leden's excellent review of the history of voice medicine (45). Galen wrote an essay on the human voice which is frequently referenced but unfortunately has been lost. He described the larynx, discussed the importance of the brain in controlling phonation, and distinguished for the first time between speech and voice. Galen's work went virtually unchallenged for more than 15 centuries, and some of it is still accepted.

Major advancement did not come until the Renaissance with the writings of Leonardo da Vinci, particularly *Quaderni d'Anatomia* in 1500. Additional important Renaissance writers who advanced knowledge of the voice included Andreas Vesalius, Bartolomeus Eustachius, and Fabricius Ab Aquapendente. Fabricius wrote three books on the larynx, including *De Larynge Vocis Instrumento*. Similar important advances occurred in the East, particularly in the ninth century, when Rhazes the Experienced in Baghdad described disorders of the voice and recommended respiratory and voice training. There are also excellent descriptions of voice production and disorders in the *Quanun*, written by Avicenna the Persian. The *Quanun* was a standard medical textbook for more than 500 years.

Additional advances occurred in the eighteenth century through the efforts of Giovanni Morgagni, who first related dysphonia to abnormalities in the larynx. Antoine Ferrein described physiological experiments on animal and human cadaver larynges and coined the term *vocal cords*, comparing the vocal folds to the strings of an instrument. Albrecht von Haller detailed the anatomy of vocal resonance. In Germany, Johannes Mueller described the mechanism of vocal-fold vibration. In the nineteenth century, Hermann von Helmholtz essentially started the science of acoustics with experiments that are still considered valid.

All of the scientists mentioned above laid the foundation for the close liaison that has existed between physicians and singers. However, the clear and widely recognized beginning of arts medicine in the voice world dates from the time of Manuel Garcia, who was born in 1805. Garcia was a world-famous opera singer in his teens. Although he was the son of an acclaimed singer and director, his apparently faulty technique and extensive operatic singing impaired his voice, causing him to retire while still in his twenties. Thereafter, he became a thoughtful, effective teacher and was made professor of singing at the Conservatoire de Paris at the age of 30. In 1854 Garcia bought a dental mirror and invented the technique of indirect laryngoscopy. The laryngeal mirror is still the basic tool for visualizing vocal folds and is used daily by otolaryngologists. Garcia observed larynges closely with his new tool and presented his findings before the Royal Society of Medicine in 1855. He was considered the greatest singing teacher of his age, and "on his one hundredth birthday in 1905 he was honored by physicians, music teachers and scientists from all over the world" (45).

Physicians and singers have enjoyed a liaison that is perhaps closer than that of instrumentalists with other specialists. Possibly because the vocalist's body is in effect his instrument, he is highly sensitive to changes and problems. Perhaps the history of medical interest in the voice, dating back centuries, made communication among singers and otolaryngologists somewhat easier and more natural. Vocal abuse, various kinds of laryngitis, vocal nodules, upper respiratory tract infections, and other difficulties came under the purview of otolaryngologists and voice therapists in this century (46).

Since 1972, the annual symposium, "Care of the Professional Voice," sponsored by the Voice Foundation, has brought together voice specialists from the fields of medicine, science, teaching, speech-language pathology, and performance. Its proceedings were originally published as a transcript, but have appeared in the *Journal of Voice* since 1987 (47). A number of other specialty journals have also featured articles on medical care of professional voice users. For example, in 1981 the *NATS Journal*, published by the National Association of Teachers of Singing, began a medical column called "Laryngoscope" (48) which appears in every issue.

In recent years many high-technology examination and measurement methods have become available, including strobovideolaryngoscopy, high-speed photography, and electromyography. In the 1980s, major advances in objective analysis of the voice dramatically improved the care of professional voice users, and voice medicine became established as a subspecialty of otolaryngology (49).

Even as early as the 1950s there were concerns beyond dental and vocal problems. Music educators placed what some might now consider unwarranted emphasis on germs from mouthpieces and other hygiene issues (50–53). A number of the medical articles published appeared to mention musicians only as interesting victims of diseases afflicting a more general population (54–57).

RISING CONCERN

The 1960s was a period of great interest in the physiology of music making. Prior to that time, as John Basmajian wrote in a discussion of vibration in trumpeters' lips, "Scientific experiments on musical performance are surprisingly sparse when one considers that neuromuscular control of skilful [sic] motor performance reaches its acme in music" (58). A Dutch researcher, Arend Bouhuys, did extensive studies on respiratory function and breathing in instrumentalists. His work discounted music making as a cause of emphysema (59–61). In the United States, scientist Kenneth W. Berger used electromyography and other technology to examine the playing of wind instruments, especially in regard to respiration and intraoral pressure (62). Many of these studies showed that what the musician thought his body was doing and what actually happened were frequently two very different things. Ironically, such confused instructions often produce the desired musical result. One writer attributed this to the musician's increased effort and abandon (63).

The 1960s also saw a rise in concern over hearing loss caused by music. Perhaps it is reflective of the musical tastes of most adult researchers that this occurred at about the same time as the advent of rock and roll. Initial studies focused on audiences at rock concerts and discos, with mixed results (64), as discussed elsewhere in this book. Most of the next group of surveys concerned rock musicians, concluding that this musical genre represents a definite risk for hearing loss.

Once researchers became interested in the orchestral environment, results were not so conclusive. Whether studies of the 1960s and 1970s attempted to measure rock or symphonic "noise," they often further clouded the issue due to the sort of sound that was measured, how far away it was, etc. However, many measurements beyond Occupational Safety and Health Administration (OSHA) standards for industry were recorded, and through OSHA standards might not be entirely applicable in a music context, these investigations did call attention to the problem (65).

In the late 1960s, several items in music journals signaled the beginning of what might be considered more serious interest in occupational diseases on the part of musicians. The May 1967 issue of the *Strad*, a British publication geared toward string players, carried an item by Dr. Frederick F. Polnauer and Morton Marks, M. D. Polnauer was a well-respected string teacher and coauthored, with Marks, *Senso-Motor Study and Its Application to Violin Playing*. After a short discussion of the importance of exploring the physiology of string playing, the authors wrote, "we are earnestly requesting the string playing public to furnish us with individualized and detailed case histories as to the nature and extent, cause and recurrences of the occupational hazards that the player has encountered" (66).

Also in 1967 the *Instrumentalist*, an American publication read by many music educators, published a letter by a trumpet professor, Maurice Faulkner. Faulkner summarized research on respiratory function and intrathoracic pressure carried out in Vienna and other European centers. He advised, "University medical schools and music departments should cooperate in wide-spread experimentation to learn the best methods of respiratory activity on all instruments" (67).

Faulkner himself had carried out experiments on the circulatory effects of trumpet playing, along with Dr. E. P. Sharpey-Schafer. Their 1959 article in the *British Medical Journal* (63) was cited in many subsequent studies (62, 68–71). In 1971 Faulkner collaborated with Alan Tucker and Steven M. Horvath at the Institute of Environmental Stress in California on a study of cardiopulmonary function in brass players. The study quoted figures showing an increased incidence of heart disease and a reduced life expectancy among musicians (70). These figures were reported widely in the medical and music literature for several years (68,69, 72–74).

BIRTH OF A FIELD

Also in the 1960s, physicians' interest in music medicine was increasing. A number of case reports appeared as letters to the editor in several of the more widely read journals, such as the *New England Journal of Medicine* (73,75–78), the *British Medical Journal* (79–85), and *Lancet* (86,87). The *New England Journal of Medicine* first printed a letter from John Dawson, M. D., of South Dakota. Dawson suggested that "Physicians across the nation, through the medium of their state medical associations in conjunction with the Association of College, University, and Community Arts Administrators, and the International Society of Performing Arts Administrators, set up a network for musical referral. . . . It takes little experience in this arena to become aware of the subspecialty one might call 'musical medicine' " (76).

This provoked an almost immediate response from Kay Cynamon, a Philadelphia medical student: "I believe that the establishment of a 'musical referral network' and the enlightenment of all members of the medical profession will add greatly to the quality of emotional and physical health care of musicians" (75). Stanley Davis of California responded with statistics regarding the physiological stress of music making: "Since physicians may encounter musicians as patients I consider it important for them to be aware of these stresses. . . . Too often, music making is considered a benign labor of love. It may be, but to the professional it can also be very hard work" (73). *Senza Sordino*, the newsletter of the International Conference of Symphony and Opera Musicians, reprinted the letters of Dawson and Davis (88,89).

Both physicians and musicians showed definite interest in music medicine, but there was as yet no real cooperation or direction. The 1972 Danube Symposium, on Neurology in Vienna, focused on the neurology of music. The success of this meeting spurred two attendees, MacDonald Critchley and R. A. Henson, to write a book based on the same subject (90). *Music and the Brain: Studies in the Neurology of*

Music, published in 1977, marked the birth of the field of music medicine, according to many experts (91,92). The first part of the book dealt with nervous system function during musical activity, and the second concerned the effects of neurological disorders on musical functions. While this was not a book on music medicine in the same way as Singer's book had been, it did include a good deal of information on the occupational diseases of musicians. The fact that the book had been published at all and was widely quoted lent credibility to the notion of a developing subspecialty (90).

During the late 1970s, interest in music medicine continued to widen. David G. Dibbell, M. D., wrote and lectured on the diagnosis and treatment of velopharyngeal stress incompetence in musicians. Perhaps surprisingly, Dibbell's work on surgical correction of the problem was published in several music journals before a more extensive article appeared in the medical literature (93–97).

Stress of all types was a major concern among musicians. In 1978 *Senza Sordino* reported a National Institute for Occupational Safety and Health study (96) that ranked 130 occupations based on diagnosed mental health disorders at a community mental health center. Musicians ranked fifth, behind health technicians and waitresses, before policemen, firemen, lawyers, and physicians (97). On several occasions previously, *Senza Sordino* had reported on European studies of stress and musicianship, especially those commissioned by the Vienna Symphony (98). The 1978 publication of *Tension in the Performance of Music*, edited by Carola Grindea, was greeted enthusiastically by musicians (99).

In 1980 the *International Trumpet Guild Newsletter* began a medical column under the editorship of Leon J. Whitsell, M. D., whose objectives were to review major research reports related to medicine and trumpet playing and to discuss medical questions (100). The *Newsletter* reprinted several medical articles, including Faulkner's and Sharpey-Schafer's 1959 study (101).

THE DAM BURSTS

Though interest in music medicine was growing among physicians and musicians, the public remained generally unaware of any real problems. Then a 1981 article in the *New York Times* detailed the hand difficulties of Gary Graffman and Leon Fleisher, as well as their problems in obtaining satisfactory answers to their concerns. Eventually they both arrived at Massachusetts General Hospital in Boston, under the care of a team led by Fred Hochberg, M. D. (102).

Though neither Graffman nor Fleisher found a complete or permanent cure, the publicity regarding their plight led to inquiries from a large, previously unknown group of injured instrumentalists. Many of these musicians had avoided physicians, preferring alternative therapies such as acupuncture, myotherapy, and various relaxation techniques. Now, as Graffman himself described it, "The dam had burst, and soon Boston was inundated with indisposed instrumentalists of every description. . . . seeking 'conventional' medical help" (103).

During the next two years, the clinic at Massachusetts General received heavy coverage in medical, music, and popular publications (104–110). *Piano Quarterly* printed a long interview with several of the physicians, as well as a questionnaire readers could complete (109). The first real report of the clinic's experience, published in the *Journal of the American Medical Association* in 1983 (111), represented a landmark in performing arts medicine.

Another item that thrust music medicine into the limelight was the controversy over performance anxiety and the use of beta adrenergic blocking drugs. Performance anxiety or stage fright has occurred among musicians as long as there has been music performance, with various relaxation techniques, psychotherapy, tranquilizers, or mood-altering substances used as treatments in the past (112). Beginning in the late 1970s, researchers began to test various beta blockers such as propranolol for performance anxiety. Developed primarily to treat angina pectoris and other cardiovascular problems, these drugs may also control the physiological aspects of the stress reaction (113). Among others, studies by Ian James in England and Charles Brantigan, M. D., in the United States showed that musicians felt less nervous and tended to perform better after treatment with beta blockers (114,115), but without the drowsiness and lack of intensity caused by other drugs (112).

Naturally, musicians were quick to note these developments. What some of them did not note were possible side effects and contraindications. Physicians and others became alarmed that musicians apparently obtained beta blockers and used them without medical supervision. Because many musicians are reluctant to say whether they use beta blockers or not, facts on how much and under what circumstances they are used have never been easy to come by. While the drugs work well for many musicians with performance anxiety, some opponents offer the philosophical argument that musicians should not have to take drugs to practice their profession (113). Adverse effects on performance anxiety have also been observed, especially among singers (116).

Despite increased attention, the prevalence of occupational diseases in general among musicians was unknown. Early reviews of the subject bemoaned the lack of solid statistics (47,66,69,102,111,117,118). Physicians and musicians believed there must be more study than had been reported in the literature, and sought to communicate with other practitioners and injured musicians. Exchange of information between health professionals and musicians became more common.

CONFERENCES BEGIN

In 1982 the National Flute Association's annual convention featured several presentations under the umbrella title "Flute Fitness." The fall issue of the *National Flute Association Newsletter* contained a questionnaire on performance anxiety and a short summary of occupational diseases related to the flute. In his last paragraph John Wion wrote, "This October the International Center for Dance Orthopedics and Dance Therapy is holding its second international symposium. . . . It is my hope that we will soon see the formation of a similar body devoted to compilation and dissemination of information about rehabilitation from, and prevention of injuries to musicians" (119).

Wion was not the only one who felt something important was about to happen. In 1983 Alice Brandfonbrener, M. D., of Chicago, organized the first "Medical Problems of Musicians" conference in conjunction with the Aspen, Colorado Music Festival. A large number of physicians and musicians shared papers, demonstrations, and discussions (120). The Aspen conference has now become an annual event and includes the problems of dancers. It is cochaired by Richard J. Lederman, M. D., and cosponsored by the Cleveland Clinic Foundation (121).

As evidence of growing interest in music medicine, 1984 saw several conferences in addition to the one in Aspen. The American String Teachers Association (ASTA) sponsored a conference entitled "Sforzando! The String Player's Stress Points—and Their Relief." The conference featured lectures on the care and prevention of injuries, along with presentations on the Alexander Technique and yoga. ASTA published the proceedings of this conference (122), as well as several articles in its journal, *American String Teacher* (123–125). While some teachers had shown interest in the physiology of string playing as early as the turn of the century, real concern increased with the growth in music medicine (124).

The "Biology of Music Making" conference in Denver also met in 1984. Besides occupational diseases of musicians, this conference included presentations on various neuropsychologic issues (126). One of the organizers of the conference, Frank Wilson, M. D., has been a strong advocate of the interrelationship of music and medicine. Wilson has lectured and written extensively on neuromusicology, especially in music publications (113–130).

In subsequent years the number of conferences multiplied to include the International Society for the Study of Tension in Performance at Westminster Choir College, "Mind, Body and the Performing Arts" at New York University, the International Society for Music in Medicine conferences (127), and "Playing Hurt," directed by cellist Janet Horvath and cosponsored by the University of Minnesota and the Minnesota Orchestra (131). There were also an increasing number of local seminars (132,133), usually including presentations by physicians as well as lectures and demonstrations by musicians who had developed techniques to deal with musicians' injuries, such as Dorothy Taubman. Ms. Taubman's techniques, involving retraining of pianistic movements, have reportedly helped many injured performers resume playing. While Ms. Taubman and alternative therapists have not always enjoyed cordial relations with physicians, many medical practitioners have begun to approach them with a more open mind (134). New technologies put to creative uses, such as biofeedback to control tension, have been considered as well (135).

Increasingly, these conferences have been covered in medical (112,118,136, 137), music (104,138–144), and popular publications (120,145), sometimes extensively. Publishing in the field has increased dramatically, with over 100 articles appearing in the 1970s and over 400 in the 1980s, nearly ten times as many as were written in the 1960s (23,24). In 1986 the *Cleveland Clinic Quarterly* published an issue dedicated to music medicine, containing papers from the 1984 Aspen conference. Richard Lederman, M. D., and Alice Brandfonbrener, M. D., wrote in their introduction to the issue, "In the past several years, there has been increasing attention to the medical problems of the performer, spurred perhaps by the climate of health awareness and consumer advocacy, as well as by the considerable publicity attending the afflictions of some renowned performers. This field of performing arts medicine, while still in its infancy, seems to be emerging as a legitimate area of interest and investigation and has obvious ties to both industrial and sports medicine" (146).

AUSTRALIA

While the United States was one active region, another existed in Australia. This was due mainly to one physician, Hunter J. H. Fry, a surgeon from Victoria. In 1983 he and other physician-musicians founded the Performing Arts Medicine Society as a section of the Australian Medical Association. This group carried out a large number of surveys at music schools and among orchestral musicians (147).

In an attempt to alleviate some musicians' problems, Fry devised several types of instrument posts which have been used by a number of instrumentalists (148). He developed a grading system for overuse which has been adopted by some music medicine specialists (149–152). Fry's articles, especially those in the *Medical Journal of Australia* (153) and *Lancet* (151), caused a deluge of letters to the editors (154–156).

DANCE MEDICINE

As interest in music medicine began to increase, a parallel upsurge occurred in dance medicine. The pioneers in the field include Eivind Thomasen of Denmark and Henry Jordan of New York City, often called "the dance doctor" during the 1950s and 1960s. Others have continued to treat a group of professionals who work under tremendous physical and mental stress.

Dancers almost always begin training while quite young, with a single-mindedness that leaves little room for a normal childhood or any activities beyond dancing. Even a dancer who succeeds in becoming a professional must continue to train constantly. The dancer's career is notoriously short and many are forced into retirement by age 35 or 40, due to declining physical abilities. Until recently scant attention was paid to this traumatic event.

Because of the extreme physical demands, most dancers are chronically fatigued and often display highly irregular eating and sleeping patterns. The constant battering and unnatural positions, especially of the lower extremities, can lead to sprains, fractures, tendinitis, arthritis, and other problems. While the history of dance medicine cannot be adequately addressed in this chapter, a relevant group of citations is included in the list of references (157–172).

CLINICS AND UNION ACTIVITY

Along with the increasing activity in music and dance medicine, a growing number of performing arts medicine clinics have developed across the United States, mainly in large cities with resident orchestras. Some treat only instrumentalists; others include singers, dancers, and actors. Some concentrate only on occupational diseases while others provide primary care for performers as well. Some are headquartered at a single hospital with extensive physical therapy facilities. Other clinics are loosely organized referral networks of physicians, allied health professionals, and alternative therapists throughout the city. A few have received outside funding, but most exist on a shoestring and the goodwill of their staffs and institutions. The majority of clinics are staffed mainly by physicians who are themselves musicians (173–175).

These developments were not lost on the musicians' unions. In 1985 the International Conference of Symphony and Opera Musicians (ICSOM) included a session on music medicine in their annual meeting. Stuart Schneck, M. D., stated in his opening remarks, "None of the meetings held to discuss medical problems of musicians had been directed specifically at the performing artists themselves. This conference is an attempt to remedy that oversight" (176). Transcripts of the lectures were sent to each of the 48-member orchestras. In the same year ICSOM did a sound level survey to highlight hearing problems, as well as possible solutions such as earplugs, plexiglass shields, and baffles (177). *Senza Sordino* continued to print information about conferences, clinics, and other music medicine activities (138, 139,178–180).

International Musician, the newsletter of the American Federation of Musicians (AFM), also began to feature music medicine. Along with summaries of conferences (141,144,181), the AFM published a very clear explanation of the major occupational disease categories (182), and a series on coping with performance anxiety (183–185). The local chapters of the AFM were not left behind. *Allegro*, published by Local 802 in New York, has included three health supplements, as well as other articles concerned with music medicine (186–188). *Hi-Notes,* the newsletter of Local 161-710 in Washington, D. C., inaugurated a health column in 1989 (189).

ORGANIZATIONS

In addition to the formation of some 20 performing arts medicine clinics and increased union activity, the late 1980s saw other developments. The January 1985 issue of *Philadelphia Medicine* included a short article by Richard Lippin, M. D., entitled "Arts Medicine: a Call for a New Medical Specialty." Lippin wrote, "Through the growth of an Arts Medicine specialty, physicians and other health professionals would be encouraged to seek a more formal scientific understanding of the artistic milieu in which the patient works. . . . Collaboration and cooperation with the professional artistic community and arts educators would be encouraged . . . An association of professionals dedicated to this specialty could be founded and would be known as the IAMA or the International Arts Medicine Association" (190).

Lippin proposed the very broadest definition of arts medicine, including all the creative arts, arts therapy, and other healing properties of the arts. Later that year he and a number of other health professionals engaged in the arts did form the International Arts Medicine Association. The organization has broad goals, including the collection and dissemination of information, prevention of dysfunction, provision of information regarding treatment resources, promotion of scientific research, and rehumanization of health education. In 1988 the IAMA decided to concentrate its efforts on information management. They have begun a liaison with other organizations interested in developing a comprehensive international arts medicine information system (191).

Instrument-specific music associations have begun to show increased interest in music medicine as well. In 1985 the National Flute Association set up a Dysfunction Committee composed of physician-musicians and flutists with interests in occupational diseases and physiology. The guidelines for the committee include receiving and answering inquiries from flutists, participating in the annual convention, and publishing material in the *Flutist Quarterly*. The committee has sponsored a presentation at each convention and a booth in the exhibit hall where questions may be addressed, hearing tests given, and other advice offered (192). Committee members have contributed summary articles to the *Flutist Quarterly* (193–201), and an occasional column usually features information on clinics and conferences (202).

Along with other instrumentalists, flutists have expressed interest in the ergonomic aspects of their instrument. Richard Norris, M. D., developed a flute rest to alleviate problems in the left index finger (197). More recently he devised an angle-headed flute which decreases rotation and tilting of the head, thus decreasing the occurrence of arm, shoulder, and neck problems. Emerson Musical Instruments has begun limited production of a model with a 30° angle (203). Other repair technicians and custom flute makers have shown interest in "rebuilding" the flute. They specialize in repositioning and reshaping various keys to fit small, less flexible, or injured hands (204,205).

High technology has begun to have an impact on instrument redesign as well. A California surgeon uses his office computer to manipulate videotaped images of musicians playing their instruments. The computer software can alter the instrument's design to avoid painful hand positions and provide a printout of the proposed redesign for an instrument maker (206).

A JOURNAL IS LAUNCHED

In 1986 a landmark event occurred in the development of performing arts medicine as a specialty. The quarterly journal *Medical Problems of Performing Artists* (*MPPA*) began publication under the editorship of Alice Brandfonbrener, M. D. It is published in Philadelphia by Hanley and Belfus, Inc. While *MPPA* is primarily a scientific journal, it has performers on its editorial board and encourages their contributions.

In her opening editorial Brandfonbrener stated, "The purpose of *Medical Problems of Performing Artists* is to promote interest in the medical problems of performing artists, to help in the search for and dissemination of information, and by these means to promote the well-being of this vulnerable and valuable segment of our society" (207). She also noted that there had been very little research in the field of arts medicine and expressed the hope that *MPPA* would stimulate such activity by providing a publishing outlet (207).

MPPA did indeed provide a forum for a surprising number of physicians, musicians, allied health professionals, and alternative therapists. The journal was widely publicized in both professional and popular publications (91,92,130,131,179,208–210). In the first year, articles included Gary Graffman's personal experience (103), a survey of musculoskeletal problems among instrumentalists (211), a discussion of tonsils and adenoids (212), a summary of the Alexander Technique (213), and many other diverse offerings. Another early contribution was "Music and Medicine: a Classification" by Robert Kurth, M. D. Though hardly recognized by outsiders as a specialty, Kurth proceeded to categorize the subject matter based on an analysis of the ever-increasing literature (214). Such a classification lent credibility to the idea of a distinct field.

MPPA's first issue contained a short article by Tom Hall, at that time editor of *Senza Sordino*, applauding the increased communication among all those interested in the developing specialty. He listed some of his concerns as: discovering healthy, physiologically sound methods of practice and performance; systematic identification and classification of occupational diseases of musicians; better understanding of each discipline's specialized terminology; and identification of competent music medicine facilities and practitioners. Hall concluded, "Above all, we do not want music medicine to be merely a fad" (215). Through the pages of *Medical Problems of Performing Artists*, the development of arts medicine as a specialty has unfolded. Many of the papers from Aspen and other conferences, as well as the results of a wide range of research studies, have appeared in this journal.

One of the most important and certainly most quoted of these was the ICSOM survey. During 1986 ICSOM distributed a questionnaire requesting detailed information on medical problems to each player in the 48-member orchestras (138). In its March 1988 issue, *MPPA* reprinted a preliminary overview of the results from *Senza Sordino* (216). The figures most quoted showed that 82% of musicians experienced a medical problem, and 76% had a problem that severely affected their performance. Other results included increased prevalence among women, the relatively high use of beta blockers for performance anxiety, and the predominance of problems with the left versus the right hand. The authors concluded: "Given the proportion of professional musicians reporting medical problems severe enough to affect performance, there can be little doubt that music medicine is a field that deserves serious attention from health professionals" (217).

While the study was not faultless, a 55% response rate gave a very large sample for continuing analysis (217). In addition to questions of prevalence, physicians and others began to address themselves to incidence. A March 1988 article in *MPPA* reported the incidence of upper extremity problems at a university music school. The author found that 8.5 new cases of disability occurred per 100 musicians per year. His findings regarding gender, site of the problem, and symptoms agreed with previous studies (218).

Another topic receiving increasing emphasis is the need to prevent the occurrence of occupational problems. A 1988 article by Crispin Spaulding described what may be the first prevention program at a conservatory, in Norway. Students are taught to understand their bodies and to monitor their practice and performance habits so that problems can be avoided or caught in the earliest stages. The student, medical professional, and teacher all work together to make playing as comfortable and adaptable to change as possible (219).

Medical Problems of Performing Artists has often given a first hearing to new topics in music medicine. In 1987 a two-part article focused on the occupational stresses experienced by rock musicians. Most previous research had focused on classical musicians, but this study showed that stress-related difficulties of rock musicians were worthy of serious study (220,221).

Another 1987 article presented some of the cost constraints on health care access for performers. It highlighted the fact that many performers have no health insurance and therefore often go without timely or needed health care (222).

A three-part article published in 1988 and 1989 by France's famed hand surgeon, Raoul Tubiana, reviewed in detail the anatomy and physiology of the hand. The final part described fundamental positioning of the arms in the pianist, violinist, and guitarist to achieve minimum stress and energy expenditure (223–225). Another 1989 article reviewed several clinical applications of the musical instrument digital interface system technology. Known as MIDI, this technology has the potential to develop norms for keyboard technique, assess the impact of injuries, and monitor rehabilitation (226).

THE FIELD ARRIVES

While *MPPA* might be considered on the cutting edge of the field, it is certainly not the only journal in which progress is being reported. The *Journal of Voice* began publication in 1987, edited by Robert Sataloff, M. D. This peer-review publication was the successor to the *Transcripts of the Annual Symposium on Care of the Professional Voice*, which had been published by the Voice Foundation since 1977 (47). *Guitar Player* has published several articles in its "Musicians' Health" series (227), and features a medical column called "Ask the Doctor" (228). Even trade newsletters such as the *Emerson Flute Forum* include medical columns (229).

Of particular significance to physicians was the appearance of an article by Alan H. Lockwood, M. D., and a related editorial by Richard J. Lederman, M. D., in the January 26, 1989 *New England Journal of Medicine* (91,230). For many, discussion of the topic in this premier forum "underscored the arrival of performance arts medicine" (231). Lockwood's eloquent review and assessment of the current situation prompted many letters to editors (232).

Beyond the published literature, several organizations acknowledged the growth of arts medicine. In 1987 the American Occupational Medical Association created an arts medicine section and offered a seminar at its annual meeting (233). During the meeting, health professionals had an informal discussion with members of a jazz group participating in the New Orleans Jazz Festival. This was a relatively new idea, but both groups came away with valuable information. While the jazz musicians had many of the same medical problems as classical musicians, they generally had less access to health care. Physicians in attendance realized that innovative approaches to education and health care delivery were needed for jazz musicians (234), even as Raeburn had earlier concluded they were needed for rock musicians.

In 1988 the Library of the Medical and Chirurgical Faculty in Baltimore set up the Music Medicine Clearinghouse. The Clearinghouse's primary mission is gathering, organizing, and disseminating information to health professionals, musicians, and researchers. Besides books and journal articles, the collection includes a large file of ephemeral material such as brochures, newsletters, and fact sheets. The Clearinghouse provides an ongoing bibliography on music medicine and prepares subject bibliographies (235).

At the 1989 Aspen conference, formation of the Performing Arts Medicine Association (PAMA) was formally announced. PAMA, the first professional medical organization in the field, is dedicated to providing quality medical care for performers. Members hope to develop guidelines for the practice of arts medicine, to encourage research, and to sponsor meetings to educate both physicians and musicians (231). That same fall, the newly formed Association of Medical Advisors to British Orchestras invited interested practitioners to apply for special training (236).

As the 1990s arrive, "the presence of Arts Medicine as a medical discipline is an accepted reality today" (231). A substantial number of clinics are now in place, and the number and variety of meetings on the subject continues to increase. The popular press and professional journals in both fields have intensified their coverage. Research efforts are widening as well, ranging from the use of motion analysis techniques in the study of upper extremity problems (237) to testing the effects of preventive programs in major orchestras (131).

With research comes the responsibility for sharing of information and education. Although there are not yet many answers to occupational problems, lessons learned must be passed onto the next generation of health care professionals and musicians. Alice Brandfonbrener, M. D., described the challenge: "If we sit back and do not take active roles in shaping the specialty, we will have only ourselves to blame when it then fails to achieve its full potential. Let us continue to be as attentive and involved as any good parents must be throughout an offspring's potentially difficult adolescence in order to assure a healthy maturation" (231).

REFERENCES

1. Stone WH. On wind-pressure in the human lungs during performance on wind instruments. *Philosophical Magazine* (series 4) 1874; 48(316):113–114.
2. Ramazzini B. *Diseases of Tradesmen*. comp H. Goodman. New York: Medical Lay Press, 1933.
3. Akgun N, Ozgonul H. Lung volumes in wind instrument (zurna) players. *American Review of Respiratory Disease* 1967; 96(5):946–951.
4. Wolff J. The treatment of writer's cramp and allied muscular affections. *British Medical Journal* 1890;2:165–166.
5. Cornet player's cramp. *Maryland Medical Journal* 1893;29:436–437.
6. Poore GV. Clinical lecture on certain conditions of the hand and arm which interfere with the performance of professional acts, especially piano-playing. *British Medical Journal* 1887;1:441–444.
7. Lederman RJ. Occupational cramp in instrumental musicians. *Medical Problems of Performing Artists* 1988;3(2):45–51.
8. Forbes WS. The liberating of the ring finger in musicians, by dividing the accessory tendons of the extensor communis digitorum muscle. *Maryland Medical Journal* 1885;12:171–173.
9. Parrott JR, Harrison DB. Surgically dividing pianists' hands. *Journal of Hand Surgery* 1980;5(6):619.
10. Anderson RH. Operation for improving the mobility and flexibility of the hand in piano playing. *Medical Record* 1893;43(9):283–284.
11. Tenotomy to increase the mobility and power of the musicians' ring-finger. *Maryland Medical Journal* 1890;23:249.
12. To facilitate piano playing: Prof. E.S. Bonelli cuts the tendon of the ring finger. *New York Times* 1890.
13. Kochevitsky G. *The Art of Piano Playing: A Scientific Approach*. Evanston, Il: Summy-Birchard, 1957.
14. Hochberg F, Leffert RD, Merriman LA. Special report: The ailments of musicians. In: *Health and Medical Annual*. Chicago: Encyclopedia Brittanica, 1984;297–301.
15. Henson RA and Urich H. Schumann's hand injury. *British Medical Journal* 1978;1(6117):900–903.
16. Gehrig RE. *Famous Pianists and Their Technique*. Washington, D. C.: Luce, 1974.
17. Ortmann O. *Physiological Mechanisms of Piano Technique: An Experimental Study of the Nature of Muscular Action as Used in Piano Playing, and its Effects Thereof Upon the Piano Key and the Piano Tone*. New York: Da Capo, 1981.
18. Singer K. *Diseases of the Musical Profession: A Systematic Presentation of their Causes, Symptoms and Methods of Treatment*. W. Lakond. New York: Greenberg, 1932.
19. Pollack R. Occupational diseases of musicians: Psychic ailments. *Hygeia* 1935;13(1):46–49.
20. Pollack R. Occupational diseases of musicians: Physical ailments. *Hygeia* 1935;13(2):132–135.
21. International Labour Office. *Occupation and Health: Encyclopedia of Hygiene, Pathology and Social Welfare*. Geneva: ILO, 1934.
22. Schullian DM and Schoen M, eds. *Music and Medicine*. New York: H. Schuman, 1948.
23. Harman SE. Occupational diseases of instrumental musicians: bibliography. Baltimore, Md.:Music Medicine Clearinghouse, 1989.
24. Harman SE. Related bibliography. Baltimore, Md.: Music Medicine Clearinghouse, 1989.
25. *Index Medicus: a Quarterly Classified Record of the Current Medical Literature of the World*. various publishers, 1879–1927.
26. *Quarterly Cumulative Index Medicus*. Chicago: Medical Library Association, 1927–56.
27. *Current List of Medical Literature*. Washington, D.C.: National Library of Medicine, 1941–59.
28. *Index Medicus*. Bethesda, Md.: National Library of Medicine. v.1:1960.
29. *Music Index*. various publishers. v.1:1949.
30. Porter MM. Dental problems in wind instrument playing. 1. Dental aspects of embouchure. *British Dental Journal* 1967;123:393–96.
31. Porter MM. Dental problems in wind instrument playing. 2. Single-reed instruments—the lip shield. *British Dental Journal* 1967;123:441–3.
32. Porter MM. Dental problems in wind instrument playing. 3. Single-reed instruments—restorative dentistry. *British Dental Journal* 1967;123:489–93.
33. Porter MM. Dental problems in wind instrument playing. 4. Single-reed instruments—partial dentures. *British Dental Journal* 1967;123:529–32.

34. Porter MM. Dental problems in wind instrument playing. 5. Single-reed instruments—full dentures. *British Dental Journal* 1967;123:590–3.
35. Porter MM. Dental problems in wind instrument playing. 6. Single-reed instruments—the embouchure denture. *British Dental Journal* 1968;124:34–6.
36. Porter MM. Dental problems in wind instrument playing. 7. Double-reed instruments. *British Dental Journal* 1968;124:78–81.
37. Porter MM. Dental problems in wind instrument playing. 8. Brass instruments. *British Dental Journal* 1968;124:129–32.
38. Porter MM. Dental problems in wind instrument playing. 9. Brass instruments (continued). *British Dental Journal* 1968;124:183–6.
39. Porter MM. Dental problems in wind instrument playing. 10. Brass instruments (continued). *British Dental Journal* 1968;124:227–31.
40. Porter MM. Dental problems in wind instrument playing. 11. Brass instruments (continued). *British Dental Journal* 1968; 124:271–4.
41. Porter MM. Dental problems in wind instrument playing. 12. Brass instruments (continued). *British Dental Journal* 1968;124:321–5.
42. Kilpinen E. *Condition of Teeth and Periodontium in Male Wind Instrument Players in the City of Helsinki: A Clinical and Radiologic Study.* Helsinki, Finland: University of Helsinki, 1976.
43. Howard JA, Lovrovich AT. Wind instruments: their interplay with orofacial structures. *Medical Problems of Performing Artists* 1989;4(2):59–72.
44. Krivin M, Congorth SG. An embouchure aid for clarinet and saxophone players. *Journal of the American Dental Association* 1975;90:1277–1281.
45. Von Leden H. The cultural history of the human voice. In: Lawrence VL. *Transcripts of the Eleventh Symposium: Care of the Professional Voice: Part II.* New York: Voice Foundation, 1982; 116–123.
46. Sataloff RT. Common diagnoses and treatments in professional voice users. *Medical Problems of Performing Artists* 1987;2(1):15–20.
47. *Journal of Voice.* New York: Raven Press. v. 1:1987.
48. Laryngoscope [column]. *NATS Journal.* v.37:1981.
49. Sataloff RT, Spiegel JR. Objective evaluation of the voice. *Medical Problems of Performing Artists* 1988;3(3):105–108.
50. Bryan AH. Band instruments harbor germs. *Music Educators Journal* 1960;46(5):84–85.
51. Bryan AH. Mouthpiece hygiene: Wind instrument mouthpieces harbor countless disease germs. *Instrumentalist* 1956;10:20–24.
52. Case F. Germs in the band room. *Music Educators Journal* 1955;42(1):61–63.
53. Koehler JK. Health and safety in the instrumental music class. *Music Educators Journal* 1961; 47(4):91–93.
54. Ashley RE. Diseases of the salivary glands. In: *Otolaryngology*, vol. 4. eds: Coates GM, Schenck HP, Miller MV. Hagerstown: Prior, 1955, 1–18.
55. Bachman AL, Seaman WB and Macken KL. Lateral pharyngeal diverticula. *Radiology* 1968; 91(1):774–782.
56. Kopell HP, Thompson WAL. Pronator syndrome: A confirmed case and its diagnosis. *New England Journal of Medicine* 1958;259(15):713–715.
57. Ward PH, Fredrickson JM, Strandjord NM, Valvassori GE. Laryngeal and pharyngeal pouches: Surgical approach and the use of cinefluorographic and other radiologic techniques as diagnostic aids. *Laryngoscope* 1963;73(5):564–582.
58. Basmajian JV and White ER. Neuromuscular control of trumpeters' lips. *Nature* 1973;241 (384):70.
59. Bouhuys A. Breathing and blowing. *Sonorum Speculum* 1962;13:1–12.
60. Bouhuys A. Lung volumes and breathing patterns in wind-instrument players. *Journal of Applied Physiology* 1964;19:967–975.
61. Bouhuys A. Airflow control by auditory feedback: Respiratory mechanics and wind instruments. *Science* 1966;154(750):792–799.
62. Berger KW. Respiratory and articulatory factors in wind instrument performance. *Journal of Applied Physiology* 1965;20(6):1217–1221.
63. Faulkner M, Sharpey-Schafer EP. Circulatory effects of trumpet playing. *British Medical Journal* 1959;1(5123):685–686.
64. Westmore GA, Eversden ID. Noise-induced hearing loss and orchestral musicians. *Archives of Otolaryngology* 1981;107(12):761–764.

65. Hart CW, Geltman CL, Schupback J, Santucci M. The musician and occupational sound hazards. *Medical Problems of Performing Artists* 1987;2(1):22–25.
66. Polnauer FF, Marks M. Occupational hazards of playing string instruments. *Strad* 1967;78:23–25.
67. Faulkner M. Experimentation in breathing as it relates to brass performance. *Instrumentalist* 1967;21(2):6–7.
68. Borgia JF, Horvath SM, Dunn FR, Von Phyl PV, Nizet PM. Some physiological observations on French horn musicians. *Journal of Occupational Medicine* 1975;17(11):696–701.
69. Harman SE. Occupational diseases of instrumental musicians, a review. *Maryland State Medical Journal* 1982;31(6):39–42.
70. Tucker A, Faulkner ME, Horvath SM. Electrocardiography and lung function in brass instrument players. *Archives of Environmental Health* 1971;23(5):327–334.
71. The way to high D. *Lancet* 1973 3;1(797):247–248.
72. Calif. Univ. medicos claim horn playing makes coronaries. *Music Trades* 1972;120:20–21.
73. Davis SD. Stressed musicians [letter]. *New England Journal of Medicine* 1975 29:292(22):1197.
74. Nizet PM, Borgia JF, Horvath SM. Wandering atrial pacemaker (prevalence in French hornists). *Journal of Electrocardiology* 1976;9(1):51–52.
75. Cynamon KB. Musical medicine [letter]. *New England Journal of Medicine* 1975;191(13):705.
76. Dawson JB. Musical medicine [letter]. *New England Journal of Medicine* 1975;292(6):322.
77. Saunders HF. Wind parotitis [letter]. *New England Journal of Medicine* 1973;289(13):698.
78. Wind parotitis [letter]. *New England Journal of Medicine* 1973;289(20):1094–1095.
79. Curtis P. Guitar nipple [letter]. *British Medical Journal* 1974;1(5912):226.
80. Dahl MGC. Flautist's chin: a companion to fiddler's neck [letter]. *British Medical Journal* 1978;2(6143):1023.
81. Gardner LD. Flautist's chin [letter]. *British Medical Journal* 1978;2(6147):1295.
82. Hindson TC. Clarinettist's chelitis [letter]. *British Medical Journal* 1978;2(6147):1295.
83. Jago JD. Medical and dental problems of musical instruments [letter]. *British Medical Journal* 1978;2(6147):1295.
84. Murphy JM. Cello scrotum [letter]. *British Medical Journal* 1974;2(914):335.
85. Shea MJ. Saxophonist's diverticulosis [letter]. *British Medical Journal* 1979;1(6172):1217.
86. Cobcroft R, Kronenberg H, Wilkinson T. Cryptococcus in bagpipes [letter]. *Lancet* 1978; 1(8078):1368–1369.
87. Stevenson D. Cryptococcus in bagpipes [letter]. *Lancet* 1978;2(8080):104–105.
88. Davis SD. Stressed musicians [letter]. *Senza Sordino* 1975;13(6):2.
89. Dawson JB. Musical medicine [letter]. *Senza Sordino* 1976;14(4):2.
90. Critchley M, Henson RA, eds. *Music and the Brain: Studies in the Neurology of Music*. London: Heinemann, 1980.
91. Lockwood AH. Medical problems of musicians. *New England Journal of Medicine* 1989;320(4):221–227.
92. Ver Berkmoes R. How some MDs help the band play on. *American Medical News* 1989;32 (12):31–32.
93. Dibbell DG. Can surgery improve trumpet playing? *NACWPI* 1978;27(1):24–25.
94. Dibbell DG. The incompetent palate: A trumpeting disaster. *Journal of the International Trumpet Guild* 1977;2:37–38.
95. Dibbell DG, Ewanowski S, Carter WL. Successful correction of velopharyngeal stress incompetence in musicians playing wind instruments. *Plastic and Reconstructive Surgery* 1979;64(5):662–664.
96. Colligan MJ, Smith MJ, Hurrell JJ Jr. Occupational incidence rates of mental disorders. *Journal of Human Stress* 1977;3(3):34–39.
97. Symphony playing stressful job says NIOSH team. *Senza Sordino* 1978;16(5):3.
98. Shaw H. Stress and musicianship. *Senza Sordino* 1972;10(4):3.
99. Grindea C., ed. *Tension in the Performance of Music*. 2d ed. London: Kahn & Averill, 1988.
100. Whitsell LJ. Why a medical column: A prospectus. *International Trumpet Guild Newsletter* 1980; 6(3):12.
101. Faulkner M, Sharpey-Schafer EP. Circulatory effects of trumpet playing. *International Trumpet Guild Journal* 1982;9(2):22–23.
102. Dunning J. When a pianist's fingers fail to obey. *New York Times* 1981.
103. Graffman G. Doctor, can you lend an ear? *Medical Problems of Performing Artists* 1986;1(1):3–6.
104. Carey J. Pianist ends 17-year silence. *USA Today* 1982.
105. Clarke G. The sound of two hands playing. *Time* 1982;20(3):75.

106. Graffman N. Leon Fleisher's long journey back to the keyboard. *New York Times* 1982.
107. Hand pain a sour note for musicians. *American Medical News* 1983;26(15):41.
108. Musicians whose hands are out of tune get a work-up by Mass General physicians. *Medical World News* 1982;23(15):98–101.
109. Silverman RJ. Physicians' views of physical problems. *Piano Quarterly* 1983;31(120):42–47.
110. Wanger F. Updates from the Aspen Symposium and Massachusetts General Hospital [letter]. *Piano Quarterly* 1983;31(123):2–4.
111. Hochberg FH, Leffert RD, Heller MD, Merriman L. Hand difficulties among musicians. *Journal of the American Medical Association* 1983;249(14):1869–1872.
112. Lehrer PM, Rosen RC, Kostis JB, Greenfield D. Treating stage fright in musicians: The use of beta blockers. *New Jersey Medicine* 1987;84(1):27–33.
113. Wilson FR. Music and medicine, 1986 II. Inderal for stage fright? *Piano Quarterly* 1986 Summer; 134:30–35.
114. Brantigan CO, Brantigan TA, Joseph N. Effect of beta blockade and beta stimulation on stage fright. *American Journal of Medicine* 1982;72(1):88–94.
115. James IM, Burgoyne W, Savage IT. Effect of pindolol on stress-related disturbances of musical performance: Preliminary communication. *Journal of the Royal Society of Medicine* 1983;76(3): 194–196.
116. Gates GA, Montalbo PJ. The effect of low dose b-blockade on performance anxiety in singers. *Journal of Voice* 1987;1(1):105–107.
117. Ziporyn T. Pianist's cramp to stage fright: The medical side of music-making. *Journal of the American Medical Association* 1984;252(8):985–989.
118. Brauer A. Musical medicine: The newest specialty. *MD* 1983;27(9):97–100, 107–108, 111.
119. Wion J. Flute fitness I. *National Flute Association Newsletter* 1982 Fall;8(1):5, 9.
120. Schonberg HC. Musicians' disabilities provoke medical study. *New York Times* 1983.
121. *The Seventh Annual Symposium on Medical Problems of Musicians and Dancers* [conference abstracts]. Snowmass, Co.: Cleveland Clinic Foundation, 1989.
122. Mischakoff A, ed. *Sforzando! Music Medicine for String Players.* Bloomington, In.: American String Teachers Association, 1985.
123. Chick D. Injury prevention for violists. *American String Teacher* 1988;38:73–75.
124. Fray DL. Physiological studies in string playing. *American String Teacher* 1981 Winter;31:33–36.
125. Irvine JK, LeVine WR. The use of biofeedback to reduce left-hand tension for string players. *American String Teacher* 1981 Summer;31:10–12.
126. Roehmann FL, Wilson FR. *The Biology of Music Making: Proceedings of the 1984 Denver Conference.* St. Louis, Mo: MMB Music, 1989.
127. Wilson FR. Music and medicine—1985. *Piano Quarterly* 1985 Winter;34(132):21–26.
128. Wilson FR. Teaching hands, treating hands. *Piano Quarterly* 1988;36(141):34–36, 38–41.
129. Wilson FR. Music as basic schooling for the brain. *Music Educators Journal* 1985;71(9):39–42.
130. Wilson FR. Music and medicine: An old liaison, a new agenda. *Psychomusicology* 1988;7(2):139–146.
131. Samples P. Music has charms (but strains muscles): specialists help musicians play without pain. *American Medical News* 1989;32(23):9–10.
132. Giuliano M. Arts medicine program scheduled at Peabody. *Peabody News* 1988.
133. Schien BL. Myotherapy: An interview with Nancy Shaw. *Maryland Music Educator* 1989; 35(4):22–24.
134. Piano school tones up the hands on the keys. *New York Times* 1986.
135. LeVine WR, Irvine JK. In vivo EMG biofeedback in violin and viola pedagogy. *Biofeedback and Self-Regulation* 1984 Jun;9(2):161–168.
136. Hinz CA. MDs meet musicians' medical needs. *American Medical News* 1984;27(31):2, 15.
137. Hinz CA. Musicians' health needs call for a medical team approach. *American Medical News* 1984;27(31):26–28.
138. Burrell M. Medical survey becomes a reality. *Senza Sordino* 1986;14(4):1.
139. Burrell M. 1986 Aspen Conference. *Senza Sordino* 1987;25(4):2, 5.
140. Howard D. The 1984 Aspen conference. *Senza Sordino* 1985;23(3):2–3.
141. Kella JJ. Experts study the role of stress in the arts. *International Musician* 1985;84:4, 20.
142. Koplewitz L. Medicine and music at Aspen. *Instrumentalist* 1984;38(6):23–24.
143. Rozek M. Musicians and medicine: Is there a doctor in the house? *Symphony Magazine* 1985; 36(1):9–12.
144. Summer conference to examine stress in the performing arts. *International Musician* 1985;84(6):5.

145. Clark M, Gosnell M. Hurt at center stage: Arts medicine and the medical arts. *Newsweek* 1986; 108(5):46–47.
146. Lederman RJ, Brandfonbrener AG. Medical problems of musicians: Introduction and overview. *Cleveland Clinic Quarterly* 1986 Spring;53(1):1–2.
147. Fry H. Australian group studies sound level problem. *Senza Sordino* 1985;23(6):1–2.
148. Fry HJH. Occupational maladies of musicians: Their cause and prevention. *International Journal of Music Education* 1984;(4):59–63.
149. Fry HJH. Prevalence of overuse (injury) syndrome in Australian music schools. *British Journal of Industrial Medicine* 1987;44(1):35–40.
150. Fry HJH. How to treat overuse injury: Medicine for your practice. *Music Educators Journal* 1986; 72(9):46–49.
151. Fry HJH. Overuse syndrome in musicians: Prevention and management. *Lancet* 1986; 2(8509):728–731.
152. Fry HJH. Overuse syndrome of the upper limb in musicians. *Medical Journal of Australia* 1986; 144(4):182–185.
153. Fry HJH. Overuse syndrome in musicians—100 years ago. An historical review. *Medical Journal of Australia* 1986;145(11–12):620–625.
154. Overuse syndrome in musicians [letter]. *Lancet* 1986;2(8512):916–917.
155. Overuse syndrome in musicians [letter]. *Medical Journal of Australia* 1987;147(2):98,100–101.
156. Overuse syndrome in musicians [letter]. *Medical Journal of Australia* 1987;146(7):390,393–394.
157. Reynolds N, Hamilton WG. On its toes: Ballet medicine. In: *Medical and Health Annual*. Chicago: Encyclopedia Britannica, 1988, 132–149.
158. Schneider HJ, King AY, Bronson JL, Miller EH. Stress injuries and developmental changes of lower extremities in ballet dancers. *Radiology* 1974;113(3):627–632.
159. Miller EH, Schneider HJ, Bronson JL, McLain D. A new consideration in athletic injuries: The classical ballet dancer. *Clinical Orthopaedics and Related Research* 1975;111:181–191.
160. Sammarco GJ, Miller EH. Partial rupture of the flexor hallucis longus tendon in classical ballet dancers. *Journal of Bone and Joint Surgery* 1979;61A(1):149–150.
161. Teitz C. Sports medicine concerns in dance and gymnastics. *Pediatric Clinics of North America* 1982;29(6):1399–1421.
162. Micheli LJ, Sohn RS, Solomon R. Stress fractures of the second metatarsal involving Lisfranc's joint in ballet dancers. *Journal of Bone and Joint Surgery* 1985;67A(9):1372–1375.
163. Warren MP, Brooks-Gunn J, Hamilton LH, Warren LF, Hamilton WG. Scoliosis and fractures in young ballet dancers: Relation to delayed manarch and secondary amenorrhea. *New England Journal of Medicine* 1986;314(21)1348–1353.
164. Schnitt JM, Schnitt D. Eating disorders in dancers. *Medical Problems of Performing Artists* 1986; 1(2):39–44.
165. Laws K. Physics and the potential for dance injury. *Medical Problems of Performing Artists* 1986;1(3):73–79.
166. Garrick JG. Ballet injuries. *Medical Problems of Performing Artists* 1986;1(4):123–127.
167. Sammarco GJ. The hip in dancers. *Medical Problems of Performing Artists* 1987;2(1):5–14.
168. Chlmelar RD, Fitt SS, Schultz BB, Rohling RO, Zupan MF. A survey of health, training, and injuries in different levels and styles of dancers. *Medical Problems of Performing Artists* 1987; 2(2):61–66.
169. Quirk R. Knee injuries in classical dancers. *Medical Problems of Performing Artists* 1988;3(2):52–59.
170. Hardaker WT, Colosimo AJ, Malone TR, Myers M. Ankle sprains in theatrical dancers. *Medical Problems of Performing Artists* 1988;3(4):146–150.
171. Greben SE. The Dancer Transition Centre of Canada: Addressing the stress of giving up professional dancing. *Medical Problems of Performing Artists* 1989;4(3):128–130.
172. Watkins A, Woodhull-McNeal AP, Clarkson PM, Ebbeling C. Lower extremity alignment and injury in young, preprofessional, college, and professional ballet dancers: part I. Turnout and knee-foot alignment. *Medical Problems of Performing Artists* 1989;4(4):148–153.
173. Brandfonbrener AG. From the editor [editorial]. *Medical Problems of Performing Artists* 1986; 1(2):iv.
174. Brandfonbrener AG. Establishing performing arts clinics: The patients [editorial]. *Medical Problems of Performing Artists* 1986;1(3):iii.
175. Brandfonbrener AG. The bottom line: Funding arts medicine [editorial]. *Medical Problems of Performing Artists* 1986;1(4):iii.

176. Medical problems of musicians. Presentations read at International Conference of Symphony and Opera Musicians Annual Conference, 1985.
177. Holland-Moritz K. Preliminary sound level survey report. *Senza Sordino* 1985;23(5):1–2.
178. Fry HJH. Overuse syndrome in musicians—100 years ago. An historical review [excerpt]. *Senza Sordino* 1987;25(4):5–6.
179. 1985 music medicine symposia. *Senza Sordino* 1985;13(4):3.
180. Torch D. Aspen music medicine conference. *Senza Sordino* 1989;27(3):4.
181. Kella JJ. Symposium on musicians' medical problems: Performing arts medical specialty continues to grow. *International Musician* 1987;86:7,19.
182. Kella JJ. A musician's guide to performing arts medicine: Musculoskeletal, neurological and dermal ailments of musicians. *International Musician* 1988;87(1):7,18–19.
183. Sternbach D. Overcoming playing anxiety—with practice/part two. *International Musician* 1989; 88(1):6–7,19.
184. Sternbach D. Overcoming playing anxiety—with practice/part one. *International Musician* 1989;87(9):16–17.
185. Sternbach D. Taking control of your stress—on stage and off. *International Musician* 1988;87 (2):9,21.
186. Kella JJ. A guide to preventing musicians' occupational injuries. *Allegro* 1989;89(4):13,15,19.
187. Kella JJ. Performing arts medicine. *Allegro* 1987;87(4):15–16.
188. Kella JJ. Performance anxiety. *Allegro* 1987;12(4):4.
189. Sternbach D. Healthy tips from Dave [column]. *Hi-notes* 45(6),1989.
190. Lippin RA. Arts medicine: A call for a new medical specialty. *Philadelphia Medicine* 1985;81:14–15.
191. *International Arts-Medicine Association Newsletter* 1988;3(2):8–9.
192. New Dysfunction Committee. *Flutist Quarterly* 1985 Spring;10(2):59.
193. Horenstein S. Hands. *Flutist Quarterly* 1987 Summer;12(3):73–74.
194. Mitchell SA. Keep it clean. *Flutist Quarterly* 1987 Winter;12(1):27.
195. Mitchell SA. The flutist and the doctor. *Flutist Quarterly* 1987 Winter;12(1):28–29.
196. Norris RN. Applied ergonomics: the angled-head flute. *Flutist Quarterly* 1989 Summer;14(3):60–61.
197. Norris R. The flute rest, or "Look, Ma, no hands." *Flutist Quarterly* 1988 Summer;13(3):28–30.
198. Weiss J. The problem and prevention of hand trouble from a flutist's viewpoint. *Flutist Quarterly* 1989 Spring;14(2):74–75.
199. Horenstein S. Caring for your hearing. *Flutist Quarterly* 1987 Spring;12(2):86–87.
200. Horenstein S. Teeth. *Flutist Quarterly* 1987 Spring;12(2):87.
201. Mitchell SA. The flutist and food. *Flutist Quarterly* 1987 Fall;12(4):76–77.
202. Dysfunction committee report. [column] *Flutist Quarterly* 1985;10.
203. Norris RN. The angle-headed flute. *Emerson Flute Forum* 1989 Spring-Summer;6(1):10.
204. Hoover K. Adapting the flute for small hands: Some proposals. *Flutist Quarterly* 1985 Fall; 11(1):50–51.
205. Wimberly D. An improved B footjoint design: Increased comfort and security for small and large hands. *Flutist Quarterly* 1987 Spring;12(2):31–32.
206. Von Biel V. SF surgeon creates memorable lessons using a computer. *California Physician* 1989;6(11):56–58.
207. Brandfonbrener AG. To celebrate a new journal [editorial]. *Medical Problems of Performing Artists* 1986;1(1):1.
208. Marbella J. Painful performances: Real show-stoppers. *Baltimore Sun* 1988.
209. New music medicine clinics, journal debut. *Senza Sordino* 1985;24(2):2.
210. Power W. How not to break a leg: "Arts medicine" helps performers stay healthy on the job. *Wall Street Journal* 1986.
211. Caldron PH, Calabrese LH, Clough JD, Lederman RJ, Williams G, Leatherman J. A survey of musculoskeletal problems encountered in high-level musicians. *Medical Problems of Performing Artists* 1986;1(4):136–139.
212. Hart CW, Logemann JA. Tonsils and adenoids and the professional musician. *Medical Problems of Performing Artists* 1986;1(2):58–60.
213. Murray A. The Alexander technique. *Medical Problems of Performing Artists* 1986;1(4):131–132.
214. Kurth R. Music and medicine: A classification. *Medical Problems of Performing Artists* 1986; 1(3):95–98.

215. Hall T. A musician's view of music medicine. *Medical Problems of Performing Artists* 1986;1(1):2.
216. Burrell M. The ICSOM medical questionnaire. *Senza Sordino* 1987;25(6):1–8.
217. Fishbein M, Middlestadt SE, Ottai V, Straus S, Ellis A. Medical problems among ICSOM musicians: Overview of a national survey. *Medical Problems of Performing Artists* 1988;3(1):1–8.
218. Manchester RA. The incidence of hand problems in music students. *Medical Problems of Performing Artists* 1988;3(1):15–18.
219. Spaulding C. Before pathology: Prevention for performing artists. *Medical Problems for Performing Artists* 1988;3(4):135–139.
220. Raeburn SD. Occupational stress and coping in a sample of professional rock musicians (first of two parts). *Medical Problems of Performing Artists* 1987;2(2):41–48.
221. Raeburn SD. Occupational stress and coping in a sample of professional rock musicians (second of two parts). *Medical Problems of Performing Artists* 1987;2(3):77–82.
222. Saxon J. Cost constraints on health care access to some performing artists. *Medical Problems of Performing Artists* 1989;4(3):105–107.
223. Tubiana R. Movements of the fingers (second of a series of three articles). *Medical Problems of Performing Artists* 1988;3(4)–123–128.
224. Tubiana R, Champagne P. Functional anatomy of the hand (first of a series of three articles). *Medical Problems of Performing Artists* 1988;3(3)83–87.
225. Tubiana R, Champagne P, Brockman R. Fundamental positions for instrumental musicians (third of a series of three articles). *Medical Problems of Performing Artists* 1989;4(2):73–76.
226. Salmon P, Newmark J. Clinical applications of MIDI technology. *Medical Problems of Performing Artists* 1989;4(1):25–31.
227. Norris RN. Overuse injuries: When practicing puts you on hold instead of onstage. *Guitar Player* 1989;23(9):94,96,98.
228. Norris RN. Ask the doctor [column]. *Guitar Player* 23(11), 1989.
229. Norris RN. Ask the doctor [column]. *Emerson Flute Forum* 6(1), 1989 Spring-Summer.
230. Lederman RJ. Performing arts medicine [editorial]. *New England Journal of Medicine* 1989; 320(4):246–248.
231. Brandfonbrener AG. Performing arts medicine: A checkup [editorial]. *Medical Problems of Performing Artists* 1989;4(3):101–102.
232. Musicians' maladies [letter]. *New England Journal of Medicine* 1989;321(1):51–53.
233. Upcoming conferences/symposiums. *International Arts-Medicine Association Newsletter* 1986 Fall-1987 Winter;2(4):1,4.
234. Brandfonbrener AG. The jazz musician: A challenge to arts medicine [editorial]. *Medical Problems of Performing Artists*1988;3(3):iii.
235. Harman SE. Music Medicine Clearinghouse—progress report. *Maryland Medical Journal* 1989; 38(9):756–757.
236. Medical care for British orchestras. *Lancet* 1989;2(8673):1232.
237. Hochberg F. Research in medical problems of performing artists. *International Arts-Medicine Association Newsletter* 1988;3(1):1.

Textbook of Performing Arts Medicine, edited
by R. T. Sataloff, A. Brandfonbrener, and
R. Lederman. Raven Press, Ltd.,
New York © 1991.

2

Epidemiology of the Medical Problems of Performing Artists

Alice G. Brandfonbrener

*Assistant Clinical Professor of Medicine, Northwestern University Medical School,
and Director, Medical Program for Performing Artists of the Rehabilitation Institute of
Chicago, Chicago, Illinois 60611*

EPIDEMIOLOGIC CONSIDERATIONS IN PERFORMING ARTS MEDICINE

Until recently, few people outside the performance communities acknowledged the existence of performance-induced injuries. Although there is still limited awareness, many more people have become concerned about the frequency and especially the prevention of these medical problems. The medical specialty concentrating on medical problems of performers is new (1); this first text is a response to the rapidly increasing demand for knowledge and training. However, in spite of this burgeoning interest, our knowledge remains incomplete. In this chapter we will discuss the roots of some of the injuries and medical problems that occur as a consequence of being a performing artist. Many of the current suspicions regarding etiology of these performance-related ailments are based on anecdotal experiences and calculated guessing. In spite of gratifying progress, many of the current assumptions on which diagnoses are made and treatments are prescribed await scientific verification. We would be less than honest if we did not make this disclaimer at the outset.

A large part of our discussion will pertain especially, although not exclusively, to classical, instrumental musicians. However, problems of other performers, such as popular musicians and those in the theater, are similar, and special comments are added in selected instances where there may be important differences or special considerations. In this book we will not concentrate heavily on those problems which occur "off the field of play." Finally, while this is a textbook, performing arts medicine is an evolving specialty. Consequently, a number of the ideas presented will be more a matter of the author's own experience and opinions in the absence of any generally accepted dogma.

Historically there have been some notable examples of career-ending or -altering injuries and illness among instrumentalists, the best known of which affected Robert Schumann (2). It has been only within the last decade, however, that these have attracted significant attention from either musicians or medical practitioners. With this heightened interest, the great frequency of other performance-related impairments, not all of them career-ending, has become increasingly apparent.

THE PREVALENCE OF PERFORMANCE-INDUCED INJURIES IN MUSICIANS

As part of the developing interest in performing arts medicine, a number of studies have been undertaken of the frequency of these disabilities. Several populations of instrumentalists have been surveyed concerning how many musicians within a given period have had problems, yielding prevalence rather than incidence data. It is interesting to note, however, that within the differing populations studied, and using differing methods, the results appear strikingly consistent.

The most comprehensive study done was that undertaken for the International Conference of Symphony and Opera Musicians (ICSOM) in 1986 by Fishbein and Middlestadt (3). From a population in excess of 4,000 from 48 American orchestras, they received 2,212 responses. Of these, 76% indicated having had a medical problem severe enough to affect performance. The majority of these problems were painful musculoskeletal syndromes, most frequent among the string players (78%). Of nonstring musicians, 75% also had a "severe" medical problem. In a 1986 study involving eight orchestras in Australia, the United States, and England, Fry (4) found a 64% occurrence of "overuse syndrome," which, when the least severe of these was subtracted, amounted to 42% with a more significant level of symptoms. Fry also noted a 63% to 69% injury rate among men and women musicians, respectively, whereas Middlestadt and Fishbein (5) found a more striking difference of 72% and 84%. In a smaller but more diverse population of "high level" musicians, Caldron et al. (6) found 59% of 378 respondents reporting a "musically related musculoskeletal problem," again with a significant preponderance of women.

The reasons responsible for the generally high rate of injury, the predilection for those who play certain instruments, and the gender differences in these occurrences are the substance of the research currently engaging many specialists in performing arts medicine. Whereas the data are not yet in, it is assumed that there are several responsible factors, including the number of repetitious actions required, playing techniques, stress, hand size, and joint condition.

Several surveys have also been done involving preprofessional musicians of secondary school age, as well as conservatory students. In Australia, Fry (7) reported up to 13% of a surveyed group of adolescent students with an overuse problem at the time of study, with a prevalence of injured girls. In Houston, Lockwood (8) studied 113 serious high school musicians, 32% of whom complained of a medical problem, 17% of which were reportedly "severe." Once again, these were noted in girls (68%) more commonly than boys (47%). Manchester (9) reported on the incidence of hand problems among 1,606 conservatory students over a 4-year period. There was an incidence rate of 8.5 episodes per 100 performance majors, with the men's and women's rates being 5.7 and 11.5, respectively.

THE FUTURE OF PERFORMING ARTS MEDICINE

These preliminary studies appear to more than justify the current level of interest in performance-related injuries of musicians. Needed are prospective studies and information concerning incidence as opposed to prevalence, as well as standardization of measurement criteria.

The development of predictably effective treatment and prevention strategies will ultimately depend on the establishment of clear-cut etiologies. Performing arts medicine is actively involved in expanding the fund of scientific knowledge to answer this need. More medical centers are being established specifically for these performer-patients, giving the opportunity for increased clinical observation and experience. The decreasing reluctance of performers to openly examine and share information about their medical problems with investigators provides research opportunities which are the essential factor for progress (10). Funding for research into these medical problems is scarce because while they may be career-threatening, they are not life-threatening. In the future, we hope that performing arts medicine will be deemed at least as important in its role as sports medicine is for professional and amateur athletes. If the great progress that has been made in the past decade continues, we may anticipate the inclusion of more plentiful data in a second edition of this text than are available for chapters in this first book.

THE APPROACH TO EVALUATING THE ETIOLOGIES OF MUSICIANS' INJURIES

Although not unique to the medical problems of instrumentalists, in many, if not most, instances there are multiple etiologies operating synergistically rather than a single factor being responsible for a given injury (11). The importance of this lies in the fact that unless all of the etiological factors are taken into consideration, successful treatments may be difficult to develop. The approach to identifying the factors contributing to the onset of a given medical problem, injury, or disability may require considerable detective work. While this can be challenging under any circumstance, it may be especially so when dealing with voice- or instrument-generated dysfunctions because they can be so subtle. Finally, as in other areas of medicine, the interrelationship of physical and emotional stresses is apparent and must be considered when examining risk factors among musicians.

Although the understanding of the musculoskeletal system has been greatly advanced by sports medicine and has been important to the development of this field, performing arts medicine is in reality a branch of occupational medicine. For the most part, not only are the injuries incurred by musicians a consequence of their work, they are of the repetitive strain variety, similar to those occurring in industrial workers, computer operators, and even grocery checkout workers! (12,13). Appropriate prevention strategies developed for factory workers (14) are likely to be directly transferable to the concert halls and practice rooms of musicians, and vice versa. Determining the multiple etiologic variants requires an analysis of: (1.) the occupation, (2.) the instrument, and (3.) the musician.

CHOOSING MUSIC AS A VOCATION OR AVOCATION

The Beginning of the Process and Its Risks: Education

The development of sufficient interest to pursue the study of a musical instrument depends on many factors. Whereas talent may determine the ultimate outcome, it is initially the appropriate and timely exposure that generates the necessary spark of interest. This must be followed by the opportunity to pursue the interest. As we tend to be drawn to the familiar, a child who hears music of any variety from an early age is more likely to develop an interest in these sounds and their reproduction. For most children it is the mother's voice which is the earliest music heard, although there are those who are convinced of the influence of sounds heard even prenatally. In any case, we know both from experience and from the biographies of successful musicians that the achievement of adequate proficiency for vocational or avocational success characteristically depends on a start early in childhood (15,16,17). This is especially true for some instruments, notably strings and keyboard. However, the ear and intellect, as well as manual dexterity, are involved in musical skill and the quality of performance; progress in all musical categories is more assured if the head as well as the hands have been trained early. Thus, the accepted methods for musical training in the western world are integrally related to early childhood education. In some western preschools and primary schools, music education may include teaching systems such as Orff and Kodaly, providing an opportunity to understand, duplicate and create simple rhythmic patterns and musical intervals long before a child is verbally or musically literate. The enormously successful Suzuki Talent Education Method, which capitalizes on the mother/child bond to introduce musical training to very young children, teaches the playing of the instrument in advance of instruction in what Suzuki proponents consider the "distraction" of musical notation. For older students, many conservatories have "preparatory" departments which serve as natural feeders into sequentially more advanced, preprofessional educational tracks.

Apart from being the basis for possible musical careers, the provision of music lessons is a source of satisfaction and status for parents, as is the vicarious sense of accomplishment that comes with their childrens' successes (17). Although parents are reluctant to give up these opportunities for their children, even at considerable personal economic sacrifice, this is not the situtation in the public school systems where all of the arts are a likely first target for curriculum reductions in the face of budgetary crises. Consequently, for most children the opportunity for the kind of early musical exposure that is required for later success is linked to the economic status of the parents, the neighborhood, and the local schools. Therefore, it is in part an accident of birth that determines the pool of prodigious and lesser talents from which come most future professional musicians.

There are many reasons why these seemingly irrelevant factors relate to the development of later medical problems. First, the ability to progress in skill on an instrument, even as a child, depends upon an unchildlike commitment of time and energy as much as it does on the support of family and environment. How a child practices (both qualitatively and quantitatively), who teaches the child, what music the child hears, whether the child gains or loses self-esteem (18), whether or not the child has an identity and status in addition to the musical one and, most importantly, whether there is adequate raw talent on which to base future progress—all of these components are crucial in determining how the musician and the instrument interact, especially in the long term (19). These diverse factors play a role in the development of injuries, both as students and later in life, when the habits which were ingrained in youth may reveal their protective or destructive side effects. We will discuss this at much greater length below.

Another important aspect of the potential conflicts arising from early identification of children as serious musicians is that, by and large, the child is a passive part of this process. At the age when these decisions are frequently made, a child cannot have a sense of their impact on his or her future, let alone judge whether those decisions are based on a realistic appraisal of talent. These initial decisions are characteristically made by parents and teachers who cannot be expected to be dispassionate in their reasoning. Therefore, through no fault of his or her own, a child may be steered into an all but irrevocable educational track through well-meaning but inadequately informed judgments. With maturity the student must come to accept or reject the decision that has already been made by coming to terms with it (20). Failure to resolve this potential dilemma may prevent the individual from achieving a satisfying career as a musician or in any field.

Talent is both native and nurtured, but without a reasonable amount of the former, young musicians may be faced with overwhelming tasks and tensions trying to live up to the competition of their peers, as well as to fulfill the expectations of the adults around them (22). It is generally accepted that the way to Carnegie Hall is to "practice, practice, practice" but, as we will discuss, both the amount and intensity of the practice may also be key to the development of musical injuries (21). A young musician attempting to overachieve is particularly at risk for injuries. We do not yet have risk data concerning musical longevity. Is it a health benefit or hazard to have played the instrument for many, many years, starting well before the body is mature and full-grown? It is likely that at least a partial answer to this question will lie in how the instrument and player interact—the technique. This, in turn, is largely a function of the teaching and the teacher.

The music teacher is commonly selected by a musically naive parent and, once again, the future musician may be a victim of good intentions but poor judgment. The nature of the music student–teacher relationship is nearly unique in our educational system, both because it is "one on one," and because it tends to carry over from year to year, unlike the classroom teacher. Thus there is the potential for the music teacher to exert an inordinate amount of influence on the musical and extra-musical life and development of a young student, at times akin to that of a parent. One may turn to almost any musical biography for confirmation of this tendency. The choice of music teacher, initially by a parent and later by the student, becomes both a musical and a personal decision of great importance to the youngster's present and future direction. It is virtually impossible to monitor the interactions in the music studio, although the development of injuries or painful syndromes in a music student may be a clue regarding playing or practice techniques, as it may also be a marker for nonmusical stresses. Like parents, teachers can hardly be liable for all of their charges' problems, but clearly they are an important factor. The "best" teacher may not be the best teacher for everyone. Expertise in playing brings with it no guarantee of teaching ability. There are many important questions that must be taken into consideration in choosing a teacher. Not only are questions of competency involved, but of at least equal importance are issues of ease of communication, style, and mutually compatible goals. Teachers and students should go through a mutual auditioning process, with parents included when young students are at issue, before a commitment is made. These commitments ought not be written in stone; if a mistake has been made by either party it should be rectified through discussion and appropriate changes.

Some final comments about students and their special risks. Although faulty technique frequently lies behind a medical musical problem, sudden changes in activity level are equally risky for students and even for more mature instrumentalists. Changing teachers, the introduction of a new technique, new repertoire, and changes in practice and playing requirements must all be considered in trying to understand the etiologies of these injuries. Increased stress, whether primarily mental or physical, is critical, and the timing of injuries is frequently an important clue. The increased practice time required for competitions, recitals, and auditions makes these times of special risk (9), as are the periods of return to playing activity after vacations or illnesses.

Age as a Risk Factor

There have been studies to indicate that conductors may have an increased life expectancy (23), but there are no comparable statistics for instrumental musicians. Although there are many factors involved in this longevity, including opportunities to deal with stress, the amount of aerobic activity that can accompany conducting has always been considered its protective feature. These data have different implications from the study of music-generated injuries, none of which appears to relate directly to life expectancy. Recent studies of young musicians appear to implicate the process of music making itself as being the principal risk factor for injury and to suggest that, unlike with sports injuries, age is neither a significant protector nor a detriment (7,8). Data from the large survey conducted by the International Conference of Symphony and Opera Musicians (ICSOM) in 1986 indicates a peak injury occurrence in orchestral mid-life (24). Assuming that, for most musicians, this is the time of peak financial and family responsibilities, this would appear to indict the total amount of activity rather than the age of the musician as the critical factor in injuries. In a study of older orchestral musicians, the time of retirement appears to be more a consequence of chronological age than of a specific disability. The failure of retired musicians to continue to play post-retirement seems due more to a loss of motivation than to a decline in physical ability (25).

It stands to reason that while they may not have an increased incidence of aging-related diseases, musicians are no less susceptible to, nor on the other hand protected from: cardiovascular disease, degenerative joint dysfunction, or the effects of aging on the central nervous system. In fact, as we will discuss later, musicians' characteristically sedentary existence theoretically puts them at increased risk for cardiovascular disease. Likewise, as a consequence of hand-intensive activities and unnatural posturing over such a prolonged time period, the joints of the upper extremity and the neck of musicians may be subject to an accelerated risk of degenerative disease (26). Therefore, with advancing age, the various activities peculiar to the lives of musicians may become more difficult to perform, the quality of performance may suffer; even without a specific injury it may become prudent for instrumentalists to withdraw from careers in professional music while they are still able to play acceptably.

Although studies have been limited, those that have been done indicate that while youth itself is not a risk factor for increased occurrence of injuries, neither is it a protector. In studies of musicians of school and college age, the injury figures are comparable to those of professional musicians. Therefore, there must, indeed, be something inherent in being a musician that accounts for these injuries, more than does age (7,8).

Performing Careers and Lifestyle as Risk Factors

In addition to the technical aspects of playing an instrument, what is it about their activities that put musicians at risk for injuries? Environmental concerns about the workplace include considerations of the social, economic, and health issues of musicians as a group. To a large extent the particulars of these relate to the individual instrument, musical style, and vocational choice within performing music. Although there are similarities among the lives of orchestral musicians, popular musicians, soloists, and those who divide their musical activities between teaching and performing, there are clear-cut differences. For a variety of reasons, including socioeconomic factors, popular musicians remain especially underserved and understudied medically. This is a problem shared by people working in the theater. Many of the discussions throughout this book will have most complete applicability to classical musicians. However, it should not be inferred from this that other performing artists are without risk, that they have no need for improved medical care, or that the origins and resolutions of their peculiar medical problems do not bear investigating.

THE OCCUPATION: THE ENSEMBLE AND THE ENVIRONMENT

It is important to recognize that there are many features relating to when, where, and what the instrumentalist is playing that affect the potential for music-related injuries. The number of rehearsals and quality and quantity of repertoire are such factors, as are the acoustic properties of the environment, its temperature, seating and lighting conditions, and the space provided per player. In addition to the number of required performances, pit orchestras are commonly regarded as among the highest risk because of the limited space, sound properties, and frequently poor lighting conditions. Playing out-of-doors brings many hazards to the musicians as well as to the audiences. The author has treated injuries related to insect bites, falling stage parts, bat bites, and allegedly from both excessive cold and heat. Many others are rare but nevertheless medically interesting and challenging. Every performer has a tendency to regard his or her situation as the most potentially perilous. Falling off the stage, while not necessarily humorous, is more likely the fault of the individual than of the environment. Falling scenery, on the other hand, is a hazard for people onstage and off, including those in the pit. There are medicolegal as well as purely medical aspects of such problems. Many of the patients seen for stage-related trauma are actors and dancers, and the variable properties of the surfaces on which they are required to perform are, indeed, a hazard. Despite good combat instruction, acting is truly a dangerous profession. Injuries may occur from various aspects of stage fights, poorly constructed scenery and props, poor lighting, and other causes. Special effects such as fogs can be risky for all, especially for those with respiratory impairments.

Musicians who spend time in the recording studio are virtually unanimous in describing these sessions as more stressful than a routine rehearsal or performance. The reader can readily imagine the reasons for this, including the need to achieve a level of perfection in performance not achievable in concert. With modern technology and splicing, it would seem that some of this tension should now be avoidable if the musician understands the technology of the studio and uses it to his or her benefit.

This discussion is far from complete, but it will serve to remind us that the environment of performance is an important contributor to the hazards to which performers are subject, and it must be considered in the medical evaluation of these patients.

ACCESSING MEDICAL CARE

Many popular musicians and people associated with the theater are identified with countercultural philosophies, and members of these communities frequently do not lead mainstream lives or access traditional medical care. Although there are inadequate data to support it, there is a commonly held notion that popular musicians are less at risk from music-induced injuries than their classical counterparts, perhaps because they are more "macho" and less neurotic. However, theatrical personnel are at least as prone to illnesses and injuries as the general population. Both popular musicians and theater people have had a long tradition of seeking nontraditional solutions to their medical problems. Whether or not this is considered a risk factor for performers is in part a question of bias, but it is another aspect of the health of performing artists which needs nonjudgmental study.

The advent of performing arts medicine as a specialty grew out of the recognition that, as a group, performers are underserved, having generally found it difficult or impossible to find affordable care that is sensitive and responsive to their needs (27). It is difficult to assess the impact this has had on the actual incidence of medical problems and their complications among musicians, or how many performance careers may have been impaired because of the lack of appropriate medical intervention. It is now accepted that there are currently many performers with performance-related injuries, and the generally enthusiastic support from the consumers of care at special artists' clinics has been largely responsible for the growth of this subspecialty. The final proof of its effectiveness as a medical subspecialty will come in the ensuing years of experience and from prospective studies of injuries and other measurements of health status.

ALTERNATIVE LIFESTYLES AND THE PERFORMING ARTIST

Substance Abuse

Preliminary studies indicate that, although the stressors may be different from those in classical music, popular musicians have their own occupation-related sources of tension (28). Although the use of drugs and alcohol is pervasive throughout society, it appears to be more common and acceptable within the pop music culture, as well as in the theatrical community, than among the general population. How much of this presumed use is tied to lifestyle and the perception that being in a mind-altered state improves performance, and how much is because drugs and alcohol provide a needed and accepted release from stress, we cannot answer. Although it represents an enormous problem for society in general and for the arts in particular, risk-taking behavior of this magnitude is beyond the scope of this chapter. Nor does the world of classical music escape substance use and abuse. In many ways, economically and socially, these performing artists are themselves not mainstream. However, generally speaking, the lifestyles of classical musicians are as traditional as are most of their backgrounds and their music, so that their use of drugs and alcohol, while still a problem, is more representative of society as a whole than of the artistic life.

Diet

It can be argued that diet is irrelevant to the medical problems of performing artists, other than dancers. However, since overall physical condition is important when looking at risk factors for injury, including stress, our epidemiologic consideration of this topic would be incomplete without a consideration of diet in the health of performing artists.

What we eat is not only the consequence of taste and availability, it is very much a matter of habit. Dietary habits come from parents' dietary preferences, whether they are based on economics, geography, religion, or personal idiosyncracies. With age these habits are altered, in turn, by circumstances—what is affordable, what one's peers eat, what is liked or disliked, and what is believed to be healthy or unhealthy. Dancers' dietary habits are themselves the subject of much writing and study and, although they may be a reflection of societal as well as personal whims, they are clearly driven beyond all else by occupational factors or risks (29,30,31). These are considered in the section of this book dealing with dance medicine. It is impossible to generalize about the dietary habits of performers, although musicians and people involved in the theater tend to encounter similar difficulties. Most people are subject to the convenience and lure of fast foods, and performing artists are perhaps even more so because of pressures imposed both by their schedules and their budgets. In general, performers are particularly negligent of their bodies and their overall health, including their dietary habits. Although their lifestyles may embrace self-neglect and self-abuse, performing artists are similar to other consumers in their vulnerability to media barrages and dietary fads. What may be the most important factor when examining the dietary habits of musicians, as well as of theater personnel, is the compromised social function of eating that is a common consequence of their professions. Both tend to work long and unusual hours with rehearsals at irregular times of day or night. Performances tend to be in the evening, sometimes in addition to a matinee. Most performers prefer either not to eat at all or at least not to consume a full meal before performing. In some instances, this is because a full stomach may cause a compromise of breathing technique. In others, it is the recognition of a level of performance anxiety incompatible with good digestion. It may be a combination of these and other factors. By the time a musician or an actor is prepared to eat, fatigue may have replaced hunger; restaurants and groceries may have long since closed; and nonmusician friends and families may have already eaten and, in many cases, retired for the night. Social life becomes more difficult to maintain outside of the workplace, and many performers appropriately prefer to limit their extramural contacts with their colleagues. Eating without a social function may serve as both an appetite suppressant and as the rationale for eating less than ideal food. It may also serve as an ongoing source of stress, which in turn may be reflected in numerous other problems, including household and family crises. Although the author is unaware of any statistics concerning divorce rates among performing artists, one gets the impression from the popular press, even at the more responsible end of the spectrum, that multiple marriages and divorces are even more a part of the accepted lifestyle of performers than of the general population, where currently one in three marriages ends in divorce. Again, whereas social habits may not be the direct etiological agents for injuries in performing artists, they may be a major source of stress, which is clearly an important factor responsible for performers' medical problems.

PSYCHOLOGICAL PROBLEMS

A much more thorough discussion of this very complicated subject appears elsewhere in this book. However, several things need to be said here in the context of discussing the etiologies of injuries and illnesses in performing artists. In addition to all of the usual stresses and psychological risks of life in general, performers are especially vulnerable to other unique occupational stresses. Job and financial insecurity play an important role (5). Whether artists as a group are more "sensitive" is debatable, but this assertion may be true to some degree, because of the demands of their artistry (32). Because of the long and intense requisite training, and because this is an ongoing process, performers may be subject to higher levels of ongoing stress than are other occupational groups. The long periods of solitude required for practicing in musical careers can foster depression at all ages and delay the development of social skills among younger players. Players of solo instruments do not have even the potential for interpersonal contacts with peers that can be a part of playing ensemble instruments. Obviously, these drawbacks represent a greater threat to some than to others, but these are factors that should be considered in making a career choice, developing coping techniques in that career, and assessing medical difficulties in performers.

Actors charged with portraying the intense feelings of their characters are subject to unique stresses, and the obligation to understand their own as well as to interpret their character's feelings can impose a heavy load (33). Although not limited to this group, there may be a reluctance on the part of performers to undergo psychotherapy, based on the misperception that the process will impede their natural spontaneity and creativity (34). Those artists who have had psychotherapy in general belie this reservation, and this attitude probably simply represents another facet of the common resistance to delve into potentially painful issues.

One cannot separate health problems into categories of those which are purely emotional and those which are physical. Because of the intensity and pervasiveness of stress in the performing arts, and the exacting demands of performance, it is especially important in performing arts medicine to consider all aspects of the performer-patient's health in assessing the etiologic factors of their medical problems.

Performance Anxiety

Although in many ways this subject more properly belongs to the section on individual risk factors, the presence of some degree of performance anxiety among performers of all types is nearly universal. That is not to say that a majority of artists are severely impaired by performance anxiety symptoms, or have not found their own ways to cope satisfactorily with it. However, the impact that various symptoms of performance anxiety have on players of different instruments and the extent to which different individuals suffer from these symptoms is highly variable.

Difficulties with concentration and the potential for memory slips are obviously a concern for all performers, musical and otherwise. Other, more specific symptoms caused by the general sympathetic discharge of anxiety that have a special effect on musical performance are: impairment of musculoskeletal control (including tremors and breathing control problems), gastrointestinal irritability, decreased salivation, feelings of imminent doom and syncope (caused by changes in blood pressure, cardiac rate, and hyperventilation), and hyperhidrosis, especially of the palms of the hands. The challenge of playing an instrument in the presence of a severe tremor is obviously greater for some instruments (e.g., the strings) than for others (e.g., the brass). Likewise, although it may be unpleasant, a dry mouth is not a potential hazard for pianists as it is for wind players. Therefore, satisfactory treatment of performance anxiety, which is discussed elsewhere, must consider the impact of both its psychological aspects and its physical manifestations (35).

THE ROLE OF THE INSTRUMENT IN THE ETIOLOGY OF INJURIES

It has been suggested by a colleague, not entirely facetiously, that all musical instruments should carry a warning from the surgeon general that their use "may be injurious to your health." Whereas, in study after study, all instruments appear to be implicated in injuries, certain instruments are associated with higher degrees of risk—namely, string and keyboard instruments. The critical factors which appear to account for this increased risk in playing particular instruments are: (1.) the posture maintained in playing, (2.) the weight of the instrument, if it is held, (3.) the pressure of the instrument at its contact points with the body of the musician, (4.) the nature of the repetitions of musculoskeletal activity required to perform on the instrument, and (5.) the individual physiologic demands of the instrument, such as breath control. Although these are general principles, the individual features of each instrument or class of instrument make it preferable to consider each of these points vis-à-vis the particular instrument (4). As this is intended as a medical textbook rather than an instrumental method book, the discussions of technique will not go into the great detail that the latter require. Nor does time or space permit discussing the fine points of different instrumental designs (e.g., the action of a Steinway versus that of other piano manufacturers), although when variable designs or modifications of instruments appear to play a role in the development of injuries or their resolution, mention of these will be made (e.g., offset G keys in the flute, shoulder rests in violins and violas, and instrumental size, when there is a choice).

The Instrument

It is crucial in determining the etiology of music-induced injuries to understand the interaction of a biological system (the musician) with an inanimate object (the instrument). We will look first at the less variable component of this relationship, the instrument. This includes examining the general, intrinsic risks of the instrumental class, and the peculiarities that may exist within an individual member of that species that may be responsible for creating challenges over and above the instrument class as a whole.

The Keyboard Instruments

Although neither the frequency of injuries nor, in many instances, the exact diagnoses of injured pianists, organists, and other keyboard players can readily be determined, the percentage of such patients presenting to the practices of most performing arts clinics is high, ranging anywhere from 40% to 60% of the musician patients. Starting in conservatories, these players appear to be especially vulnerable. Why this is so is a matter of conjecture at this time, but it would appear to be multifactorial.

Few would argue that the most logical explanation for the high incidence of neuromusculoskeletal injuries in pianists is directly related to the number of repetitive activities of small musculoskeletal units, i.e., the fingers. All activities in which there is repetitive use of tissues entail such a risk, depending in part also on the amount of effort expended. Using these units over and over again produces fatigue and stresses many tissues beyond their reasonable limits, inducing states of overuse, whether the work be industrial or musical. There is no known formula for predicting the tremendous individual vulnerability in this regard. The existence of multiple and seemingly diametrically opposed schools of piano technique which have always abounded are testimony to there being no "one and only" way to produce the optimal result at the keyboard, either musically or medically. There simply are too many variables of instruments, repertoire, and especially of the human body and psyche, to develop steadfast formulas in this regard. In medicine, we are taught from the beginning the importance of the individual in assessing and treating patients and diseases, and to rarely, if ever, say "never" or "always." There is a difference between having strong convictions that one's methods are generally correct and believing that they are invariably correct. Good teaching, as good medicine, necessitates good critical judgment, but inflexibility has no role in either (22,36). On the other hand, there are too many examples of musicians with unorthodox technique who have injury-free and successful careers, while on the other hand, people who have studied with all the "right" teachers and have faultless technique have had injury-plagued careers that may ultimately need to be abandoned. For purposes of this discussion, we will consider the following factors: (1.) posture at the instrument, (2.) the special musculoskeletal demands of keyboard performance, and (3.) individual repertoire and practice technique risks (from a medical, not pedagogical, point of view). There will be an assumption, as a matter of practicality, that medical problems presenting in pianists, organists, harpsichordists, and other keyboardists are variations on a theme.

Posture

With very few exceptions (e.g., entertainers, classroom teachers, and choir directors), a sitting position is required both for practice and performance in keyboard playing. In fact, there is a tendency for persons who do attempt to play standing for any length of time to develop problems with the hands and wrists due to the hyperextended wrist position. Although we will largely confine this discussion to the piano, it must be acknowledged that organ benches and posturing present a special set of problems, especially for organists of small stature or disproportionately short extremities. In selecting a bench or chair for the piano, prolonged comfort will be achieved only when the seat height and the distance from the keyboard are appropriate for the individual player. The chair must be adjustable both vertically and horizontally. These adjustments are important considerations from both medical and pedagogical viewpoints, although it may have to be a choice among the lesser of evils if there are mutually conflicting needs to satisfy. The pianist who is exceptionally tall or long-legged will have problems different from those experienced by a person of short stature, adult, or child. There are mechanisms to build up the pedals for the latter, but what to do with very tall individuals is an acknowledged problem without a satisfactory solution. The use of a padded versus nonpadded bench is an individual choice, although for those not endowed with much padding of their own, a hard surface is more likely to produce symptoms of compression of the sciatic nerves, especially after prolonged practice. Although relatively few players select a chair with a back support, the entire back is at issue, especially considering the lengthy time periods that many pianists remain seated in less than ideal positions.

The maintainance of a "good" posture is important, but if tension and rigidity are required to maintain this position, they get transmitted to the rest of the body, including shoulders, arms, and hands. In order to avoid this potential problem, one should consider the following points: (1.) the need for overall good muscle tone, especially of the paraspinal muscles (this will come only with appropriate exercising, away from the instrument), (2.) the need to maintain flexibility in posture and therefore a balance between excessive tension and total collapse of the back musculature, and (3.) the need to avoid excessive back fatigue. The player must recognize the need to get up and move about periodically during long practice sessions (these principles, of course, also apply not only to other musicians but to computer operators, secretaries, and people in other relatively sedentary occupations). The neck is also a frequent location of pain and tension among pianists, as it is in other musicians and occupational groups. The length of the neck is especially important in the musician. Unusually tall individuals, or those with longer than average necks, tend to play hunched forward over the keyboard, creating tension in the paraspinal muscles and the trapezii. Many consider contending with chronic neck, shoulder, and upper back tension and pain to be an inevitable part of playing a keyboard instrument. For some it is unrelated to body size and proportion and simply a function of muscle tension and fatigue. Maintaining mechanically unsound postures, as with the neck excessively flexed and rigid, is frequently the underlying cause of these pains. Likewise, poor generalized muscle tone and inadequate large proximal muscle support for the upper extremities also play a role.

Since the keyboard height is fixed, the most critical factor in chair height is the position of the arms vis-à-vis the keyboard. Individuals with "nonstandard" body proportions (e.g., shorter or longer relative lengths of upper versus lower arm segments) must be considered. The ideal (i.e., physiologically and mechanically) is for the lower arms and wrists to be level with or slightly above the keyboard, while at such a distance that the hands are neither crowded into the keys nor so far away that the arms must be extended at the elbows to reach the keyboard. The upper arms should hang naturally and relaxed from the shoulders, slightly anterior to the trunk, with the elbows partially flexed. For most pianists this allows for optimal integrated functioning of the hands, wrists, arms, shoulders, and back.

Many schools of piano technique regard the position over the keys and posturing of the fingers as singularly important. Some recommend invariably curved fingers, especially at the proximal interphalangeal joints, others a more modified flexion, and very few a technique similar to Vladimir Horowitz's fully extended fingers! How the wrist is held is also partially a function of one's pedagogical school, although as physicians, we generally recommend that the wrist be maintained as closely as possible to a neutral position—in a relatively straight line with the forearm, neither bent toward the thumb (radially) nor toward the small finger (ulnarly). Obviously, it is both a function of repertoire and individual construction that will largely determine these choices, no matter what pedagogical school is represented. How one stretches to reach octaves, the choice of fingerings, and how the arms are extended for distant notes will, in most cases, be an amalgam of what has been taught, and adaptations to the individual pianist's particular physical characteristics (36).

Most questions of injuries and repertoire will be discussed with individual risk factors, but there are a few other generic risks to be included here. First, for most individuals, easier music means less technically challenging, more limited stretches, fewer series of octaves or chords, slower tempi, less complicated rhythms, and shorter periods of forte, legato, or prestissimo playing. However, even relatively uncomplicated music can, if practiced inappropriately or excessively, produce injuries in vulnerable persons. While not invariably true, it is by and large relatively advanced players, or at least those playing advanced repertoire, who sustain most of the significant keyboard-induced injuries. How practicing is done is important for instrumentalists at all levels of playing in all genres of music. If the musician, trying to master a difficult passage, plays the same series of notes in an unvarying rhythm for a particularly long time, those tissues being used repetitiously, without an adequate opportunity for rest and recovery, are subject to injury. There can be no formula that dictates how many times a phrase can be repeated safely, even for the same individual, and repetition is integral to most learning. It is honesty, rather than begging the question, to suggest the use of common sense in practicing for a "reasonable" period of time. There simply is no way to accurately gauge or predict the effect of the many relevant variables. However, it is clear that practice sessions are times of great risk for instrumentalists, so teachers should assume the responsibility for discussion and planning of practicing as much as for development of safe technique and repertoire.

There are many types of keyboards, including piano, clavier, harpsichord, organ, synthesizer and even accordion! There is an ever-increasing array of variants: electric and acoustic types, different action systems, instrument models, keyboard lengths, and individual instrumental properties. Most professional pianists have preferences based on what they are accustomed to—individual style, repertoire, training, and comfort. Unquestionably, some keyboards are more difficult and hazardous to play than others, and for some performers there can be tremendous variations in those on which they are expected to play. Unlike animals, pianos that may be especially vicious are not mercifully disposed of, so that they will do no further harm. However, attempts should be made to match a player's technical characteristics with the instrument, and efforts should be made to modify troublesome pianos with the help of competent technicians. Weather and other conditions may change the action of an instrument from day to day, and instruments should be monitored for such deviations. Only the top piano soloists have the luxury of traveling with their own instrument, or playing on a preselected piano while on tour. The vast majority must accept the instrument at hand, ranging from fine to virtually unplayable. (In fact, Gary Graffman, who was forced to abandon a successful performance career of two-handed repertoire because of a crippling dysfunction of his right hand, ascribes the injury which may have laid the groundwork for this to a problem inflected years before by a faulty instrument.) Accommodating to the idiosyncrasies of individual piano actions is simply a fact of life for the vast majority of pianists at all levels. Although forewarned may be forearmed, it is difficult to make these instant adaptations while immersed in performance. An adequate practice period on an unfamiliar instrument may help (37). Nevertheless, it may be prudent, if unpopular, for a pianist to, on occasion, refuse to play on a faulty instrument or under other adverse conditions. These are frequently overlooked risk factors, and patients who are keyboard players should always be interrogated about unusual postures (e.g., standing while playing), as well as about a history of playing on a variety of pianos.

Perceived differences between the risks posed by different repertoire, such as classical versus jazz, are also interesting. In many instances, popular and classical pianists have had similar training. Whereas the access to medical care may be a factor, it does appear that there are fewer injuries among nonclassical pianists than classical. It remains to be determined whether this is because of different technique, demands of repertoire, psychological factors (e.g., the relative unimportance of note perfection), or a combination of all of these. The difference is not likely due to inability or reluctance to access medical care. In our clinic, we see significant numbers of popular musicians, especially guitar and bass players, but keyboard players are notable by their comparably fewer numbers.

Summary of Keyboard Risks

In spite of the conjectural nature of some of what is said here, it is nevertheless difficult to be all-encompassing. Based on current experiences within the context of instrument-induced injuries, pianists and other keyboard players are among those at highest risk. It appears this is due to factors which are indigenous to the instrument, the repertoire, and the mechanical features required to play them. From a psycho-physiological point of view, the acquisition of the required independent, finely coordinated actions of both hands is a remarkable feat, and it is not surprising that this delicate mechanism is so vulnerable to injury.

String Instruments

In considering the risks posed by instruments, one must separate bowed from plucked instruments. Although there are medical problems common to all bowed string instruments, there are also some notable differences—among them, the violin, the viola, the cello, and the bass. These important differences are related to posture, instrument size, string calibre and tension, bow grip, and additional factors. In most clinical practices in which instrumental musicians are seen, string player patients constitute a number comparable to that of keyboard players. When there are similarities between the problems of bowed and plucked strings, we will indicate this, but generally we will discuss these instruments separately.

As is true in keyboard pedagogy, there are many schools of string playing and many variations in how methods are actually implemented. This is not the place to enter into the relative merits of the Russian versus other schools of violin technique. However, physicians and others treating these musicians should familiarize themselves with the various string-playing techniques and associated postures and hazards. Again, the issue is not so much what is "right" or "wrong" but what works best for a particular musician, both musically and technically (22). Given the requirements for mastering string instruments, there is a wide range of subtle but important choices to be made. Although certain postures and hand positions tend to serve the needs of some players better than others—including their potential for inducing injuries—there are numerous exceptions to any rule.

Special Postural Requirements for Playing String Instruments

The Violin and Viola: The Head, Neck, and Left Shoulder. I will apologize in advance to those instrumentalists, especially the violists, who will quite accurately point out that the viola is a different instrument with playing demands quite different from the violin. It is not simply a large violin, but for the purposes of this text we will knowingly commit the sin of discussing them together, for the most part (38).

When we discuss the postural requirements of playing a particular instrument, this includes not only the positioning of the trunk musculature, but also that of the neck, arm, wrist, hand, and fingers. The modern violin or viola customarily has attached to it one or two aids for supporting the instrument, although the required position is still not musician-friendly for the left upper extremity. There is a chin rest on the top surface of the instrument, and, more variable and subject to individual tastes and philosophies, usually a shoulder support underneath the body of the instrument. The chin rest is rigid (wood or plastic), comes in different contours, can be placed centrally or more laterally over the tailpiece, and is also obtainable in different heights to suit individual preference and structure of the neck, shoulder, and chin. To minimize the irritation of the chin rest against the neck and jaw, it can be padded by using a handkerchief, chamois, or other soft cloth, or by pasting a soft rubber and cloth pad on its surface (e.g., *Strad Pad*). Many players incline their neck and head to varying degrees to the left to assure stability of the instrument, as well as enabling them to occasionally watch their left hands. The baroque equivalents of the modern violin and viola were and are played without a chin rest. The position in which they are played is more anterior, with the left arm much less elevated than the modern version, hence there is less need for the additional support of a chin or shoulder rest.

How far laterally or centrally the left hand supporting the neck of the instrument is positioned is a function of teaching, as well as of arm length (right as well as left). If the violin is held too far to the left, the right arm will have obvious difficulty placing the bow on the strings, especially the lower strings, which are the farthest to the left.

Sitting and Standing. Violins and violas may be played standing or sitting, with soloists traditionally standing and ensemble players sitting. However, when practicing, many choose to stand, whether or not they are soloists, because of the freedom it gives the upper body. When sitting, the choice of seating is one of individual preference, except in those orchestras in which, for the sake of uniformity, there is little or no choice. Aside from the importance of having the chair height adjusted so that the feet can be placed fully on the floor for maximum stability and balance, the ideal angle of both the seat and the backrest of the chair vary according to instrument and individual dimensions. Most violinists and violists tend to sit back against the back of the chair, or at least inclined toward the back. For them, a slight backward tilt of the seat may therefore be most convenient. However, the ideal depth of the seat is more a function of individual size. Some players, while preferring to sit back, are most comfortable with added lumbar or shoulder support on the seat back. In general, seating choice is much more a function of the individual's needs and comfort than of instrumental requisites. It has been only in the relatively recent past that orchestras have recognized the nonuniform seating needs of their players and that chair manufacturers have responded. However, while individual preferences for seating may be acknowledged in principle, for a number of reasons, including economic and aesthetic ones, relatively few ensembles have taken advantage of these options.

Size of the Instrument

A critical factor in many injuries encountered in string players is the relationship between the size of the instrument and that of the player. While there are a limited number of choices to be made, there is some variety possible, and size is an important consideration in understanding the etiologies of many medical problems. Within a very limited range, there are variations in individual instruments and in how they are fitted up to play that may help adapt them to musicians with different bodily proportions. The crucial measurement for most string instruments relates to string length. With that as the limiting factor, some modifications can be made which take into account different hand and finger size, arm length, and so forth, to enhance the instrument's "playability" for an individual player.

There is some choice in the instrument size of all string instruments but, by and large, with the exception of instruments designed specifically for children, the sizes and proportions of most violins are fairly constant. It is beyond the scope of this text to discuss the fitting of instruments for children. String instruments range from as small as $^1/_{16}$ size to full size in violins, with somewhat less selection in the lower strings. Although they are not entirely equivalent, violins can be strung as violas for children too small to play the smallest viola. Cellos also come in fractional sizes, while basses for the very small child are not available. There is a lovely story which Yo-Yo Ma tells about his own choice of instrument. When he was four years old and selecting an instrument, he really wanted to play the bass, but had to settle for the cello instead, much to the benefit of his subsequent audiences! Some instruments are overall of slightly smaller proportions than others (there are some so-called ladies' violins that are approximately $^7/_8$ of a more fully proportioned instrument), and there can be some variation in things such as the thickness of the neck of the instrument, accommodating different hand sizes and proportions.

In the case of violas, there is a much wider range in size, including string length, length of the entire instrument, depth, height, and neck proportions. Although the quality of sound may vary and therefore be the limiting factor, there is in general much greater latitude in finding a viola to fit an individual's size needs (38). Again, it is not simply a question of size and reach. In the hand, for instance, many players with otherwise full-size hands have relatively short "pinkies," or fourth fingers, as they are designated by string players. Some hands are very broad, others narrow, so that one needs to look at the ability of the hand to play in all of the playing positions on the violin or viola to evaluate the fit between the instrument and the musician. Although questions of size more frequently relate to inadequate proportions of players versus the instrument, on occasion the problem is one of arms or hands that are excessively large for the instrument at hand, and players may actually be impeded by their size.

It is critical for all people, including children, to have an instrument that is playable for them. The time for advancing the size of the instrument must be dictated by the growth of the child and not the convenience of availability or considerations of sound quality. The difficulty in finding the string instrument of choice, including the cost, is a major limiting factor for many string players.

Cello. There are fewer postural choices to be made in playing the cello than for the violin or viola. Sitting is the universal position for playing the cello except when playing the national anthem, when many will temporarily stand. Although there are variations in the individual player's style of playing, arm and shoulder height, the angle at which the instrument is placed, and the individual demands of a particular cello's proportions, the range is relatively narrow. The player must be able to reach around the cello with both arms and hands, so that a sitting position against the back of the chair, especially one that is tilted backwards, is decidedly disadvantageous. Therefore, in addition to planting both feet squarely on the floor in a secure position in front of them, allowing the cello to rest between the knees, most cellists favor a chair that is either completely flat in the seat, or in some instances actually tilted slightly forward. The height at which the cello is held is also a function of the length of the end pin which comes from the base of the instrument and supports the instrument against the floor. A very tall player who has a small instrument is able to compensate for this by elevating the cello with an especially long end pin. Conversely, a cellist of short stature can position the instrument lower by not fully extending the end pin. Baroque predecessors of the modern cello were not supported by this device but depended on the pressure of the adducted knees against the instrument. Although some modern players do use knee pressure against the sides of the instrument, in reality this is superfluous and produces tension.

As with violas, cellos come in a sufficient variety of dimensions that the individual with particular needs has some leeway in selecting an appropriate instrument.

Double Bass. The bass—double bass, string bass, upright bass, bass viol—is, by whatever name it is known, a challenge to musicians to play. Although, as mentioned above, it, too, comes with some limited choices of size and proportions, these choices are even more limited than in the case of the cello. The relative paucity of female bassists is in part a corollary of this fact as well as that the bass has not traditionally been regarded as a "feminine instrument." It is an instrument rarely considered an option for girls choosing a string instrument unless they are outstandingly tall. Among the ICSOM population surveyed, there was a total population of 331 bassists, of whom only 34 were females. This contrasts with the 440 cellists, of whom 181 were females (3). In fact, there is a wide variety of sizes and shapes of male bass players, short and tall, having long or short arms, etc., so that size alone is not the criterion, even for males, in selecting this instrument.

Largely because of the unwieldy size of the bass, players have chosen a limited number of playing postures, largely a matter of comfort and facility. Some sit on a high stool with both feet off the floor. The problem for them, as well as others, comes when they must play in the "high" positions, which are in physical reality down low, that is, both the bow and the fingering arms must be extended to reach them. Other players prefer to stand while playing, using the same high stool for rests only, while others lean, more than sit, against the stool. The vast majority of classical bassists opt for a compromise posture in which they partially sit on the stool, with the left knee bent and supported on a rung of the stool, while the right leg is extended and partially weight-bearing. This may be responsible for compression of the left sciatic nerve in bassists as in cellists. However, without any question, the most universal medical problems in bass players are with the back—upper, middle, and in particular the low back. There are clear-cut advantages as well as disadvantages to height for bassists, but the back problems that are seen occur in musicians of all heights. Simply put, as we know from general health figures, the back is a weak link in our evolutionary process, and is a frequent cause of disability in a wide range of occupational groups, including musicians. Again referring to the ICSOM study of 1,378 respondents indicating a severe musculoskeletal problem, 241 were cellists and 192 were bassists. Among the cellists, 26 (11%), and 40 of the bassists (21%), implicated the low back as the site of their primary problem (3). There is no evidence that associates these problems in musicians with an unusual incidence of degenerative disc disease. That is, the majority of the low back pain seen in these patients is muscular or ligamentous in origin. As in the general population, most of the back problems seen are a consequence of strain, inadequate muscle support, poor physiological posturing, fatigue, and excess tension. Given the high prevalence of back problems in bassists and the efficacy of exercise, this would appear to be an ideal situation for various forms of exercise to prevent injury, including swimming and the Paul Williams type of program.

Transporting the Instrument

Never to be forgotten are the problems with the back and other body parts which are incurred more as the result of moving the instrument from place to place than of playing it per se. It is both educational and a source of continuing amazement to observe the many ingenious devices used—especially by players of large and ungainly instruments—to transport them, both on foot and for loading them into a car. In fact, the model of car driven is often dictated for musicians by their instrument's dimensions rather than their own. With very large instruments such as the bass and the harp, there are a limited number of options, although single wheels can be placed on the bottoms of bass fiddles, and moving dollies can be used for harps. Golf carts can be used for somewhat smaller instruments such as the cello, contrabassoon, and others of intermediate size, while shoulder straps and harnesses serve for violins, violas, and wind instruments. A never-ending variety of Rube Goldberg creations to attach an instrument, more or less securely, to a back or to a bicycle can be seen, particularly on campuses and around summer festivals.

The Right Hand and Arm Problems of String Players

Although often not appreciated by nonmusicians, the sound quality of string performance is largely a function of the right, or bow, arm (22), rather than the left hand of the string player. The left hand does more finely coordinated and repetitive actions with the fingers. Whereas the same degree of complicated activity and independence of the hands needed to play the piano is not required in playing string instruments, there is nevertheless little relationship between the physical activities of the right and left arms and hands of string players. The fingers of the left hand are in relatively constant movement, flexing and extending, abducting and adducting, while the fingers of the right hand are in continuous flexion but are relatively stationary in guiding the bow's traversal of the strings. The arms do not move through the same planes, at the same speeds, or require equal amounts of tension and motion. Left hand and arm problems are seen more commonly in younger players, and right hand, arm or shoulder problems in older players, although there are many exceptions. Hand dominance does not appear to be a factor, and although left-handed string instruments do exist, they are rarely used except by guitar players, regardless of hand dominance. The ICSOM study revealed approximately twice the problems with the left versus the right hands of string players, whereas problems with the right and left shoulders were of similar prevalence (3).

By and large the right shoulder problems are mechanical in nature, frequently causing tendinitis of the rotator cuff, with or without an impingement syndrome. The medical consultant should become familiar with the range of options for bowing positions of the shoulder, arm, wrist, and hand in evaluating string-playing patients. The problems seen appear to result from a number of different causes, the most frequent of which is excessive playing and/or poor mechanics of the shoulder. Although bowing does require right-arm pressure, proper distribution of the work of the right arm to include the larger proximal muscles will assist in the required endurance more than will brute strength. Although bows come in subtly different weights, balances, and pliability, these differences may elude the untrained observer while at the same time requiring considerable adjustment on the part of the musician. The string player overpracticing, using excessive tension in any of the involved muscle groups, or with limited range of motion at any of the involved joints, stands to injure associated tissues: muscles, tendons, ligaments, and joints. One must also bear in mind both acute and chronic processes, especially when evaluating older patients who may have primary or associated degenerative joint conditions.

It is worth noting, without going into the technical details of bow grips, that cellists tend to have a greater frequency of painful problems with their right thumbs than do other string players. The cello bow is larger, heavier, and requires the use of somewhat greater pressure than is used to play the violin or viola. There are a variety of permissible bow grips, and unorthodox positions may work well for those musicians who use them. However, those using an extended right thumb are prone to problems, especially pain, which appears to be the consequence of excessive tension on the metacarpophalangeal and basal joints.

The work of the bow arm, including the shoulder, is in part a function of how the bow is held or gripped in the fingers of the right hand. In fact, probably the most frequent problems encountered in the right hand are a reflection of how much tension is created by this "grip." Every school of string playing has a favorite and "unchallengeable" hand position. The nonmusician needs to understand that whereas the bow is indeed directed and controlled by the right hand, undue pressure will not only influence the sound quality of the bow drawn over the strings, but will also create excessive tension throughout the right arm. If the bow is inadequately controlled through finger position and tension, both the sound quality and the ability to draw the bow will suffer, and injuries may occur. There are options within the bow holds for each string instrument, and it is well worth the time of the medical examiner to become at least conversant with these variables. Likewise, the physician needs to become familiar with the different methods of using the bow for different sound effects, e.g., spiccato (bouncing off the string), legato (drawn out), etc.

While it is beyond this text to enter into technical detail concerning bow grips, special mention must be made in regard to bass players, who have two very distinct alternative hand positions. These are referred to as the "French" and "German" bow grips, one of which is roughly comparable to a cello bow hold, and the other which involves the hand and arm being partially pronated. The author has not found the bow grip to be a clear-cut incriminating factor in the etiologies of the medical problems presented by bass players. However, they do involve vastly different muscle actions of the entire upper extremity and not simply of the involved hand, and more study is needed to determine the medical implications of these different techniques.

An important consideration which must always be kept in mind is that a symptom may be particularly troublesome because the patient is a performer, but it may have resulted from an entirely unrelated activity. Several players treated by us had shoulder injuries, some career-ending, which probably were brought about by a combination of occupational and nonoccupational processes. It is essential to understand the details of the work requirements of the instrument played in order to understand the etiology of an injury, the impact of an injury, and the rehabilitative needs of the injured musician; nonoccupational activities must be similarly scrutinized.

Bass Guitar. In our clinic we see a disproportionate number of electric bassists, comparing them with both classical and upright bassists and with other guitarists. Although many electric bassists also play acoustic bass, the reverse is not true. Furthermore, these dual-function bassists are apt to use a plucking technique rather than the traditional bowing of the classical bassist. It appears that this increased vulnerability is in part a function of supporting the instrument's weight, as well as related to the calibre and resistance of the strings used on all types of bass instruments. The electric bass is played standing, with the instrument held almost horizontally, and with a neck strap to help support the considerable weight of the instrument. There is a wide range both in bulk and in weight, depending on the type and thickness of the wood or woods used in guitars, but these dimensions are factors in many of the medical problems seen with various instruments.

Predictably, the strings on basses are thicker than those on comparable but higher-pitched string instruments and require proportionately greater effort to depress against the fingerboard with the left hand, or to pluck and pull with the right. The style of playing used by many popular genre bassists entails a great deal of pulling and displacement by the right-hand fingers, as well as depression of the relatively heavy strings with the left-hand fingers. This frequently results in right and left hand and arm symptoms. There are strings available which have greater and lesser compliance, and a change in string construction may be the solution to a bassist's medical problem, in spite of any undesirable effect on the sound quality.

Guitars. Although belonging to one large family, there is such a wide variety of instrument types and styles of playing that, in general, one cannot simply address the subject of "guitar" without being more specific. We will continue the discussion of guitars as a group, pointing to the similarities and important differences between electric guitars—used largely for popular, jazz, rock, and country western repertoire—and classical and folk guitars. Even though all may use acoustic instruments, the style of playing is as different as the repertoire. Consequently, we see many more classical guitarists than folk guitarists as patients. We will not have separate discussions of banjo players, zither players, or other ethnic and less common instruments. However, most of what is said here about guitarists can be applied readily to other strummed string instruments.

As already detailed in the bass guitar section, electric guitars are by and large played standing, held more or less horizontally, with the left hand coming from underneath and behind the neck, the fingers being held against the struts, or depressing the strings directly against the fingerboard. The right hand comes over the top of the instrument with the fingers either holding a thin pick between the thumb and index fingers, or strumming with bare fingertips. Classical guitarists maintain long fingernails of the right-hand fingers to get a sound quality similar to that from a pick. While use is occasionally made of the fleshy pulp of the fingers, the sound produced is of another quality entirely. Electric and occasionally folk guitars are partially supported by the use of a neck strap, although some players will, while standing, use a flexed knee on a chair for additional support. The classical guitarist, who plays seated, uses a small stool under the left foot to elevate the knee, which also places the guitar at a more user-friendly angle. Occasionally, a guitarist may use a small, firm pillow to additionally elevate the angle of the neck toward a more upright position.

From the point of view of the risk of medical problems, in spite of these minor adjustments in the position of the instrument, the critical risk factor common to all guitarists relates to the playing position of the arms, especially that of the wrists. Although to some extent varying with finger length and with the angle that the neck of the instrument is held above the horizontal, there is a tendency for both wrists to be held in marked hyperflexion. This appears to be a critical factor in many of the musculoskeletal problems encountered in guitarists, whatever their style of playing. The more that the guitarist is able to reduce this hyperflexed position toward a neutral wrist position, the less vulnerable the musician appears to be to suffer hand, wrist, and arm problems. In the fingers of the left hand, aside from the question of repetitive activity, there is a varying but ever-present need for strength in the flexors of the fingers to be applied against the strings and struts. Especially with classical repertoire, considerable dexterity is necessary in addition. The right-hand fingers require moderate strength, especially in the aforementioned popular technique of pulling against the strings. In the case of classical guitarists, their finely coordinated, independent, repetitive actions require great control and endurance as opposed to brute strength of the fingers. The use of a pick in the right-hand fingers, whatever the style of playing, tends to take a toll on the pinch muscles of the thumb and forefinger. Because the picks are both thin and of a slippery plastic, we have found it helpful to build up the held edge of the pick with tape to make it easier to grasp.

To some extent with electric guitar, but even more so in the playing position assumed by classical guitarists, the downward and foreward slope of the shoulders and arms has a tendency to produce the compressive symptoms of a thoracic outlet syndrome, correctible in most instances by postural readjustment rather than surgery. Perhaps more than with any other class of instruments, the proportions of the individual player have a great deal to do with the degree of risk of injury in playing the guitar. Hyperlaxity of the finger joints, another important factor for guitarists as well as other musicians, will be covered with individual risk factors.

The Dermatological Effects of String Instruments

Although to some extent these problems properly belong with individual risk factors, some are so close to universal that they may be fairly described as risks of the instrument. Characteristically annoying but not devastating, on occasion these dermatological problems are of such severity that they affect a career.

Practice Points, Fiddler's Chin. One of the relatively few dermatological problems seen in musicians comes as a result of the pressure of the chin rest against the neck and chin. Many players have variably sensitive spots on their necks, known as "practice points," and, particularly for novice players, it is a kind of badge of honor, indicating how much they have practiced! Some players have similar areas where the clavicle is rubbed by the instrument. However, for most players it is a source of annoyance as well as being unaesthetic. In many players it becomes cystic and secondarily infected, requiring drainage and/or antibiotic therapy, and occasionally necessitating a rest from the instrument. Excision should rarely, if ever, be performed because of the inevitably continued friction at the site. The potential problems caused by a scar in the area may be worse than those posed by the original dermatitis. Although there are individual factors of susceptibility, the common causes of this problem may confront all violin or viola players. Excessive tension of the relatively soft neck tissues held against the rigid chin rest is probably the critical factor. This comes about not so much from pushing the instrument into the neck with the left arm as it does from the efforts to cradle the instrument securely between the neck and left shoulder. This is especially true of individuals who have relatively long necks and small shoulders (see discussion of shoulder rests). In addition, although there are many exceptions, women tend to be more vulnerable to this problem than are men, perhaps for two reasons: (1) the beard of the male chin and upper neck produces a natural protection, (2) many women have necks that are long relative to their smaller shoulders and are, therefore, more inclined to press excessively with their necks against the chin rest. In general, violinists and violists regard the practice point as a sign of excessive tension used in playing, or simply as an unfortunate but unavoidable consequence of the instrument.

Allergies. Occasional players have a contact allergy to the resin used on the bow hairs to enhance contact with the strings. There are varieties of resin available and occasionally a person who is allergic to one is not hypersensitive to the other. However, there is no alternative to the use of resin, and if the reaction to it is severe, it is conceivable that the musician might find it necessary to abandon playing a string instrument.

Calluses. Calluses are so universal as to be regarded a risk of the instrument, rather than of the individual. In general, calluses, primarily on the fingers of the left hand, are considered a normal and welcome consequence of playing a string instrument. For a few, they represent a small but significant problem. The calluses which string players characteristically develop on the skin of the fingertips of the left hand, like "practice points," are a consequence of chronic friction. While they may be a problem when they build up excessively, they are even more of a problem if they fail to develop, or when they diminish after a period of nonplaying. Calluses are generally considered advantageous because they render the skin of the fingertips less vulnerable to trauma and less sensitive to pain. Calluses with grooves (matching the site of indentation of the skin on the fingertip by the string) develop as a consequence of the pressure of the usually metal or metal-wrapped string against the finger as it pushes down against the rigid fingerboard of the instrument. Although in most players these develop into useful structures by virtue of their thickness and insensitivity, in some players they may continue to develop and hypertrophy, becoming impediments because of their size and because they catch against the strings. As they are avascular, once calluses become cracked from trauma or excessive drying, they rarely heal. Many players will carefully trim the callus when it becomes excessively large, understanding that if they do this they must not jeopardize the entire callus. With prolonged vacations, or excessive exposure to water, as from swimming, even the firmest of calluses have a tendency to soften or even disappear. When players return to musical activity they must play carefully while waiting for their calluses to reform.

There are individuals who, even though they play a great deal, simply do not develop this tissue. Although for some this is not problematical, for others it can cause sufficient distress and pain to force the abandonment of careers or of serious studies and avocations. The use of commercially available protectants (e.g., Nu Skin®) may be of help to some individuals, as may a variety of skin tougheners, such as tincture of benzoin. However, even though players characteristically swear by their own methods of callus enhancement and preservation, natural calluses are the best and most satisfactory (39).

The Temporomandibular Joint in Violinists and Violists

Temporomandibular joint (TMJ) problems are encountered commonly in violinists and violists as a result of displacing the left side of the jaw against the chin rest, thus also stressing the right TMJ. Because this is such a common phenomenon, and because, like all TMJ problems, it can be resistant to therapy, it is well to be alert to the problem before it becomes highly symptomatic or does permanent damage to the integrity of the joints. The approach is generally dual—a technical one by reducing the pressure and the displacement of the instrument against the jaw, and a dental approach through the use of a splinting device and exercise.

Hearing

Hearing is a problem of tremendous proportions in all performers because of their extreme dependence on this special sense, and because their work and environment may place it in jeopardy. This is discussed in detail in Chapter 9, but we would make two points in the context of discussing the risks of string players. In the case of popular musicians, including guitarists, the acute and chronic hazards of greatly amplified sound systems cannot be overemphasized. While no one has in fact done an in-depth study of the incidence of serious auditory damage to popular musicians (and their audiences), it is widely acknowledged as a fact of their lives, and, unfortunately, in many instances simply accepted as such.

The other point to be raised here is the apparently cumulative risk to the hearing of the left ears of violinists and violists due to the proximity of that ear to the sound, both airborne and vibratory, through the instrument. Again, there are no satisfactory studies of the frequency of this impairment, but left-sided hearing loss is widely reported to be disproportionate as compared with the right ear or with deterioration expected with age (40).

Summary of String Instruments

While there are no reliable statistics concerning the frequency of medical problems in guitar players, all of the studies on orchestral players indicate the highest frequency of such problems among string players. In the ICSOM study they accounted for from 65% to 70% (3). Having detailed the large variety of risks, and through understanding the long hours of repetitious playing that are required, these are not surprising figures. Over and above these considerations, there are some gender risks, especially in the case of certain instruments, that will be described in the section on individual risk factors.

Wind Instruments

It is conventional to separate instruments played using the breath into the woodwinds and the brass. Although for the sake of literary ease we will adhere to that convention here, the differences in the requisites for playing (especially between the different woodwinds), and hence the medical problems, are tremendous. In addition, we will confine the discussion to contemporary wind instruments, although there are earlier, especially baroque, instruments played in western culture (exclusively, in the case of some musicians), that have somewhat different associated medical problems. Likewise the bagpipes, a variety of brass instruments, and those from other cultures, will be deleted. We will first examine separately the systemic and theoretical problems encountered as a result of the air flow requirements of these wind instruments in general. Embouchure, dental, and other musculoskeletal aspects of wind playing will be covered in separate discussions of each instrument.

Cardiovascular and Pulmonary Aspects of Playing Wind Instruments

Whereas the respiratory mechanics of playing different wind instruments are vastly different from one another, certain principles concerning air flow and pressure requirements have both some real and theoretical similarities. It can be readily understood that more pressure is required to breathe through a narrow tube than through a wide one. Likewise, it is clear that not only the bore of an instrument but its total volume will determine the amount of air requisite to producing a given sound.

Brass instruments are classified as high brass (namely, the trumpet and the French horn), and low brass (the trombone and the tuba). Although there are many differences between them, the most significant from a medical standpoint are the differences in air volume and pressure which are required. This can be a limiting factor from the outset in the selection of players, and it can be the decisive factor in limiting playing as a musician ages. Investigators dispute whether the playing of a wind instrument positively affects pulmonary function, especially the vital capacity. Generally, the smaller the instrument, the smaller the requisite air volumes, but the greater the pressures needed.

Looking at the extremes at the one end is the trumpet, with rather small air volumes but with the greatest intrathoracic pressures caused, especially in playing high and sustained notes. However, even these high pressures are lower than those attained with a hefty cough. The tuba, at the other end of the brass spectrum, needs a large air volume to contend with its larger bore tubing, requiring relatively less air pressure. Among woodwinds, the extremes are the flute at the low end and the oboe at the high end. In fact, the problem encountered in this smallest of double-reed instruments is keeping the air contained while generating small volumes at high pressures (41,42). The effects are those of a Valsalva maneuver, which theoretically can cause a host of difficulties for the player (43), not the least of which is syncope.

Hemorrhoids and inguinal hernias are both anecdotally reported to occur in increased numbers among wind players, but while this makes theoretical sense, as with so many other problems, this has not been documented. There are no reports in the literature of an increased incidence of cerebrovascular accidents in this population. However, in the presence of severe cardiovascular or cerebrovascular disease it would be prudent to avoid the potential risk of these abrupt changes in pressure in the cerebral and systemic vessels, as well as the risk imposed by the reduced cardiac output secondary to the decreased filling. Horvath et al. (44,45) described the induction of cardiac arrhythmias (including wandering pacemaker) in French horn players. Although the arrhythmias produced were not of clinical significance, it would seem prudent to periodically evaluate the cardiac and pulmonary function of players as they age.

Smith and Levine reviewed the literature (46) and reported a case of hypopharyngeal dilatation in a young male trumpet player, as opposed to the more frequently noted laryngoceles in wind players, which are frequently asymptomatic. In our clinic we have treated three cases of large hypopharyngeal defects in young male trumpet players, in some instances causing discomfort, in others causing difficulty in generating adequate air pressures to play because of the large volume of the defect.

Another potential problem which has not been reported or studied, but which the author has seen several times, is pneumothorax. One patient, a tubist, sustained three or four recurrences of collapse in both the left and right sides of the chest over a period of several years. He subsequently abandoned a performance career. Two other patients, one a female, were both bassoonists with apparently unilateral disease, and they fared better. Although a pneumothorax can and does occur in the absence of a ready explanation, it is not difficult to understand that persons with congenital lung defects who are wind instrumentalists might be especially subject to such problems.

Players with intrinsic or extrinsic asthma which is controlled are capable of playing wind instruments. However, clearly, significant bronchospasm represents a major impediment to playing any wind instrument, especially those requiring large volumes of expired air. A significant number of persons who have otherwise asymptomatic or exercise-induced bronchospasm may encounter difficulties. These players do very well by using an inhaled bronchodilator prior to playing.

A discussion of other respiratory pathology and the playing of wind instruments is beyond the scope of this book. These problems are also vastly understudied, considering the potential of such investigations for yielding important basic information.

One hazard which cannot be overlooked is smoking, for musicians and nonmusicians alike, but especially for wind players and singers. The deterioration of pulmonary function, the reduced resistance to infection, as well as the compromise in cardiovascular status, make it clear that smoking is especially risky for this population. Once again, there are no statistics concerning smoking among performers, but one need only be backstage during breaks, whatever the nature of the production, to witness that smoking appears to be at least as common here as elsewhere. Of all the forms of self-abusive behavior for performers, smoking seems especially inappropriate.

Brass Instruments

The Embouchure. The significant musculoskeletal risks encountered in performing on brass instruments involve primarily the facial musculature, or the embouchure. Although there was a 35% occurrence of "severe" musculoskeletal problems among the brass players reported in the ICSOM survey (3), in comparison with other musicians, they appear to deserve their common designation as being the "macho" players of the orchestra (this is not intended as a slight to the 8% of brass players who are female) (3). Postural problems, especially involving the upper torso, shoulders, and neck are frequent but usually resolve with symptomatic treatment.

Much more common are the embouchure problems of all wind players; for now we will confine the discussion to brass players. Although players and practitioners (medical and dental) alike report a high percentage of problems with some portion of the embouchure, most of these refer to one component (e.g., the teeth, the TMJ, the lips), and not to an overall occurrence rate. The customary complaints are of pain and/or loss of control in some part of the apparatus. Therefore, in evaluating brass players with embouchure complaints, one has to examine each anatomic component as well as the technical aspects of the instrument.

The mouthpiece of each class of brass instrument is somewhat peculiar unto itself. That is, mouthpieces for the trumpet come in an assortment of circumferences, depths, and rim contours within a rather narrow range. Likewise, for each brass instrument there are a limited number of choices to be made, subject to the repertoire being played, the characteristics of the individual embouchure, including size, lip and teeth positions, and comfort. Where the mouthpiece is held (centrally or eccentrically), the proportions of upper to lower lip used, the pressure with which it is held against the mouth, the integrity of the underlying teeth, and breath control are some of the many factors contributory to embouchure problems.

Many of the problems encountered in wind players require the services of a skilled and knowledgeable dentist (47,48). If a player is full-grown and has a well-functioning embouchure, it behooves him or her to have a cast of the teeth made as a permanent record, should reconstruction become necessary following trauma or degenerative conditions. Dental procedures in wind players must be conducted with special reference to any potential damage to the embouchure. Other dental problems that need special consideration in wind players are orthodontic problems and permanent dental structures, which need meticulous protection. How much the teeth, especially those in front, are jeopardized by long-term pressures of the mouthpiece against them is not known, but pressure is, once again, commonly accepted as a potential hazard. As always, prevention is preferred to finding a solution once the damage has been done, involving the combined efforts of musical and dental experts.

Lip Problems of Brass Players. Lip problems are common in all wind instrument players, but are especially frequent among brass instrumentalists. These problems may be mechanical, traumatic, infectious, neural, or allergic, and involve both the skin and mucosal surfaces.

The external problems relate to the pressure of the mouthpiece against the lips, and the position of the lips relative to the mouthpiece. In addition are the problems on the muscosal side of the lips, which may be subject to trauma by the underlying teeth, especially if they are jagged or protruding.

Mouthpieces come in a variety of metals, with and without plating. A major constituent is nickel (in the brass), to which a number of persons are allergic. The solution to this generally lies in the silver or gold plating of the mouthpiece. As in the evaluation of other medical problems in musicians, the examiner must have at least a cursory knowledge of the technical aspects of playing, or have access to someone that does. Generally the symptom produced by allergy is swelling of the lips, but this is also a common reaction to the sustained pressure of the instrument, usually directly related to the length of time of playing. In most instances swelling resolves within a short time, although ice may speed this process. Occasionally the swelling during playing is so severe as to impair the function of the embouchure, primarily because of the failure of the edematous lips to vibrate properly. A fortunately rare but serious problem is rupture of the orbicularis oris muscle. Although it can be repaired, the effect of this on the embouchure is unpredictable (49).

Infections in and about the embouchure, especially of the lips, represent a frequent and painful problem. It is interesting to note the coincidence of particularly stressful playing (or singing, in the case of vocalists) with the appearance of herpes simplex lesions in these musicians. Once again, there are no statistics available, but both musicians and physicians charged with their care will affirm this observation. The explanation appears to be that there is a combination of physical and psychological stress that increases the individual's susceptibility to the virus. Although the use of oral acyclovir is not generally considered for minimal lesions, it may be justified in these performers to abbreviate the duration of the outbreak.

Old traditions do not readily die, and such is the case of sharing or passing mouthpieces among players, as well as between teachers and students. This occurs with all wind instrumentalists, but seems especially customary with brass players. There is no evidence that the HIV virus can be transmitted through saliva, even though it may be present. However, this is not true of herpes viruses, those of the common cold, or of bacterial and spirochetal infections. With that information in mind, it seems superfluous to suggest that sharing of mouthpieces is a risk that need not be taken. As far as infections from the body of the instrument are concerned, there is evidence of fungal infections harbored in bagpipes, but, although it is theoretically possible to transmit pulmonary infections, this has not been documented.

Sensation of the lips is supplied by the third division of the trigeminal (V) cranial nerve. The motor supply to the orbicularis oris muscle is provided by the facial (VII) cranial nerve. The most common neurological problems of the embouchure are disturbances of sensation resulting from compression by the instrument. Neurological complications are discussed in Chapter 5. We would add a reminder that systemic neurological diseases may present with symptoms affecting the playing of an instrument, particularly because musicians are sensitive to minute alterations of these functions. We have seen two patients in whom the presenting complaint of myasthenia gravis related to an impaired embouchure. The evaluation of musicians having embouchure problems should include full neurological as well as dental and otolaryngologic examinations. Further information about these problems is in Chapter 5.

The Woodwinds

With the exception of the flute, the mouthpieces for this group of instruments are contained within the lips as compared with the brass, where the mouthpiece is held externally. The reader is referred to a thorough review of this subject as well as the dental ramifications of wind instrument playing, by J. A. Howard (47). As in the case of the brass instruments, the medical hazards of woodwinds occur at the mouthpiece, or blowing end, of the instrument in pulmonary aspects, and in both the required support of the instrument and the mechanical aspects of playing that involve the upper extremities, the neck, and the back.

The Embouchure of Woodwinds. Although inevitably involving the same structures, embouchure problems among woodwind players are somewhat different from those among the brass players. The flute and piccolo category must be considered separately, and to some extent reed instruments must be divided into single and double reeds. Not only are the intraoral pressure requirements vastly different from one another, as from the brass, but the differences in the ways that the embouchure is formed and maintained involve very different uses of the teeth, jaws, and facial muscles. Once again we are at a loss for incidence statistics, although the dental and orthodontic literature contains some information, especially regarding tooth development and alignment vis-à-vis the various kinds of mouthpieces (47).

The lip position of reed players involves curling over the teeth of the lower lip. This is called a single embouchure as opposed to the more rarely used double embouchure, in which the lips are held around both the upper and the lower teeth. This can cause direct trauma, especially to the mucus membrane of the lips, as can irregular, prominent, or sharp teeth. Many players habitually use a guard such as thin paper (cigarette paper) folded between the lip and the teeth, or substances such as dental wax. Others use these only in case of need, such as for young musicians wearing orthodontic appliances. The teeth are clamped against the mouthpiece of single reed instruments, but the reeds of woodwinds must be able to vibrate, so the lips, rather than the teeth, are used to grip the reed. It is apparently because of the tension involved in all of these positions that so many woodwind players present with a variety of TMJ complaints. As with other TMJ problems, these frequently represent a therapeutic challenge, which involves technical adjustments in playing as well as dental treatment. Flute and piccolo players hold the instruments against the skin below the lower lip, with both lips drawn back against the teeth under varying degrees of tension. Embouchure problems most commonly seen in these players are secondary to the pressure of the instrument against the lower lip and chin. These range from sensory symptoms such as pain, anesthesia and hypesthesia, to motor dysfunction of the lip secondary to trauma of the sensory and motor nerves, including branches of the mandibular division of the trigeminal (V) and facial (VII) nerves. More difficult to diagnose and of unknown origin are focal dystonias which, although less commonly than in the hands, do occur in the lip and other facial muscles of advanced wind players, both wood and brass. The symptoms caused by these are usually of such severity that a satisfactory embouchure cannot be maintained, and reliable and successful treatment has not yet been developed.

Hand Problems of Woodwind Players. As indicated above, hand and ar... problems do occur in all wind players, but are much more common in the woodwinds than in the brass. This is presumably a consequence of the greater demands of both the postural requirements and the repetitive activities of these instruments.

Flute and Piccolo

Although there are exceptions, characteristically the hand problems of these woodwinds are in the left-hand fingers, wrists, arms, and shoulders. The reason for this is the position used to support the horizonal flute, in which there is a tendency for marked hyperextension as well as radial deviation of the left wrist. Depending on many factors, including arm proportions and teaching, this may be more or less exaggerated. The thumb is involved not only in support but also in using the keys on the underside of the instrument. Many players tend to wedge the flute between the thumb and the flexor surface of the proximal phalanx of the left index finger. Although some players adjust to this position, many have problems arising from the tension this creates in the hand. In addition, the radical deviation that accompanies this hand position makes the reach to the keys by the ring and small fingers much more difficult, especially if the flute is not fitted with an offset G key, or if these fingers are disproportionately short, as is not infrequently the case. The problems seen most frequently in flutists stem from this awkward hand position, and may affect the left shoulder and neck as well as the hand, wrist, and arm. Therefore, the common satisfactory resolution of medical problems among flute and piccolo players will require a joint medical and musical technique approach (50–52).

Single and Double Reed Woodwinds

It is more common for these musicians to present with right hand rather than left hand problems. In large part this is a function of the supportive role of the right thumb, especially in clarinets and oboes. The English horn, bassoon, and bass clarinet have neck and other straps that aid in their support. In the case of the oboe and the clarinet, the greatest portion of the static load of the instrument is on the right thumb, held under a small (¹/₂ inch) metal rest on the back on the instrument. The rests are put in a fairly standard position of the instrument, which may or may not leave the thumb in appropriate opposition to the index and middle fingers. Another problem with these thumb supports is that with varying hand size, especially thumb length, the fingers may be in a difficult position vis-à-vis the keys, in order for the thumb to be sufficiently under the thumb rest. Ideally, this is in the vicinity of the interphalangeal joint; if it is distal to the joint there is excess stress on both the interphalangeal and the metacarpophalangeal joints of the thumb. This will be discussed at greater length in the sections on joint laxity and individual risk factors. There are a number of approaches to solving this problem. These include moving the position of the thumb rest, resting the instrument on the knees (if playing seated), and using a neck or other support device.

Other problems with the right hand of flutists and the left hands of clarinetists, oboists, bassoonists, and others, occur because of the general problems of repetitive activity (overuse), or because of some individual medical or technical aberration. Some alterations in these instruments which facilitate playing are possible, such as closing the open holes of flute keys and using offset keys of differing lengths. Student and other flute models are being tested in which the mouth piece is curved, easing the position of the arms (50,52).

Summary of Wind Instruments

Although the overall frequency of the medical problems of wind instrumentalists is less than that of keyboard and string instrument players, the problems they do have are as diverse as are the instruments included in this category. In addition, they can be especially challenging from the medical point of view, because they may involve such discrepant disciplines as orthopedics, neurology, otolaryngology, dentistry, pulmonary medicine, and psychiatry. It will clearly require investigation by persons with all of these skills to offer optimal medical services to brass and woodwind players.

The Harp

There are many medical problems that can occur to harpists, of which we will mention only a few here. These start with the previously mentioned logistical problems of transporting this unwieldy instrument. Likewise, the frequent tuning of the many strings of a harp not infrequently causes problems of the right wrist and hand, secondary to the repetitive turning motions of operating the tuning key. Although the instrument is tipped back into its playing position, the intent is to have it balanced without actually resting any weight against the right shoulder. Occasionally this balance is not achieved, creating a number of subsequent muscular problems, primarily with the right shoulder and upper arm. There are different schools of harp playing, with opposing views of the degree to which the elbows are held abducted from the body. In the strict Salzedo approach, the elbows are at almost a right angle with the body, whereas in modified techniques the abduction is less extreme. Further, some pedagogues teach that the wrists of both hands be hyperextended, with the fingers doing their required pulling (flexing) action from this relatively disadvantageous position. Others maintain the wrists in a much more neutral position, usually with less risk of injury.

The position of the harpist in relation to the instrument can also, at times, present a problem, depending somewhat on the size of the musician. The sitting height of the musician should be determined by what is comfortable rather than by the height of the bench which may come with the harp!

There are no studies of frequency of injury among harpists, and even the much quoted ICSOM survey did not include enough harpists to be of statistical significance. In our practice at Northwestern, we see only 2 or 3 harpists a year out of a population of about 600 patients. Among the 52 harpists then in ICSOM orchestras, 45 were women and only 7 were men; this reason alone makes them an atypical population as far as the orchestra is concerned (3).

Percussion Instruments

By way of contrast with the harpists, among 194 ICSOM percussionists, 179 were men as compared with only 15 women (3). The numbers are not large enough to make far-reaching conclusions, but the role that gender may play as a risk factor is among the many subjects awaiting investigation regarding these and all other instrumentalists. This question has already been examined by Middlestadt and Fishbein for string players in orchestras (5), and will be discussed somewhat further in this chapter with individual risk factors. There is a wide range of instruments played by most percussionists, including a variety of drums, the triangle, gongs, marimba, and cymbals. Each instrument has its risk, but those associated with the drum family are far and away the most frequently encountered. Although the techniques can be vastly different, we will in general not refer to classical and popular percussionists separately. Whereas the potential risk of hearing impairment is clearly greater among popular musicians, classical percussionists are anecdotally reputed to be at greater risk than other musicians. Orchestra members would add that this risk applies to those sitting adjacent to the percussion section as well. This is yet another risk which, although it seems to be logical, must be measured and studied before it can be resolved as a potential problem (this will be discussed in greater depth in Chapter 9).

The musculoskeletal risks of tympanists among classical percussionists, and drum-set players among the popular ones, directly relate to the repetitive actions of the hands, wrists, arms, and shoulders as well as to the resistance, impact, and vibratory characteristics of the material of the drumsticks against a variety of drum head surfaces. How the sticks are grasped, with which fingers and how firmly, how much manipulating of the sticks there is by the hands, the size, weight, and balance of the sticks are all considerations when looking at risk factors. In turn, the way that the arm is used as a whole, the size and intensity of the excursions, and what kind of impact is taken by the arms and body are other important variables. In the case of tympanists, some stand and some sit while playing—largely a question of personal preference as well as height. Neither seems to greatly affect the risk of playing.

There are no studies of the medical problems of percussionists, but it has been my experience that while many have musculoskeletal complaints of the arms, shoulders, neck, and back, relatively few are disabled by their symptoms. Popular drummers who play a greater percentage of the playing time than do classical percussionists appear to be at greater risk. In addition, it appears that those players who have not had the advantages of technical training are especially at risk of injury.

Other Instruments

There are a number of kinds and varieties of other instruments that have not been discussed. The author has had patients who played harmonica, banjo, zither, accordion, recorder, bongo drums (played with the bare hands), and has been consulted by letter by a saw player, among others! However, their numbers do not justify their inclusion here, where we have attempted to discuss the characteristic risk factors of the more commonly played instruments. In the case of some of the more exotic instruments, the medical consultant will be served by the same approach as has been used here: the analysis of the risks arising from the profession, the instrument's playing demands, and the individual musician.

This discussion is also incomplete without at least mentioning conductors. We have already referred to their alleged longevity, but they have their own set of medical problems, nevertheless. Most of their problems are a consequence of the work that is performed on the podium, although we should also mention falls from the podium as a risk. Conductors, especially those in their later years, may use a railing around part of the podium to serve as a guardrail. The author will always remember seeing and hearing Toscanini, when he used such protection. Needless to say, that was not the most memorable part of the concert! Leonard Bernstein fell off the podium while conducting the Chicago Symphony, but fortunately the only injury he incurred was a contusion caused by the large gold medallion he was wearing.

The baton itself has its hazards—to conductors, musicians and audience—and stories, many true, about stabbings and flying missiles have been recorded. Probably the earliest such is said to have been responsible for the demise of Jean-Baptiste Lully, also a composer, who, following the custom of his time, used a large post to keep the tempo. In so doing, he apparently missed the floor, injuring his own foot, which ultimately resulted in fatal gangrene.

More everyday medical problems of conductors are musculoskeletal ones with shoulder, neck, and back strains, sprains, and inflammation being fairly routine. Very tall conductors must have the score appropriately elevated. Many, if not most, conductors use a stool for rehearsals, or at least for rest periods during long sessions. Conductors who continuously keep the beat with their heels may develop a plantar fasciitis.

INDIVIDUAL RISK FACTORS

In the course of the preceding portions of this chapter we have already referred to some of the risks of playing a musical instrument which are a consequence of the individual, including lifestyle, diet, tobacco and substance abuse, education, asthma, the configuration of the teeth, neck length, height, and thumb length, to mention but a few. In this section we will examine some other individual characteristics that appear to impose additional risk factors to those already discussed. These can be divided into those risks which come about as the result of the individual's physical characteristics (including gender), how that person copes with the many psychological and physical stresses of the occupation, as well as those which are extraoccupational. Also to be considered is the relationship of the individual's total health status to the problems of being a performing artist. We have already considered many of the important aspects of this, including age, the size and proportions of the individual, diet, and dental problems. We will confine our discussion here to several other physical variables.

Concurrent and Intercurrent Illnesses and Injuries

While the thrust of this text is to point out the special health risks of being a performer, it is essential to remember that in addition to these special risks, performers are subject to all of the other vagaries of life. In taking the history and conducting the physical examination of these patients, one should not be blinded by one's own bias or the patient's, and all possibilities must be considered. For instance, medications a perfomer-patient may be taking for some unrelated problem may or may not impact on the medical problem of the moment. Similarly, the fact that a person is an insulin-requiring diabetic may or may not be responsible for a neuropathy, but until proven otherwise, it probably is.

Vision

The special needs of musicians must also be considered when prescribing corrective lenses. They must be able to read the music directly in front of them, as well as to occasionally glance at the conductor. Therefore, when correcting for presbyopia, the standard bifocals are unsatisfactory, and musicians require a lens in which the bifocal lens is in the line of direct vision. Pianists generally will use a lens that is just for reading music, as other people have other types of reading glasses. Conductors who use a score have other focal length requirements with which to deal, uneven lighting conditions, and the glare of reflected stage lights. Severely visually impaired musicians may have great difficulty getting satisfactorily corrected for their musical needs (53).

Aids and the Arts Community

In considering the impact of AIDS on the performing arts community, several factors should be borne in mind. One is the previously mentioned fact that, not unlike other patients, performers in particular may have more on the agenda in visiting a physician than the presenting complaint. In addition, they may have fallen through the medical cracks and may not have seen a physician within recent memory. AIDS anxiety is an understandable fact of life for this population, and virtually all have been touched by it in some way. It is not the intent to suggest that all performer-patients be subjected to a complete physical examination and interrogation as to their sexual and other preferences. One should be sensitive to the potential concerns of each patient.

General Medical Needs

Other neurological and medical illnesses should be considered in the differential diagnoses of performers with any neuromusculoskeletal complaint. I have already mentioned wind players with myasthenia gravis who initially presented with embouchure problems. Similarly, all forms of arthritis can and do occur in instrumentalists, and whereas their careers may not have to suffer, neither will they be benefited if they are inappropriately treated as an "overuse syndrome." Whether or not instrumentalists are at increased risk for premature or more severe forms of degenerative arthritis remains a question. There are studies from industry that would suggest this is so. There are a variety of reasons for this suggestion, some of which will be discussed below in a consideration of joint laxity.

Although we are no more able to cure the common cold, gastroenteritis, or other everyday viral infections in performers than in anyone else, it is easy to understand the crisis atmosphere that envelops a performer with even such minor afflictions. While not offering a sure cure or using inappropriate treatment, it is frequently possible to patch up a performer sufficiently to allow the "show to go on" without compromising one's medical standards. This in many cases refers simply to being sympathetic and imaginative in devising symptomatic treatment for performers. For instance, treatment of upper respiratory infections with agents that are drying or sedating, while not contraindicated for other patients, may cause increasing disability to the musician. We will not belabor this point, but it is part and parcel of treating performing artists that one understand their special variety of physical and psychological stresses and be able to accept their perspective that minor impairments can pose major impediments to performance.

Performers are subject to all of the daily potential catastrophies of other people, including breaking of bones in falls, sports injuries, kitchen accidents, and so forth. Once again, their treatment may have to be modified in some way, once the obligatory medical necessities are out of the way, by taking into account their exacting physical performance needs. This may involve the use of removable splints, or it may call for the services of a plastic surgeon as opposed to an emergency room intern for the suturing of wounds (54).

Most importantly, however, performers of all kinds may require special rehabilitation and therapy before returning to work. In addition, certain types of injuries in performers may require more aggressive treatment than in other patients. For instance, the not uncommon injury of tearing the ulnar collateral ligament of the thumb (gamekeeper's thumb) may pose a problem for many people, but in musicians it represents a therapeutic challenge. For string players, if the thumb is unstable, it causes pain due to the stress on the other thumb supports. Likewise, in clarinetists and oboists there is pain when the unstable thumb attempts to support the weight of the instrument. Therefore, prompt immobilization and/or surgical repair is essential for musician-patients with this type of injury (55).

Approximately 8% of the "normal" population has a condition known as "benign" laxity, as compared with conditions such as Marfan's syndrome and its variants, with vascular and other connective tissue complications. Benign laxity ("double-jointedness" or hyperextensible joints) has been associated with an increased number of rheumatic-type complaints, even in children (56), as well as with an increased incidence of athletic injuries. The condition stems from the increased elasticity of the ligaments, giving more play to the joints. In turn, the muscles surrounding the joints are forced to compensate for the inadequate support of the excessively elastic ligaments. Musicians with hyperextensible finger joints appear to stress both the intrinsic and extrinsic muscles of the hand as they attempt to compensate for their joint instability in addition to their movement functions. We and others have found a notably increased percentage of musician-patients presenting with hand and arm pain having significant laxity (57,58). As opposed to 8% of the general population, in excess of 20% of our instrumentalist patients are hyperextensible, especially in the interphalangeal and metacarpophalangeal joints of the hand. Characteristic of most persons with this condition, our patients, too, are young and female.

Although the condition may become more severe as the result of playing an instrument (the elastic ligaments become even more stretched out), it appears that the process is essentially a genetic one. With careful history-taking, including that of the family, a clear inherited pattern can usually be identified. A number of famous musicians, most notably Niccolo Paganini, have had their virtuosity attributed to their joint laxity. Although I cannot dispute that, joint laxity in our patients has appeared to be detrimental. For instance, whereas the hand span may be increased by a lax fifth metacarpophalangeal joint, it is accompanied by a tendency to compensate by inappropriate use of the abductor digiti quinti, and a continuing compromise of the metacarpophalangeal joint structure. While painful and disabling in the short run, there is also concern that with intense hand activity over a prolonged period, persons with excess laxity may be subject to premature degenerative arthritis (59).

Therapeutically, since the condition is both genetic and generalized, a surgical approach of tightening the lax ligaments does not appear advisable in most cases. We have established individualized programs for our patients, designed to strengthen the muscles around the joint as well as to correct the frequently noted muscular imbalances.

THE ROLE OF EXERCISE FOR MUSICIANS

Whereas there are, as yet, no statistics to prove this, clinical experience reinforces the notion that an important factor in the etiology of many medical problems of musicians is a lack of adequate overall muscle tone and conditioning. Strength per se is not so much the issue, although marked discrepancies between the strengths of opposing muscle groups are frequently noted and may be a problem. The ICSOM and other studies, where there is no clear association between age and injury occurrence, supports the observation that the problems may be a consequence of inadequate conditioning. However, there may be psychological factors, including alterations in stress levels associated with different times of a musician's life, that also need careful study.

The 1980s preoccupation with exercise has not fallen on deaf ears among performers. However, as part of their early training, many young musicians are protected or prohibited from participation in sports activities for several reasons. First, most youngsters who are seriously involved in music or dance lessons have very little time for anything else in addition to their obligatory school work. Dance is considered elsewhere in this book but we will just mention here that although there is assuredly more intrinsic physical activity in dance than in musical performance, it remains an open question whether young dancers, primarily girls, do in fact get optimal opportunities for overall healthy musculoskeletal growth. Among musicians, very few children who are involved in serious or preprofessional musical studies are allowed sufficient time or otherwise encouraged to engage in activities that will offset their otherwise sedentary lifestyles. The equally strong message communicated to musically talented children is that they must approach athletics with apprehension lest they risk their special hands and bodies in the ordinary rough and tumble of sports, even those which involve neither contact nor competition. As a result, many musicians permanently incorporate this admonition into their lifelong habits, and exercise of any sort remains an anathema to them.

A discussion of the multiple benefits of exercise for general good health is not germane to this text. Suffice it to say that for most musicians, in addition to the cardiovascular and pulmonary benefits of exercise and the mood-elevating value of the endorphins generated by strenuous physical activity, there appears to be a correlation between generalized fitness and overall good muscular tone with injury resistance at the instrument (60). While it is evident, as we have discussed under the hazards of individual instruments, that there is physical work associated with performance on any instrument, most require more extensive musculoskeletal support than is derived from the body parts which are immediately contiguous with the instrument. As anyone who has attempted to master the violin, viola, or the flute will attest, there tends to be fatigue and discomfort in the arms, upper back, and shoulders from supporting the instrument. For most musicians the kind of endurance and strength that is called for from the larger proximal muscles does not come automatically by mastering the playing of the instrument, but requires additional activity such as that derived from swimming, from racquet sports, or from working with light weights. When there is inadequate support from the muscles of the shoulder and back, there will be added stress on the arms and hands which may lead to injuries. Overall fitness and good muscle tone are essential to healthy musicianship. The particular form of exercise engaged in must be an individual choice, although certain sports, such as volleyball and basketball, with their relatively high potential for "jammed" fingers, should probably be on the prohibited list for instrumentalists. However, just as more accidents occur at home, life in general has its risks, and musicians must make their own peace with decisions involving risk-taking behavior, including sports. One hopes that artists will make appropriate choices for themselves which allow them to function in a relatively nonneurotic and healthy yet realistic fashion. As medical advisors to instrumentalists, we must be familiar with the risk/benefit ratios of different forms of exercise so that we can assist in these decisions. Once again, one should rely on informed common sense as much as on statistics for guidelines.

As a general principle, the type of strength needed by musicians is more akin to the long-distance runner than to the weight lifter. Therefore, exercises which are of the low-resistance high-frequency variety are indicated in preference to high-resistance ones designed to produce muscular mass. In fact, musicians who do participate in weight training may be hampered not only by the bulk of their muscles but by their excessive tone, or tension, which may interfere with the finer, more highly controlled and coordinated movements needed to play an instrument (61).

Therapeutic Exercises

Therapy of artists' injuries is discussed elsewhere. However, in discussing the role of exercise in this population, one does need to draw a distinction between that which is to promote health and prevent injuries and that which is necessary for an injured musician's rehabilitation from an injury or illness. In this respect, musicians are comparable to athletes who must recondition not only the injured part but the entire apparatus before reentering the field of active play following an absence. We have already noted that, to some extent, musicians must utilize their entire bodies to play—not just their hands, fingers, and forearms. Just as overuse is a concept that can be carried from sports medicine to performing arts medicine, so it is that musicians must consider what may have happened to their bodies during a period of rest—whether from choice, as on vacation, or as a consequence of illness or injury. Adequate rehabilitation is as essential to minimize the risk of reinjury for musicians as it is for athletes.

As referred to earlier in this chapter, a number of studies of musician populations have documented that rapid changes in quality and quantity of practice and playing bring increased risk of injuries. A gradual increase in activity level allows for physiological, as well as psychological, conditioning. This involves not only the total time spent at the instrument and the repertoire played, but also practice techniques. As mentioned previously, the repetitive practice of difficult passages, or the use of recurrent patterns, as in certain minimalist music, may bring special risks. In practice it is preferable to repeat the same excerpts for a limited time period than to persist doggedly until they are perfected. Alternating practicing a difficult sequence with playing other passages using different fingers, rhythms, or technique, serves a protective function.

Warm-Ups, Cool-Downs

Although it is near to heresy to say this, there is little scientific evidence mandating warm-ups and cool-downs. While most trainers, exercise physiologists, athletes, and musicians, feel that warm-up exercise does help get prepared for playing, whether it does, in fact, reduce the incidence of injuries is open to question. Interestingly enough, in a recent survey of music teachers belonging to the Music Teachers' National Association, while the majority stated that they recommended warm-ups to their students, few followed their own advice (62). The rationale behind warming up is that warm muscles contract more effectively than cold muscles, and that active muscles are warmer than inactive ones. In fact, imagining warm-ups may be as effective as doing them, and it may be the psychological boost that comes from such preparation that explains the apparent effectiveness of warm-ups more than the actual process of doing them! Whereas there is scant evidence of the positive effect of warm-ups neither is there evidence that they are in any way harmful. Questions regarding the usefulness of warm-ups and their specifications are among the many in performing arts medicine that await resolution through careful research. However, until such a time as those data become available, since the principle behind warm-ups is rational and they should be beneficial, warm-ups should be used in the practice room as much as they are in the locker room.

CONCLUSION: EPIDEMIOLOGY OF PERFORMERS' INJURIES

Tremendous progress has been made in the past decade toward understanding the multiple variables which serve as risk factors for performers' injuries. In large part these advances have been made by the simple acknowledgement that there are frequent problems, and that while they are infrequently threatening to overall health, they can have significant impact on the quality of performance, job security, and career longevity of artists. The birth of the specialty has been healthy, and endurance is assured. The adolescence of performing arts medicine, with its initial enthusiastic reception by performers, joined by an uncharacteristically committed and adventurous medical establishment, is in its final phases. The adult period, for which these earlier years have been a preparation, is ahead. During the coming decade this new medical specialty must establish its long-term viability. This can be done by further tapping all the available resources to systematically study and understand the basis for the many risk factors associated with performance. The commitments essential to developing the talent of performing artists have been recognized for generations. Now the medical task is to match that commitment and develop the means to preserve and enhance the health of these artists through dedication to the scientific evolution of performing arts medicine.

One of the most eloquent spokesmen for the arts and for quality education in the arts is Joseph Polisi, president of the Juilliard School in New York (here joined by James Sloan Allen). Their statements, which follow (63), seem a fitting end to this chapter.

". . . if art does not improve life, it cannot be worth the sacrifices it demands. And if it actually makes people worse, we had better run it out of town, as Plato had recommended doing with most art.

If art can make life better, it should make people better, artists no less than other people. But this will happen only if the appropriate place of art in the lives of artists— and in the life of culture—is openly examined by all who have a stake in the outcome. This means not only artists and art educators but everybody."

REFERENCES

1. Lederman RJ, Brandfonbrener AG. Medical Problems of Musicians. *Cleve Clin Q* 1986;53:1–2.
2. Ostwald P. Schumann. *The Inner Voices of a Musical Genius.* Boston: Northeastern U. Press, 1985;86–94.
3. Fishbein M et al. Medical Problems Among ICSOM Musicians. *Med Probl Perform Art* 1988;3:1–14.
4. Fry HJH. Incidence of Overuse Syndrome in the Symphony Orchestra. *Med Probl Perform Art* 1986;1:51–55.
5. Middlestadt SE, Fishbein M. The Prevalence of Severe Musculoskeletal Problems Among Male and Female Symphony Orchestra String Players. *Med Probl Perform Art* 1989;4:41–48.
6. Caldron P et al. A Survey of Musculoskeletal Problems Encountered in High Level Musicians. *Arth and Rheum* 1985; 28(suppl 4):597.
7. Fry HJH. Prevalence of Overuse in Australian Music Schools. *Brit J Indust Med* 1987;44:35–40.
8. Lockwood AH. Medical Problems in Secondary School-Aged Musicians. *Med Probl Perform Art* 1988;3:129–132.
9. Manchester RA. The Incidence of Hand Problems in Music Students. *Med Probl Perform Art* 1988; 3:15–18.
10. Lederman RJ. Performing Arts Medicine, Editorial. *N Eng J Med* 1989;320:246–248.
11. Lockwood AH. Medical Problems of Musicians. *N Eng J Med* 1989;320:221–227.
12. Barnhart S, Rosenstock, L. Carpal Tunnel Syndrome in Grocery Checkers. *West J Med* 1987; 147:37–40.

13. Blair S, Bear-Lehman J. Prevention of Upper Extremity Occupational Disabilities [Editorial Comment]. *J Hand Surg* 1987; 12 A #5 Part 2: 821–822.
14. Smith BL. Inside Look: Hand Injury-Prevention Program. *J Hand Surg* 1987;12 A#5 Part 2: 940–943.
15. Gardner H. Musical Intelligence. In: *Frames of Mind*. New York: Harper, Basic Books, 1985;99–127.
16. Gardner H. Unfolding or Teaching: On the Optimal Training of Artistic Skills. In: *Art, Mind and Brain*. New York: Harper, Basic Books, 1982;208–217.
17. Sosniak L. Learning to Be a Concert Pianist. In: *Developing Talent in Young People*. Bloom B, ed. New York: Random, Ballantine Books, 1985;19–89.
18. Pruett KD. A Longitudinal View of the Musical Gift. *Med Prob Perform Art* 1985;2:31–38.
19. Sosniak L. Phases of Learning. In: *Developing Talent in Young People*. Bloom BS, ed. New York: Random, Ballantine Books, 1985;409–438.
20. Bloom BS. Generalizations About Talent Development. In: BS, ed. *Developing Talent in Young People*. Bloom BS, ed. New York: Random, Ballantine Books 1985;507–549.
21. Newmark J, Lederman RJ. Practise Doesn't Necessarily Make Perfect. *Med Probl Perform Art* 1987;2:142–144.
22. Galamian I. *Principles of Violin Playing and Teaching*. Englewood Cliffs NJ 1985: 2nd ed: 11–12,105–108.
23. Mortality of Symphony Conductors. *Statist Bull* 1980; Oct-Dec.
24. Middlestadt SE, Fishbein M. Health and Occupational Correlates of Perceived Stress in Symphony Orchestra Musicians. *J Occup Med* 1988;30:687–692.
25. Smith DWE. Aging and the Careers of Symphony Orchestra Musicians. *Med Probl Perform Art* 1989;4:81–90.
26. Peyron JG. The Epidemiology of Osteoarthritis. In: *Osteoarthritis: Diagnosis and Management*. Moskowitz RC et al. Philadelphia: Saunders, 1984;9–27.
27. Brandfondbrener AG. The Jazz Musician: A Challenge to Arts Medicine [editorial]. *Med Probl Perform Art* 1988;3:iii.
28. Raeburn SD. Occupational Stress and Coping in a Sample of Rock Musicians, Part I. *Med Probl Perform Art* 1987;2:41–48.
29. Stephens RE. The Etiology of Injuries in Ballet Dancers. In: *Dance Medicine*. Ryan AJ and Stephens RE eds. Chicago: Pluribus, 1987:16–50.
30. Hamilton LH, Brooks-Gunn J, Warren MD. Sociocultural Influences on Eating Disorders in Dancers. *Int J Eating Dis* 1985;4:465–477.
31. Loosli AR, Benson J, Gillien DM. Nutrition and the Dancer. In: *Dance Medicine*. Ryan AJ and Stephens RE eds. Chicago: Pluribus, 1987:100–106.
32. Aaron S. *Stage Fright: Its Role in Acting*. Chicago: U of Chicago 1986;1–16.
33. Gedo J. Some Differences in Creativity in Performers and Other Artists. *Med Probl Perform Art* 1989;4:15–19.
34. Plaut ED. Psychotherapy in Performance Anxiety. *Med Probl Perform Art* 1988;3:113–118.
35. Brantigan CO, Brantigan TA. Effect of Beta Blockade and Beta Stimulation on Stage Fright. *Am J Med* 1982;72:88–94.
36. Gerig RR. The Perspectives of an Enlightened Piano Technique. In: *Famous Pianists and their Technique*. Bridgeport Ct.: Robert B Luce, 1974;507–517.
37. Graffman G. Piano in the Basement. In: *"I Really Should be Practising."* New York: Doubleday, 1981.
38. Primrose W. The Viola. In: *Violin and Viola*. Menuhin Y and Primrose W. New York: Schirmer, 1976:173.
39. Burr T. Calluses—How to Get Them and Keep Them. *Frets Mag*. In press.
40. Hart CW et al. The Musician and Occupational Bound Hazards. *Med Probl Perform Art* 1987;22–25.
41. Boyhuys A. Lung Volumes and Breathing Patterns in Wind-Instrument Players. *J Appl Physiol* 1964;19:967–975.
42. The Way to High D. Editorial. *Lancet* 1973;247–248.
43. Faulkner M, Sharpey-Shafer EP. Circulatory Effects of Trumpet Playing. *Brit Med J* 1959;685–686.
44. Borgia JF et al. Some Physiological Observations in Horn Players. *J Occup Med* 1975;17:696–701.

45. Nizet PM, Borgia JF, Horvath SM. Wandering Atrial Pacemaker in French Hornists. *J Electrocardiol* 1976;9:51–52, 53:33–37.
46. Smith R, Levine H. Hypopharyngeal Dilitation in Musicians. *Med Probl Perform Art* 1986;1:20–23.
47. Howard JA, Lovrovich AT. Wind Instruments: Their Interplay with Orofacial Structures. *Med Probl Perform Art* 1989;4:59–72.
48. Mortenson GC, Kolar LW. Understanding the Procedures and Risks Involved in the Extraction of Third Molars. *Med Probl Perform Art* 1988;3:199–122.
49. Planas J. Rupture of the Orbicularis Oris in Trumpet Players. *Plast Reconstr Surg* 1982;69:690–693.
50. Cooper A. My Work on Flutes. In: Galway J. Flute. New York: Schirmer, 1986;49–57.
51. Galway J. Physical Aspects. In: Galway J. Flute. New York: Schirmer, 1986;65–86.
52. Norris R. Applied Ergonomics: The Angel Head Flute. Sixth Ann Symposium Med Probl in Musicians and Dancers. Aspen Co. 1988.
53. Marmor MF. Vision and the Musician. *Med Probl Perform Art* 1986;117–122.
54. Dawson WJ. Hand and Upper Extremity Problems in Musicians. *Med Probl Perform Art* 1988;3:19–23.
55. Nolan WB, Eaton RG. Thumb Problems of Professional Musicians. *Med Probl Perform Art* 1989;4:20–24.
56. Kirk JA, Ansell BM, Bywater EGL. The Hypermobility Syndrome: Musculoskeletal Complaints Associated with Generalized Joint Hypermobility. *Ann Rheum Dis* 1976;26:419–425.
57. Brandfonbrener AG. Hyperextensibility in Musicians. Fifth Ann Symposium on Med Probl of Musicians and Dancers. Aspen Co. 1987.
58. Patrone NA et al. Benign Hypermobility in a Flute Player. *Med Probl Perform Art* 1988;3:158–161.
59. Bird HA, Tribe CR, Bacon PA. Joint Hypermobility Leading to Osteoarthritis and Chondrocalcinosis. *Ann Rheum Dis* 1978;37:203–211.
60. Klafs CE, Arnheim DD. Physical Conditioning for the Prevention of Sports Injuries. In: Modern Principles of Athletic Training 5th ed. St. Louis: Mosby, 1981;95–139.
61. Karpovich PV, Sinning WE. Physiology of Muscular Activity. 7th ed. Philadelphia: Saunders, 1971.
62. Brandfonbrener AG. Preliminary Results of Medical Survey of MTNA Teachers. *American Music Teacher* 1989;39:14–15.
63. Polisi JW, Allen JS. Music and the Good Life. *The New Criterion* 1988;1–4.

Textbook of Performing Arts Medicine, edited by R. T. Sataloff, A. Brandfonbrener, and R. Lederman. Raven Press, Ltd., New York © 1991.

3

Musculoskeletal Problems in Instrumental Musicians

*Richard A. Hoppmann and †Nicholas A. Patrone

*Associate Professor of Medicine, University of South Carolina School of Medicine, Chief of Rheumatology, Dorn Veterans' Hospital, Columbia, South Carolina 29201; and †Associate Professor of Medicine and Pediatrics, Section of Rheumatology, East Carolina University School of Medicine, Greenville, North Carolina 27858

Musculoskeletal problems in instrumental musicians are common at all levels of performance and in all age groups (1–4). Occasional minor aches and pains while practicing or performing are not unexpected considering the demands that instrumentalists frequently place on the musculoskeletal system. However, persistent musculoskeletal problems, especially pain, should not be considered "part of being a good musician or music student" and advice should be sought concerning the problem. The music teacher should be made aware of the pain or discomfort related to playing and if changes in technique, practice time, or repertoire do not result in relief, further consultation with someone in the field of arts medicine may be needed. Most problems, when addressed early, stand an excellent chance of resolution with minimal intervention and disruption of performance. Unfortunately, as has been shown by several large survey studies (1,5,6), many of the musculoskeletal problems of instrumentalists are chronic problems and can adversely affect careers in music. Both financial and personal reasons have kept musicians from volunteering musculoskeletal problems to teachers or performing arts management, but it appears the climate surrounding the performing arts may be changing to tolerate, if not encourage, musicians to seek help for their problems (7,8).

The common musculoskeletal problems affecting instrumentalists are listed in Table 3.1. Of these, musculotendinous overuse is the most frequently reported and will be discussed both in terms of a generalized "overuse syndrome" and as specific entities of tendinitis and bursitis. Hypermobility, fibrositis, osteoarthritis and other arthritides will also be discussed but nerve entrapment, thoracic outlet syndrome, and motor dysfunction are more appropriately covered in the chapter on neurological problems.

71

TABLE 3.1. *Musculoskeletal problems in musicians*

Musculotendinous Overuse
Hypermobility
Osteoarthritis
Fibrositis
Nerve Entrapment
Thoracic Outlet Syndrome
Motor Dysfunction

Before discussing specific problems, a general approach to the history, physical examination, and treatment of instrumentalists with musculoskeletal problems will be presented.

HISTORY

A brief general medical history should be obtained initially on all patients. Systemic diseases such as diabetes mellitus are associated with an increased frequency of musculoskeletal problems and musicians are as susceptible to these diseases as the general population. A history of previous trauma or surgery may be relevant to the particular problem and should be outlined in detail. Allergic reactions, renal disease, gastrointestinal symptoms, and hearing problems should be noted in anticipation of possibly using a nonsteroidal antiinflammatory drug.

Occupational history, if other than musician, should be obtained and if pertinent to the present problem should be elaborated in detail. Many of the musculoskeletal problems seen in musicians have their counterparts in industrial medicine (9). Thus, a history of many hours at a word processing keyboard in a pianist or a violinist with hand or wrist pain would aid in the diagnosis and management of the problem. Hobbies and other physical activities are also a source of musculoskeletal problems and may cause or contribute to the musician's injury. Common activities that contribute to musculoskeletal problems include gardening, craft work, and a variety of sporting activities. In fact, traumatic hand problems in musicians have been shown to be sports-related in a high percentage (10).

Table 3.2 outlines the areas of the practice performance history that have been shown to be associated with the development of musculoskeletal problems in instrumentalists. Many musicians play more than one instrument regularly and a practice history should be obtained for each instrument. The contributions to the injury may be additive, as might be expected in someone with right-shoulder pain who plays violin and flute. Pain with one instrument and not another might help elucidate the source of the problem, as in the saxophone player who has little trouble with the right shoulder while playing the alto sax, which is supported by a neck strap, but has considerable difficulty when playing the soprano sax, which is held in position by the musician and not by a neck strap.

It is not uncommon for musicians to take up a new instrument, and it is, there-

TABLE 3.2. *Practice/performance history*

A. Instrument(s)
    Instrument(s) played and for how long
    Any recent change in instrument
B. Practice habits
    Length of daily session(s)
    Warm-up, cool-down periods
    Rest periods within sessions
    Difficulty with practice pieces
C. Lessons
    Frequency, length
    Change in teacher
D. Performances
    Frequency
    Difficulty
E. Symptoms
    Duration
    Onset—while playing or delayed
    One site or multiple sites
    Limited to playing or with other activities
    Effect on performance
    Paresthesias
    Motor control problems

Data from Hoppmann and Patrone (25).

fore, important to know how long each instrument has been played. Differences can also exist in the mechanics of the instruments even though they may be of the same class. For example, the distance traveled and force required to depress a key and produce the same volume of sound can be quite different in different pianos, the harpsichord, or organ. Therefore, the history should include details about the instruments used, especially if they are new or borrowed.

Practice time accounts for the majority of the total time musicians spend with their instruments and it is a likely source of musculoskeletal problems. Practice should be analyzed in terms of total time spent per week, per day, and per session. Any recent change in either time or intensity of these should be noted. With appropriate technique and a steady but gradual increase in practice sessions, most musicians can expect to practice 30 to 40 hours or more per week without significant risk of developing problems.

Several studies have shown that all levels of musicians are at increased risk of injury with an abrupt increase in practice time (2,5,11). The rapid increases in practice often preceding juries or recitals or occurring during music camps may precipitate injuries. The length of individual sessions and the number of rest periods within a session also appear to be important factors in the development of musculoskeletal problems. Good practice habits should include a warm-up and cool-down period at the beginning and at the end of the session. Muscles, tendons, and other supporting structures function more efficiently and are less likely to be injured if they are first warmed up and put through the range of motion required for the activity to be undertaken. A warm-up period need not be 10 or 15 minutes of scales.

The warm-up period should be discussed with the teacher and can be either specific exercises or easy pieces that can be varied in tempo and dynamics to take the joints through the required range of motion and safely prepare the student for the difficulty level of the pieces to be practiced. It should also be noted that a brisk walk or other light aerobic exercise prior to the actual practice session probably has beneficial effects, both physically and mentally. Posture and whether the musician stands or sits during practice should be noted as well as the height of the music stand. If seated, the height and design of the chair, especially with regard to the back support, should be determined.

A review of the practice history should include the pieces being performed, whether they are new pieces, if one causes more problems than another, and what physical movements in the piece exacerbate the problem. There are certain pieces that are physically more demanding than others, such as piano compositions by Rachmaninoff and Liszt, for the pianist with small hands. It is an important role for the teacher to help students select pieces that are within their capability. This is just one of the many reasons why communication among the teacher, the health care provider, and the student is so important.

Although lessons do not account for a great deal of total playing time per week, they should be factored into the total time. Probably more important to note would be a change in the number or length of lessons per week. In addition, a change in teacher quite often means a change, however subtle, in technique. Technique changes can stress different muscles and supporting structures. These changes should be incorporated into the student's technique gradually and in a stepwise fashion if possible.

Performances per se do not usually contribute significantly to injuries unless they are very frequent or place greater demands on the performer, such as playing on an unresponsive piano in a large concert hall. However, performances are quite often preceded by long and frequent rehearsals and total weekly practice time can increase by 50% to 100%. This rapid increase makes some musicians vulnerable to musculoskeletal injury. Performances should therefore be planned sufficiently in advance to allow a gradual increase in practice and rehearsal times.

Pain is by far the most common complaint of instrumentalists seeking medical attention. Symptoms of paresthesia or motor control should suggest the possibility of nerve entrapment or focal dystonia. The onset, duration, sites, and aggravating factors of the pain should be sought in considerable detail. The site of pain at presentation may be the result of a change in technique in response to an earlier problem elsewhere. For example, a neck problem in a violinist may have resulted from a change in neck position that was brought about by initial discomfort with the left shoulder that has since resolved. Thus, a history should be obtained of pain or discomfort at any site within the preceding months. Description of the pain is often of a dull ache but occasionally the pain is sharp and localized, and this should suggest a specific tendinitis or bursitis.

Fry has developed a grading scale for severity of injury based primarily on pain and the effects of rest and activity on the pain (12). The severity of the pain will usually dictate the intensity of therapy, and in many cases the prognosis. Table 3.3 outlines a grading system that we have found particularly useful in managing musculoskeletal injuries. In addition to how long a problem has existed, the duration of individual painful episodes is important. Pain that is felt only temporarily after playing or that resolves shortly after playing generally indicates a mild process and is likely to respond to a decrease in practice time and/or minor changes in repertoire or technique. Pain that persists for hours after playing or progresses during a session indicates a more serious problem and generally requires more than just relative rest. Pain that never resolves between sessions or prevents playing is obviously a serious problem and may require prolonged absolute rest from playing in addition to multiple modalities of therapy.

The obvious immediate goal of treatment should be to eliminate pain and its effect on performance. Pain-free performance can be attained in most musicians, especially if the musician takes an active role in the rehabilitation process. This approach has been emphasized in a conservatory setting with excellent results (13). For that small group of musicians that do not become pain-free despite rest and other therapy, a more realistic goal may be to minimize pain, maintain function, and prevent progression of the injury. This would especially be true for the older musician who has developed osteoarthritis or another chronic musculoskeletal problem, but would like to continue to perform.

PHYSICAL EXAMINATION

The physical examination of the musician begins when the examiner first enters the room and notes the posture and overall condition of the injured musician. Both posture and conditioning can impact on many musculoskeletal problems, regardless of the specific problem or instrument played. The examiner should perform a brief, general exam, looking for evidence of underlying disease, and then perform a detailed musculoskeletal exam with the upper trunk and extremities exposed and appropriately draped. The exam should first be done without the instrument and then observation should be carried out while the patient is performing. Important points in the exam are outlined in Table 3.4. Back problems have been noted in a high percentage of professional orchestra musicians (1) and examination of the spine with emphasis on curvature, symmetrical musculature, tenderness, and evidence of paraspinal muscle spasm should be performed. The neck should be examined

---

TABLE 3.3. *Grading system for severity of injury*

Grade 1 Pain while playing or for a short period after playing
Grade 2 Pain that persists for a longer period (hours) after playing
Grade 3 Pain that progresses while playing and requires the practice session to be shortened but resolves between sessions
Grade 4 Pain that progresses while playing and does not totally resolve between sessions
Grade 5 Continuous pain that markedly reduces or prevents playing

TABLE 3.4. *Examination of the injured musician*

Inspect the spine for scoliosis, loss of cervical or lumbar lordosis, note any muscle atrophy or asymmetry in shoulder height
Test range of motion of the neck—flexion, extension, right and left rotation, right and left lateral movement
Compare arm span to the height of the patient
Test range of motion and strength at the shoulder, elbow, wrist, and hand
Test light touch sensation in the upper extremities
Note calluses on the chin, neck, and fingers
Observe the musician perform and note posture, muscle tone and movement

through its three basic movements, and range of motion and tenderness should be noted. Arm span relative to height of the patient should be noted, and span exceeding height should suggest a possible hypermobility syndrome. Range of motion and strength should be tested in all upper extremity joints on both the injured side as well as the non-injured side to detect asymmetry. Light touch sensation should be tested in the upper extremities. Sensory deficits would suggest possible nerve entrapment such as carpal tunnel syndrome or even nerve root compression in the neck. The fingers, neck, and chin should be examined for location and thickness of calluses. Unusual location or extreme thickness of calluses may suggest a technique problem or the use of unnecessary force to perform. While observing the musician perform, particular attention should be paid to body position, muscle tension, and tendon movement of the injured part. When consultation and review of the physical exam and technique with the music teacher is not possible, videotaping the musician's performance and reviewing the tape later may be a suitable alternative.

TREATMENT

Treatment for the injured musician must be individualized; however, there are general principles to consider in developing a treatment plan for most musicians (Table 3.5). It has been known for almost 100 years that rest is the most important point in the treatment of injured musicians (14). Although there has been debate as to the degree and duration of rest needed, the first step in the treatment of most musculoskeletal injuries should be rest. For severe (grade 4 or 5) injury, at least a

TABLE 3.5. *Treatment of musculoskeletal injuries in musicians*

Rest—Absolute or relative, incorporate rest periods into sessions
Technique—Correct problem, reduce static and dynamic loads
Nonsteroidal antiinflammatory drugs
Physical/occupational therapy—Splints, ice, exercise, adaptive devices
Relaxation training/Alexander technique/Feldenkrais method
Local injections—Steroids
Surgery

Data from Hoppmann and Patrone (25).

brief period of absolute rest from playing until the pain resolves or is minimal should be recommended. When performing resumes, it should be a gradual process with small increments in practice time. This is best accomplished by keeping a log of practice time each day and noting any discomfort that develops. This record should be reviewed with the teacher and health care provider regularly. For less severe problems, relative rest in the form of decreased total playing time with more frequent, shorter sessions is often effective.

It is not uncommon for instrumentalists to get quite depressed when instructed to stop or cut back appreciably in playing. This depression should be openly discussed with the musician. It should be explained that depression is a natural response to the injury and its effect on lifestyle and potential career. For some musicians, getting more involved in conducting or nonperforming musical activities such as arranging or research, although not a totally satisfying substitute, can often lessen the impact of not performing on an instrument during the recovery period. Both teacher and health care provider need to keep this emotional effect of the injury in mind when working with the injured musician, and be supportive and encouraging.

Poor technique, for whatever reason, must be identified and corrected, or recurrent problems are likely even if the present problem resolves. Technique can be a very delicate issue for the musician, the teacher, and the health care provider. There must be an attitude of cooperation and mutual respect, and not one of blame, if the desired outcome is to be achieved. With all the technical research underway (15–18) there may come a day when one technique will be shown to be more bio-mechanically efficient and less likely to result in injury without compromising quality of performance. Until that day comes there should be a relatively liberal attitude about different techniques and even individualized techniques, unless obviously harmful. A health care provider knowledgeable in musculoskeletal function and the music teacher, working together, are more likely to identify potential problems in technique than either working alone.

When evaluating technique, it is important to consider both dynamic and static loads on the musculoskeletal system. Static load is continuous muscle contraction and stress across a joint and its supporting structures. Instruments such as the violin or clarinet that must be held in a particular position to be played require constant muscle contraction in certain muscles such as the shoulder and hand for considerable periods of time. This results in static loading to these muscles and joints and can lead to problems. Reducing this load by using devices such as straps and posts can often provide immediate relief for the instrumentalist. If aesthetically acceptable to the musician, these devices can continue to be used and help prevent recurrence of the problem as well. There have also been some attempts to redesign instruments to relieve static load and to improve the ergonomic relationship of the musician to the instrument. An example is the curved-head flute that reduces neck and shoulder strain. Instrument repair shops and music schools are usually good sources of these devices or personnel that can make individualized modifications to the instrument.

Dynamic load refers to the stress to joints and supporting structures resulting from movement, especially high-frequency, forceful movements. Musicians' movements are not typically of great force, but high-frequency, repetitive movements are the rule while performing. Dynamic load can be reduced by more effi cient movements and reducing unnecessary muscle tension. Making changes in the instrument to improve the movement of the keys or decrease the distance keys or strings must be moved conserves energy and decreases load on the arms and hands.

Nonsteroidal antiinflammatory drugs are used for a wide variety of musculoskeletal problems, both acute and chronic, and have been used with some success in musculoskeletal problems of instrumentalists. We typically use nonsteroidal antiinflammatory drugs if pain is significant or if the injury appears to have an inflammatory component, such as with tenosynovitis. Possible complications of the nonsteroidal antiinflammatory drugs, such as gastrointestinal and renal toxicity, should be discussed with patients prior to starting therapy. There is one report to suggest that topical salicylate cream may be beneficial to musicians with localized pain (19). Nonsteroidal antiinflammatory drugs should not be used without also instituting either relative or absolute rest and evaluation of technique, for nonsteroidal drugs may simply mask the pain as the injury progresses.

Physical and occupational therapists, especially those with an interest in instrumentalists, are important members of the health care team managing the injured musician (20). Hand and wrist splints can be very useful early in treatment, and functional splints that allow for performing can be used for extended rehabilitation and prevention of recurrence. Individualized adaptive devices can also be made by the therapist. Ice and/or heat are sometimes effective in reducing pain. Whether to use heat or ice should be determined empirically by having the musician try both and continuing whichever seems to be the most helpful. Range-of-motion exercises and low-resistance strengthening exercises are helpful for rehabilitation and prevention. Strengthening exercises should be used with caution in the early stages of the treatment, however. Some patients have reported worsening of symptoms with strengthening exercises (12).

Standard relaxation techniques as well as more sophisticated techniques such as electromyographic feedback have been used in musicians to reduce unwanted muscle tension (21). Several approaches to teaching and treating performers, such as the Feldenkrais method and the Alexander technique, have been quite successful in some patients (22,23). These will not be discussed here, but the importance of awareness of body position, muscle tension, and efficiency of movement, which is a central theme to these approaches, should always be kept in mind when treating musculoskeletal problems. In addition, carryover of this awareness to nonperforming activities, such as writing or gripping the steering wheel while driving, should be encouraged. In fact, watching the patient write can often be instructive with regard to identifying unnecessary muscle tension in the hand. It can also serve as a model to teach muscle tension awareness. The patient can see the muscles contract, can see the fingernail beds blanch from too much pressure, and can feel with the other hand the contracted muscle. These signs can be used as feedback to develop a more relaxed and efficient way of writing and hopefully of performing. When conservative methods fail to produce satisfactory results, steroid injection or surgery may be reasonable alternatives for certain musculoskeletal problems. The risk of both of these approaches should be explained to the patient, and procedures should be done only by physicians with extensive experience in the specific procedure to be performed. Everything should be done to ensure the best results possible, for the instrumentalist places great demands on his or her body, and to perform at a high level requires optimal recovery of musculoskeletal function.

MUSCULOTENDINOUS OVERUSE

The term "overuse" has been used in sports medicine and in industrial medicine for many years and was borrowed almost since the inception of performing arts medicine, to describe musculoskeletal problems in instrumentalists. Overuse is felt to occur "when a tissue is stressed beyond its anatomic or physiologic limit"(24). The comparison of dancers with athletes is probably reasonable, but to compare instrumentalists with athletes is not. Even though athletes and instrumentalists are both highly skilled performers and spend a great deal of time performing and practicing, many of the injuries in sports medicine result from high-impact movements and physical contact, neither of which are a part of performing music. The comparison with overuse in industry is somewhat more accurate, even though the repetitive movements of assembly line workers have definite quantitative and qualitative differences from playing the piano or violin.

We classify injuries as musculotendinous overuse if the injury appears to result from excessive use, has pain as a major component, has minimal motor dysfunction, and is not due to nerve entrapment or thoracic outlet syndrome (25). This classification includes specific, localized inflammatory entities such as bicipital tendinitis and less specific diffuse injuries that we group together and call "overuse syndrome." When possible, the more specific diagnosis should be used to facilitate communication among those interested in arts medicine.

OVERUSE SYNDROME

For such a widely accepted and apparently self-explanatory concept as overuse, there is considerable controversy about the underlying mechanism of injury, and there is a paucity of pathological studies (26–29). Inflammation is rarely apparent on physical exam in patients with overuse syndrome, and it is often not clear if the injured structure is tendon, muscle, ligament, joint capsule, or a combination of these. Dennett and Fry have demonstrated muscle changes in overuse syndrome in keyboard operators (30). They biopsied the first dorsal interosseous muscles of the hand and found an assortment of changes in muscle-type grouping, mitochondria and ultrastructure. The significance of these changes is not clear, for they are nonspecific. At this time a histologic diagnosis of overuse cannot be made, and the diagnosis remains a clinical one.

In the appropriate setting, such as an acute increase in practice time prior to a recital, an instrumentalist may develop a diffuse aching sensation in the forearms. Initially this may be felt only for a short period after practicing. If the practice time and intensity continues, the achiness is likely to progress to pain that may be noticed during practice and persist for some time after practice. This pain may progress to the point of prohibiting any performing. Little may be found on physical exam except some mild tenderness in the forearm muscles, especially the wrist extensors, and the intrinsic hand muscles. Motor and sensory function are usually normal. If special maneuvers do not identify a specific tendinitis or bursitis, the diagnosis of overuse syndrome is made. The following two cases demonstrate the spectrum of the problem.

A 34-year-old pianist presented with a 1-week history of diffuse achiness in both forearms noticed shortly after practicing. She was in graduate school pursuing a nonmusical degree but had previously received a degree in music performance, and she was now accompanying voice students in order to pay her way through graduate school. She had recently increased her practice time, as two of the voice students were preparing for recitals. Her physical exam was entirely within normal limits, and there were no major problems with her technique. She was instructed to keep a log of her practice and performance time, perform stretching exercises, take breaks within sessions, and limit sessions to 45 minutes each. In order to get through the upcoming recitals, she was advised to limit her practicing to only what was required to prepare for the recitals. The achy sensation decreased appreciably over the next week. After the recitals, she continued to keep a log, maintained good practice habits, and planned to accompany only when adequate preparation time was possible. She had no recurrence of symptoms after 1 year.

The second patient was also a pianist but he presented with 4 months of severe forearm and hand pain that virtually prevented him from playing. He was a 30-year-old professional musician who worked multiple jobs that required long hours of playing and included solo piano performance, as well as participating in big band and jazz ensembles. The demand for playing increased over several months, and he was performing up to 6 hours per day, 7 days a week. On exam, tenderness was noted in the forearm muscles. Absolute rest was instituted with avoidance of all unnecessary activities involving muscle contraction in the forearm and hand. He was also started on a nonsteroidal antiinflammatory drug, moist heat, and stretching exercises. After 2 weeks and every week thereafter, a short trial of performing was attempted. Once these short sessions became pain-free, a schedule of practicing starting at 5-minute sessions twice a day was instituted. These were gradually increased over the next 6 months. Occasionally the playing time had to be temporarily decreased due to mild recurrence of symptoms. In addition, his technique was evaluated by a music faculty member who began a retraining program to improve the efficiency of his finger movements and decrease unnecessary muscle tension. At the end of one year he was regularly playing up to 3 hours per day with no significant problems.

These are fairly typical examples of the two extremes of overuse syndrome and emphasize the need for early diagnosis and intervention. If identified early, resolution of symptoms is likely with little disruption of performing schedule. In addition, teaching the musician to recognize the symptoms of the overuse syndrome and the situations in which they are likely to occur, combined with good practice habits, should markedly reduce the incidence of this syndrome.

SHOULDER PROBLEMS

Shoulder problems are relatively common among all musicians, especially string and wind players. An intricate network of muscle, bone, ligaments, and bursae make the shoulder joint the most mobile in the body. In instrumentalists it is a joint that can be under prolonged static and/or dynamic load, as in the case with the violinist whose left shoulder is under static load and whose right shoulder experiences dynamic and static loading.

Three potential shoulder problems in instrumentalists will be presented: impingement syndrome, subacromial/subdeltoid bursitis and bicipital tendinitis. Figure 3.1 depicts diagrammatically the shoulder joint and structures to be discussed.

Impingement syndrome occurs when the supraspinatus tendon is pinched between the humerus and the coracoacromial arch. A "painful arc" of abduction of the arm from 60° to 120° is noted, and there may be tenderness over the greater tuber-

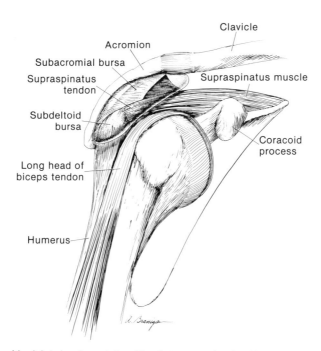

FIG. 3.1. Shoulder joint showing relationship of structures involved in problems of musicians.

osity of the humerus. If identified early, as in the case of a 16-year-old flutist who presented with two weeks of mild right shoulder pain, relative rest, range-of-motion exercises and a short course of a nonsteroidal antiinflammatory drug may lead to prompt resolution of the pain.

If the problem is not identified early, impingement can lead to chronic supraspinatus tendinitis and become quite refractory to treatment. In this case, steroid injection and absolute rest may be needed. If steroid injection is performed, a radiograph of the shoulder should be obtained to look for calcification, erosions, or arthritis of the shoulder. In addition, complications of steroid injection should be explained to the musician. These include pain, bleeding, infection, and tendon rupture. With all shoulder injuries, range-of-motion exercises such as swinging the arm in a pendulum fashion and finger-walking up the wall are of paramount importance. If range-of-motion exercises are not done, capsulitis can develop with restriction of shoulder movement ("frozen shoulder") and prolonged disability. Removing or reducing static load should be attempted. This can sometimes be accomplished by use of posts, straps, or other devices that support the weight of the instrument and relieve the shoulder of part, if not all, of the static load.

The subacromial bursa can be one large bursa or divided into two bursae. When divided, the bursa under the deltoid muscle is designated the subdeltoid bursa. These bursae separate the rotator cuff muscles of the shoulder (supraspinatus, infraspinatus, teres minor, and subscapularis muscles) from the overlying acromion, teres major, and deltoid muscles. Pain is noted more on active abduction than passive abduction by the examiner. It can be difficult to distinguish subacromial bursitis from impingement, and the two can occur together. Calcium may be seen on a shoulder radiograph in the bursa, especially if the problem is chronic. Treatment should begin conservatively with rest, heat, range-of-motion exercises, and a nonsteroidal antiinflammatory. If these are unsuccessful, steroid injection should be considered.

The long head of the biceps muscle originates on the supraglenoid tubercle of the scapula, passes through the shoulder joint, and extends down the anterior humerus to traverse the bicipital groove. The biceps muscle helps abduct and flex at the shoulder and flex and supinate the forearm. These are common movements in playing certain instruments. String players are probably at highest risk of developing bicipital tendinitis, especially on the right side, and bilateral bicipital tendinitis has been reported in a cymbal player (31).

On physical exam, pain can be elicited if the biceps tendon is rolled under the examiner's thumb. The results of this maneuver should be compared with that on the opposite side to detect a significant difference. In addition, the examiner should test for Yergason's sign, which is pain on resisted supination (Fig. 3.2). A conservative approach to treatment, as with the other shoulder problems, should be initiated; if unsuccessful, steroid injection should be considered. The injection should not be directly into the tendon but in the peritendinous region to decrease the risk of tendon rupture. The steroid preparation should flow freely from the syringe and not be forced against resistance.

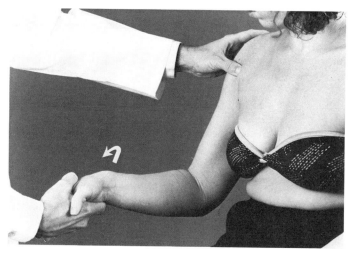

FIG. 3.2. Yergason's sign: pain at the biceps tendon on resisted supination (arrow).

LATERAL EPICONDYLITIS

Pain at the lateral epicondyle of the elbow where the wrist and finger extensors originate is called lateral epicondylitis, or "tennis elbow." Most patients with this entity do not play tennis but are usually involved in activities that require frequent use of wrist extensors. We have seen lateral epicondylitis in two percussionists who played a variety of percussion instruments, most of which required a great deal of wrist flexion and extension.

On examination, there is tenderness over the lateral epicondyle that may extend several centimeters distally. Pain is felt on resisted wrist extension (Fig. 3.3). Treatment consists of rest, nonsteroidal antiinflammatory drugs, and ice. "Tennis elbow" bands placed just distal to the elbow and devices that prevent wrist extension have been used with some success. If these measures fail, steroid injection may be necessary. Surgery is rarely needed for epicondylitis. Once the pain resolves, exercises to develop the wrist extensors can be used to help prevent recurrence.

DEQUERVAIN'S TENOSYNOVITIS

Stenosing tenosynovitis of the abductor pollicis longus and the extensor pollicis brevis at the radial styloid of the wrist is called deQuervain's tenosynovitis. Pain can be felt on the radial side of the wrist when the fingers are spread as far apart as possible, thus actively using the tendons. Pain can also be felt if the thumb is flexed into the palm and the wrist deviated in an ulnar direction (Fig. 3.4). Sharp pain over the radial styloid with this maneuver is called Finkelstein's sign. Pianists, clarinetists, and oboists develop deQuervain's tenosynovitis most commonly. In pianists, a

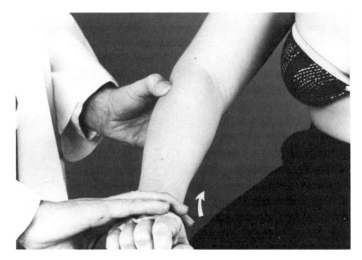

FIG. 3.3. Lateral epicondylitis: pain at the lateral epicondyle of the elbow on resisted wrist extension (arrow).

clue to the diagnosis is a history of pain with "cross-over" movements of the thumb under the fifth finger to play the next note. We have successfully treated deQuervain's tenosynovitis with rest, splinting, nonsteroidals, and steroid injection. Others have advocated early surgery in musicians since the stimulus for the injury remains and recurrence after conservative treatment is frequent (32). Surgery consists of decompression of the first dorsal compartment. This and other hand ailments are discussed in greater detail in a separate chapter.

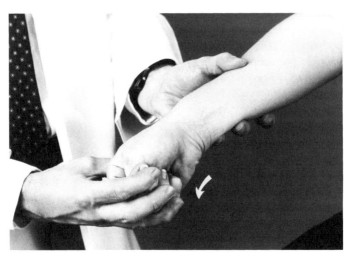

FIG. 3.4. Finkelstein's sign: pain over the radial styloid when the fist is deviated in an ulnar direction (arrow).

TRIGGER FINGER

The tendons of the fingers involved in flexion pass through a fibro-osseous pulley system and tendon sheaths that allow smooth biomechanical action. Nodule formation and/or stenosis of the tendon sheath can cause the finger to get hung up in flexion, thus producing the classic "trigger finger." Instrumentalists that develop this problem will usually report normal flexion of the fingers but increasing difficulty extending the fingers from a flexed position. They may report a snapping or popping sensation once the resistance to extension is forceably overcome. On examination, asking the musician to make a fist and quickly open it will usually identify the finger or fingers involved, because they will lag behind the other fingers or lock in flexion. A nodule may be felt on the involved tendon. Nonsteroidal antiinflammatory drugs and rest may result in a reduction in tendon and synovial swelling and return the flexion apparatus to normal. Occasionally, steroid injection followed by rest is needed. If these measures fail, surgery can successfully open the area of constriction to allow tendon movement. If done by an experienced surgeon, this procedure carries minimal risk.

GANGLION

A ganglion is a cystic structure found most commonly on the dorsum of the wrist (Fig. 3.5). It is believed to originate from an underlying tendon sheath or joint capsule and is filled with viscous fluid. It is usually asymptomatic but can cause mild discomfort due to its space-occupying nature. If the ganglion is causing a problem for the instrumentalist, it can be aspirated with a large bore needle and then injected with steroids. If the ganglion recurs and is symptomatic, it can be removed surgically. If not causing a problem, it should be left alone, for many will resolve spontaneously. Contrary to folk medicine, it should not be ruptured.

HYPERMOBILITY

Interest in articular hypermobility has expanded in the recent years with several articles and an extensive monograph (33) adding to the knowledge base of classic literature. Nevertheless, little attention has been paid to musicians and problems associated with abnormally flexible joints. Recent case reports and epidemiologic studies have begun to widen our understanding of problems in performing artists.

Though Hippocrates is credited with the first description of hypermobility, detailed descriptions of individuals or families were lacking until the early twentieth century. Finkelstein (34) and Key (35) described families with joint laxity in the first quarter of the century, but Sutro (36) in 1947 was the first to associate joint laxity and rheumatologic disease. In a study of 435 adult outpatients, he found a 4% prevalence of hypermobility and described 13 young men with joint laxity who suffered from a recurrent knee pain and effusions during military training. Finally, in 1967, Kirk et al. (37) described 24 patients in defining the hypermobility syn-

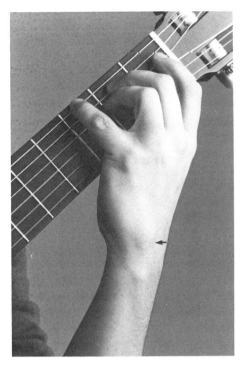

FIG. 3.5. Ganglion on the dorsum of the wrist (arrow) in a guitarist.

drome as joint laxity and arthritic symptoms in individuals who have no primary underlying disease to account for either problem.

Though several groups have looked at the prevalence of hypermobility, exact figures are difficult to determine since the definition of laxity and age of patients vary from study to study. Sutro's original description found a 4% prevalence of hypermobility in 3 or more pairs of joints, while Carter (38) found increased joint laxity in 7% of 285 schoolchildren. Arroyo et al. (39) examined 192 children, ages 5 to 19, and found a 34% prevalence of hypermobility, but noted that as children aged, the frequency of joint laxity dropped dramatically from nearly 50% during ages 5 through 18 to a frequency of 15% to 18% at ages 12 through 19.

Biro et al. (40) noted that 5.7% of their pediatric rheumatology patients had hypermobility, but no general population studies were available. Two studies have examined the frequency of joint laxity in musicians, but these, too, give scattered results. Larsson et al. (41) examined 660 students at a music school and found from 27% (if only one body part was affected) to 3% (if five body parts were affected), while Bejjani (42) found an astounding 60% prevalence of hypermobility in 72 musicians and 65% in 17 nonmusicians. Details of this study are lacking and make comparison to others difficult. Graham (43) compared 53 ballet dancers with 53 nursing students and found a definite increase in hypermobility in dance students, with an average of 35% compared to 15%. These data may be skewed by selection of individuals to dance who are able to use their hypermobility to increase the range of motion so needed in ballet. As varied as these studies are, some results are consistent. Each showed an increased female to male ratio varying from 8:1 to 2:1 depending on the age of the patients, a decreased frequency of hypermobility as the population aged, and a much earlier loss of hypermobility in males compared to females. Family histories were often positive for hypermobility, but many individuals could find no evidence of familial hyperlaxity. In addition, each study described a wide variety of the number of joints affected in individuals, with some having changes limited to small joints in the hands while others showed changes in hands, wrists, elbows, back, and knees.

Not all individuals with hypermobility develop rheumatologic problems. The patient's family members often exhibit the same changes of joint laxity and give no history of joint discomfort. Similarly, musicians with hyperextensibility and joint pain may share an orchestra section (e.g., strings) with similar individuals who have never had arthritic complaints. Arroyo's study of 192 children, ages 5 through 19, revealed that half of the study group with hypermobility gave a history of arthralgias, where 20% of those without joint laxity described joint discomfort (39). Under extreme conditions, joint laxity predisposes to injury. Nicholas (44) examined 139 professional football players and identified 39 with changes suggestive of hypermobility. Of these individuals, 72% sustained knee ligament rupture requiring surgery, compared to 4% with no changes in joint laxity. In a similar vein, Klemp et al. (45) found a higher rate of joint injury in ballet dancers with hypermobility than in control subjects. Studies of musicians with hypermobility and rheumatologic complaints have been limited to case reports and brief series with no control groups. Brandfonbrener (46) described 43 violinists or violists and 32 pianists who presented with hand pain. One-third of these showed changes of hypermobility, suggesting a relationship between joint stress and hypermobility, and the onset of rheumatologic discomfort. That musicians with hypermobility have more problems than individuals with no increased joint laxity appears likely, but to what extent or severity is yet to be determined.

In assessing hypermobility, standard measures have evolved which allow uniformity of evaluations and better comparison between studies. Beighton et al. (47), in an epidemiologic survey of rheumatologic and orthopedic disease in rural Africa, combined previous systems and developed a point system easily used by clinicians in an outpatient setting. Joint motion is measured in five anatomic areas and points are awarded for the presence of hyperextensibility. The overall scores vary from 0 to 9, with hypermobile adults showing scores from 4 to 9. Since joint laxity decreases with age, the lower score is more appropriate for men over the age of 25 and women over the age of 45. Points are awarded as follows: (1.) passive dorsiflexion of the fifth digit beyond 90°—one point for each hand, (2.) passive opposition of the thumb to the flexor surface of the arm—one point for each hand, (3.) extension of the elbow beyond 190°—one point for each arm, (4.) extension of the knee beyond 190°—one point for each leg, (5.) anterior flexion of the back with knees extended, allowing the palms to rest flat on the floor—one point (Fig. 3.6). When evaluating musicians with hypermobility, physicians must observe joint motions

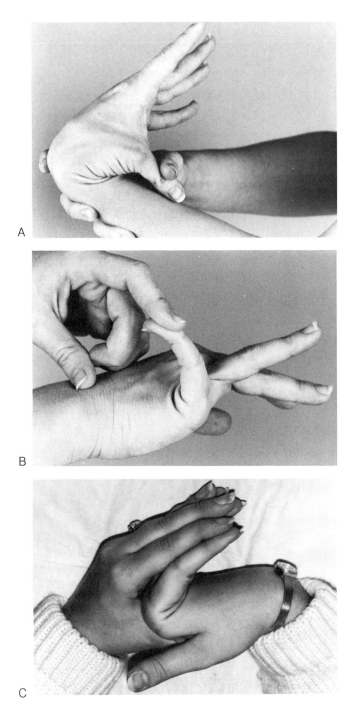

FIG. 3.6. Hypermobility of the thumb (A), fifth digit (B), MCP (C), elbows (D), and knees (E).

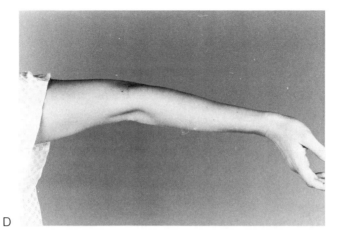

D

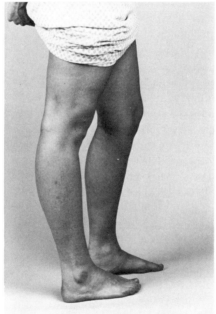

E

FIG. 3.6. *Continued.*

while the patient plays etudes which emphasize various components of technique. Playing at slower tempo may allow close and detailed observation of abnormal laxity. In addition, the help of a music teacher or performer well-versed in good technique will aid in identifying subtle alterations in motion used to compensate for increased joint laxity. Use of a goniometer aids in angle measurement.

Whether hypermobility represents an extreme range of normal joint motion or a pathological state is debatable. Silman et al. (48), in a study of 364 normal adolescents and adults, concluded hypermobile individuals represent an extreme of normal distribution, and that global hypermobility appears at the extremes of the distribution curve. Beighton's study of 502 rural African adults showed that 4% of men and 80% of women scored less than 2 on the hypermobility scale, but at the same time showed a gradual decline in frequency of joint laxity as scores increased, adding to the suspicion that hypermobility is on the extreme of normal rather than a distinct disease entity. Nevertheless, a family history is often present in patients with hypermobility, suggesting a genetic component in some individuals. In addition, studies suggest racial variation in joint laxity, with Indians showing more than Africans, who in turn show more than Europeans.

Normal joint motion is a function of muscle tone and the stretch of joint capsule and ligaments. Athletic training may either increase joint motion with stretching of the joint capsule or decrease range of motion with increase in periarticular muscle mass and tone. The dominant hand is likely to have more muscle mass and tone than the nondominant hand, and Beighton's study showed decreased range of motion in the joints of the dominant hand compared to the nondominant hand. The study of Silverman et al. (49) in children disputes this finding with no increased mobility of the nondominant metacarpophalangeal joints. Our experience with adults would agree with that of Beighton, and therapeutic exercises have been used to increase muscle tone, decreasing joint laxity in affected hands. Little is known about the underlying tissue alterations allowing joint laxity. With use of electron microscopy, Shah et al. (50) have shown a coiling or crimping of collagen fibrils. One theory of joint laxity suggests that the initial wave length of the crimp determines the capacity of the joint for stretching, with the difference in wave length between individuals accounting for differences in extensibility. Biochemical defects have been described in variants of Ehlers-Danlos, and recent studies by Handler et al. (51) suggest an increase in the ratio of type III to total type III and I collagen in individuals with benign hypermobility. Electron microscopy revealed a decreased proportion of thick collagen fibers and increased fine fibers, elastin, fibrocytes, and ground substance compared to controls.

Patients with hypermobility may present with various rheumatologic problems ranging from acute traumatic synovitis to chronic monarticular inflammatory arthritis.

Acute monarticular arthritis secondary to synovial or ligamentous stretching with tear most often affects small joints of the fingers, wrists, knees, and ankles. Overuse of the affected area or acute trauma may precipitate arthralgia, joint effusions, and increased joint instability. Active bleeding within the joint space may lead to pannus formation with a subacute to chronic monarthritis. Musicians with hypermobility who practice for hours each day may present with chronic synovitis due to repeated trauma of the affected joints. Bird and Wright (52) described a 31-year-old male guitarist who presented with synovitis of the left wrist characterized by effusion, soft tissue swelling, and pain present during playing and exacerbated by daily practice of 5 hours. Though the patient was initially thought to have rheumatoid arthritis, his examination revealed a 4 out of 9 hypermobility score and arthritic changes limited to his left wrist. His studies and laboratory results were normal and he responded well to a single corticosteroid injection. Repeated episodes of traumatic arthritis may lead to marked synovial hypertrophy, at times necessitating surgical synovectomy; with early diagnosis and intervention, this is a rare occurrence.

Individuals with hypermobility are prone to joint dislocation with minor trauma. Areas affected include the patella, shoulder, temporomandibular joint, and, in musicians, the metacarpophalangeal joints. Violinists and violists with hypermobility may be at an increased risk for spontaneous dislocation of the temporomandibular joint secondary to abnormal stress placed on the right mandibular articulation. Use of a centrally placed chin rest may decrease this stress load and decrease a tendency of stretching of the joint capsule. Wilson (53) described a clarinetist with benign hypermobility who developed chronic temporomandibular joint discomfort but responded well to orthotic treatment and a midline apparatus.

Spontaneous dislocation of the fifth metacarpophalangeal joint has been described in a violinist with benign hypermobility. Each time she lifted the fifth finger off the string, the metacarpophalangeal joint would dislocate; the process eventually led to a digital nerve compression (54). Use of a finger splint and exercises to strengthen flexor tendons led to full recovery. Musicians with benign hypermobility will often relay the history of intermittent patellar dislocation; from a performer's point of view, this anatomical dysfunction rarely hinders instrument playing, but may cause problems in dancers.

Polyarthralgias without evidence of chronic synovitis occur frequently in patients with hypermobility. Though weather fronts and at times menstruation may lead to increased symptoms, the most consistent precipitating factor is an increase in joint use. Music students with hypermobility returning from holiday often relay the history of polyarthralgias in the first few weeks with return to normal practice. Objective findings are minimal and discomfort resolves in two to three weeks. If symptoms persist, the patient should be evaluated for the onset of other disorders such as overuse syndrome. Though no controlled studies have been performed, most rheumatologists note an increased incidence of soft tissue rheumatism (bursitis and tendinitis) in patients with hypermobility, the origin thought to be similar to that of acute traumatic synovitis. Spinal complications, hip dislocation, and increased bone fragility have been reported to occur in patients with increased joint laxity, but these problems do not seem to affect musicians.

In addition to well-recognized syndromes, musicians may develop other problems related to their hypermobility. String players may find vibrato difficult to perform secondary to hypermobility of the metacarpophalangeal or distal interphalangeal joints. Hyperextensibility of the third metacarpophalangeal joint may lead to frequent drooping of the bow in string players, and at times recurrent metacarpophalangeal dislocations may lead to digital nerve entrapments. Pianists with increased laxity of the distal interphalangeal joint may have difficulty controlling finger strike. At times, hypermobility is so severe as to cause detrimental changes in technique in order to bypass the increased motion from joint laxity. Though such measures may temporarily improve play, long-term abnormal stresses across joints may lead to increased pain, loss of dexterity, and poor playing—as in the case of a flutist with benign hypermobility who modified her playing to minimize her hypermobility (55). Though she and her teacher had recognized the "double joints" at an early age in her musical education, both had accepted adaptive changes in technique. As she advanced to college level play, rapid intricate passages led to marked pain in the fingers of the right hand and extensor compartments of the left hand. Hyperextensibility of her distal interphalangeals led to air gaps in several stops. Examination while playing the flute revealed several modifications of technique to compensate for hypermobility. Her left thumb touched the flute stop with the ulnar aspect of the thumb rather than the pulp of the finger; this change caused discomfort along the abductor pollicis longus tendon while playing. The external rotation of the thumb resulted in 70° extension of the second metacarpophalangeal while playing. This abnormal position of the metacarpophalangeal caused an increased tightening of the flexor tendons over the radial aspect of the wrist and discomfort after playing even brief passages of moderately difficult music. A saddle splint had corrected the hyperextension to approximately 30° but did not reduce the discomfort of the tendons of her thumb. Alternate thumb fingering of the left hand was nearly impossible to perform secondary to the pressure being transmitted by the medial aspect of the thumb rather than the pulp of the finger. Examination of the second through fifth fingers while playing revealed a 30° hyperextensibility of the distal interphalangeal joints with the wrist in the neutral position but no hyperextension of the distal interphalangeal joints with the wrist extended to 30°. Examination of the right hand revealed no problems with slow- to moderate-tempo passages but 30° hyperextensibility of the distal interphalangeal joints during rapid passages leading to air leakage through stop holes. Adaptive devices and an exercise and education program led to recovery.

Long-term follow-up in large numbers of patients with hypermobility has not been reported. Several case reports warn of the possibility of early osteoarthritis in the metacarpal joint, knees, and shoulders. Scott et al. (56) compared 50 control individuals with 50 age-matched individuals with osteoarthritis and found a significantly higher frequency of osteoarthritis in patients with hypermobility. Early diagnosis, intervention, and close follow-up may reduce the likelihood of joint damage leading to such changes.

Treatment of hypermobility in musicians must be multidisciplinary, with close cooperation between physician, physical therapist, occupational therapist, and teacher. Patient education is paramount to effective treatment. Reassurance as to the benign nature of the condition and overall excellent long-term outcome often alleviate anxiety associated with the diagnosis of "arthritis." Demonstration of an individual's hypermobility in comparison to a normal individual helps in understanding the condition of joint laxity. Concrete explanation as to the results of trauma or repetitive use often helps with the acceptance of the need for good practice habits and avoidance of marked stresses across joint spaces. Musicians with hypermobility should change practice schedules so that sessions last no more than 45 minutes with at least 10 to 15 minutes of rest between sessions to prevent excess use in relaxed joints.

An exercise program directed at strengthening the flexor muscles will oftentimes decrease the extent of hypermobility by increasing muscle tone. Such exercises will not decrease capsule laxity but will increase tone along the flexor plane, decreasing the tendency toward hyperextension. A strengthening program for intrinsic hand muscles should be designed by a knowledgeable occupational therapist and should include composite flexion exercises for individualized profundus, superficialis and intrinsic muscle-strengthening regimens. Use of putty may aid in the completion of exercises and over a 3-to 6-week course, the patient will note a decreased ease of hyperextensibility.

At times, adapted devices may be constructed to prevent spontaneous dislocation or allow transfer to proper playing technique when rapid change is needed to continue scheduled classes or performances (Fig. 3.7, Fig. 3.8). At the same time the patients begin hand exercises, they should also begin general flexion muscle-toning programs which can be developed by a physical therapist, or may be available through private "health clubs." In general, patients should receive support to continue with the musical activity. Though some have suggested changing instruments to avoid problems in patients with hypermobility, patients will often respond to maximizing their individual abilities with education, splinting, and exercising rather than pushing for a transfer to a different musical instrument.

Episodes of acute arthritis often respond to nonsteroidal antiinflammatory drugs and splinting as indicated. Since all nonsteroidal antiinflammatory medications may be associated with tinnitus in high dosage, the daily dosage should be decreased to a moderate range when symptoms have improved, and then discontinued altogether in 5 to 7 days. At times, intraarticular steroids are indicated for chronic monarthritis, but only after a complete rheumatologic work-up has been completed.

In the case of students, close communication with teachers is absolutely necessary for proper short-and long-term outcome. Often, a teacher will be able to identify factors precipitating problems in the student who is unaware of the cause-and-effect relationship. In addition, explanation of the disease process to the teacher will increase student compliance and add an ally to the patient's therapeutic regimen. As in other patients with hypermobility, musicians should be screened for other problems, such as mitral valve prolapse, Marfan's syndrome, or Ehlers-Danlos syndrome, and treated accordingly.

OSTEOARTHRITIS

Osteoarthritis is a common rheumatologic condition with varying anatomical and clinical presentations. Prevalence figures are difficult to interpret since various definitions of disease lead to markedly different data. While autopsy studies and roentgenographic changes in individuals may show arthritic changes in up to 25% of individuals by age 30, symptomatic disease is unusual prior to age 35 but increases

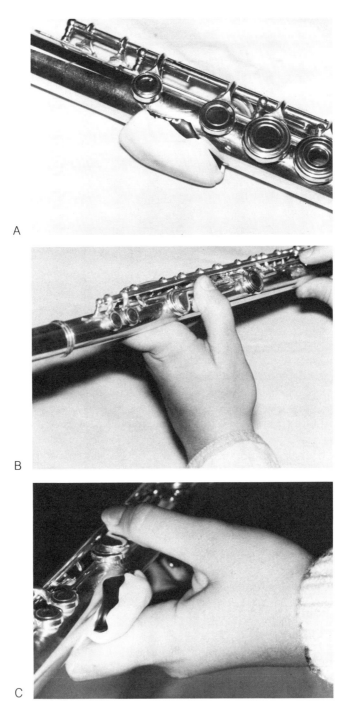

A

B

C

FIG. 3.7. Saddle splint to barrel of flute reducing abnormal MCP extension. (Reproduced with permission from Hanley and Belfus, Inc.)

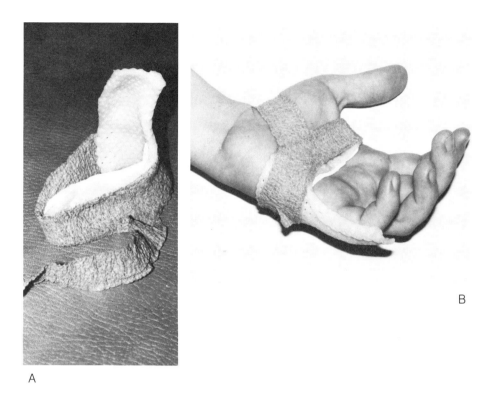

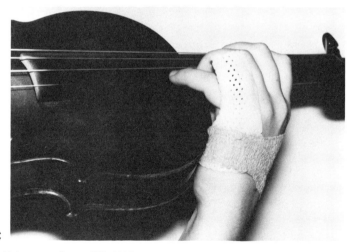

FIG. 3.8. Extensor splint to fifth MCP allowing normal lift and position of fifth digit. (Reproduced with permission from Hanley and Belfus, Inc.)

to 40% of the population by age 80. Osteoarthritis is a disease of cartilage disintegration with a change in balance between cartilage synthesis and degradation toward cartilage destruction. With degradation of cartilage, abnormal stresses are transmitted to the underlying bone; resultant structural changes are identified on x-ray as joint space narrowing, cystic lesions, eburnation, and osteophyte formation.

The pathogenesis of osteoarthritis is multifactorial with the aging process no longer thought to be the most important component. Recent studies comparing the rate of keratin to chondroitin sulfate in cartilage suggest that aging in itself has little to do with the onset of osteoarthritis. Repeated trauma, however, is thought to be a major factor in several anatomical variants of osteoarthritis. Hadler's et al. (57) study of Virginia mill workers suggested that various anatomic patterns of osteoarthritis in hands parallel the repetitive use in the same anatomic distribution. Similarly, repetitive wringing motion may lead to osteoarthritis of the scaphotrapezial joint. Pneumatic drill operators and baseball pitchers show a marked increase in the frequency of osteoarthritis in the shoulders and elbows, ballet dancers may show early destructive osteoarthritis in ankles and toes, and boxers show similar changes in the metacarpophalangeal joints. Whether the playing of musical instruments leads to an increased frequency of osteoarthritis is difficult to determine. Surveys do not seem to show an increased prevalence, though details are lacking and osteoarthritis is often clumped with "arthritis" with little clinical description of signs or symptoms. One case report of a violinist with hypermobility is of interest and would suggest that repetitive motion in some musicians may lead to osteoarthritic changes. The authors described a 68-year-old violinist concert master who had played violin for 50 years (33). For 13 years, she had complained of symptoms of osteoarthritis, and x-ray changes showed progressive disease compatible with the diagnosis. Examination of her hands revealed Heberden's nodes and "typical osteoarthritic deformities." Of particular interest were the x-ray changes showing advanced osteoarthritis of the right carpometacarpal thumb joint, the area most affected by use of the bow, and the left distal interphalangeal joints, the area most often involved in the stress of fingering notes. The left carpometacarpal joint and right distal interphalangeal joint showed little evidence of osteoarthritis. Though osteoarthritis may present in nearly any joint, five anatomic areas most often affect musicians: the distal interphalangeal and proximal phalangeal joints, the carpometacarpal joint of the thumb, the cervical spine, the temporomandibular joint, and the lower back.

Osteoarthritis of the fingers may present in one of two fashions, an acute erosive osteoarthritis most often found in women with a positive family history, or a slow, indolent course leading to Heberden's and Bouchard's nodes. Pain is the usual presenting complaint and is described as dull and aching, exacerbated by use of digits. On occasion, especially in erosive osteoarthritis, the pain may be quite severe. Morning stiffness or stiffness with inactivity improves in 10 to 15 minutes and is rarely disabling. As time passes, osteophytes form around joint spaces and the patient may note a decreased range of motion. Most individuals show little if any loss of function as the osteoarthritic nodules form. Older musicians may show changes of Heberden's and Bouchard's nodes in their fingers, and occasionally they complain of functional problems caused by these changes. The slow progression of disease and minimal symptoms usually allow gradual technique change to accompany the anatomic deviations. Bard's et al. (58) roentgenographic studies of 20 pianists showed x-ray changes of radial rotation of the third, fourth, and fifth metacarpals and rotation of the fifth phalanx in 19 of 20 individuals. Changes were most pronounced in the right hand compared to the left. Osteophyte formation involved the second and third metacarpal joints and fifth distal interphalangeal joints of the right hand with metaphyseal periosteal thickening in 14 of 20 in the metacarpophalangeal region. Only 1 of 20 individuals had symptoms suggestive of osteoarthritis. This survey suggests that though anatomic changes suggestive of arthritis may occur, the functional disability is quite minimal. Recent studies by Harding et al. (15), examining biomechanical tension in joints during piano playing, may allow for the development of prospective studies to examine in detail the relationship between joint stress and osteoarthritis in the distal interphalangeal and proximal interphalangeal joints of musicians.

As opposed to Heberden's and Bouchard's nodes, involvement of the first carpometacarpal joint may be quite disabling for both the general population and musicians. The thumb has three joints: the carpometacarpal, the metacarpophalangeal, and the interphalangeal joint. Though the latter two areas are often spared, the carpometacarpal joint is subject to large compressive forces occurring during the pinch grasp, and long-term problems include osteoarthritis with symptoms leading to hand dysfunction. Morning stiffness, pain with use of the thumb, and localized pain on pressure are characteristic with advanced changes leading to a box deformity of the joint (Fig. 3.9). Minimal trauma can lead to a marked intensification of symptoms

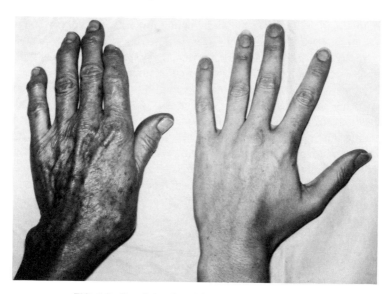

FIG. 3.9. Box deformity of CMC joint in osteoarthritis.

and temporary but nearly complete loss of hand function. Pain and weakness of the thumb are exacerbated by use and relieved by rest, though prolonged periods of nonuse may lead to an increased stiffness in the early "use period." X-rays can be used to stage the disease and help determine the need for medical or surgical therapy. Few musicians fail to recognize the stress placed on their thumbs regardless of their particular instrument. Pianists recognize the discomfort of carpometacarpal osteoarthritis with rapid scale passages as the thumb hooks under the hand advancing up the scale, clarinetists recognize the weight of the barrel of the instrument on the thumb, and string players feel the discomfort in various aspects of the bow arc, especially as the frog approaches the bridge. Though warm-up activities may increase the ease of playing during the first few minutes of a practice session or performance, as playing continues, discomfort may become quite severe, leading to loss of dexterity, facility in rapid passages, and worsening pain to an intensity precluding any further play. The discomfort may be quite severe after playing and lead to difficulty with other day-to-day function, loss of sleep, and more difficulty with the next practice session or scheduled performance.

Treatment for stage I osteoarthritis, where the joint shows less than one-third subluxation and normal articulation contours, consists of use of nonsteroidal antiinflammatory medications, molded splints, and an occupational therapy program aimed at generalized joint protection. Stage II changes will show more than one-third subluxation, and calcific fragments along the joint spaces may be managed in a similar manner. In stage III, joint space narrowing may be associated with early osteophyte formation. Oftentimes, nonsteroidal antiinflammatory drugs will control the majority of symptoms, but minor trauma may lead to severe exacerbations of discomfort, necessitating judicious use of corticosteroid injections, as in the case of a pianist/cellist who exhibited changes of advanced osteoarthritis involving the first carpometacarpal joint (Fig. 3.10). She presented with symptoms compatible with osteoarthritis, which had advanced to the point of interfering with her piano teaching and cello playing. She could not finger rapidly rising scales on the piano, and as the frog approached the bridge while bowing, she experienced marked thumb discomfort. Conservative therapy with low-dose ibuprofen had allowed her to continue to teach and perform, but a recent exacerbation of the disease had led to an inability to complete her piano lessons throughout the day. A single corticosteroid injection into the carpometacarpal joint, use of a thumb splint for nighttime and daytime use when not teaching or performing (Fig. 3.11), and an increment in the dosage of a nonsteroidal antiinflammatory drug markedly relieved her discomfort and allowed her to return to a full teaching and performing schedule. She returned 5 months later with a severe exacerbation of the disease which had occurred after she had lifted a garbage can, which had been too heavy for her. The relatively minor trauma of grasping the garbage can handle had placed undue stress on the carpometacarpal joint and worsened her problem to the point of nearly total loss of hand function. A second corticosteroid injection again markedly relieved her symptoms and allowed her to return to her previous functional status. Patients with severe stage IV disease with pantrapezoarthrosis of the scapulotrapezial joint may be responsive to medical therapy but may ultimately require surgical intervention. Volar ligament reconstruc-

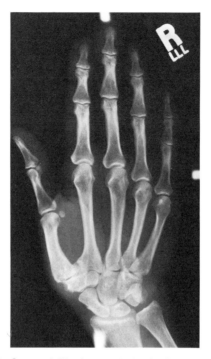

FIG. 3.10. Osteoarthritic changes in the CMC joint of a pianist.

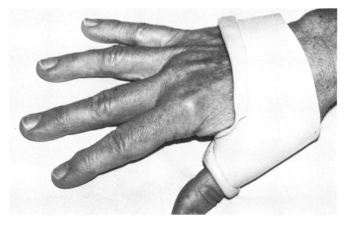

FIG. 3.11. Thumb splint worn to reduce CMC motion when not involved in musical activities.

tion followed by cast immobilization and physical therapy may allow complete return of function for the musician, but such intervention should be performed only by hand surgeons who are familiar with the intricate hand motions of musicians.

Osteoarthritic involvement of the cervical spine may result in discomfort and muscular spasm with disease of the apophyseal joints, cervical nerve root compression by osteophytes growing into the neuroforamina, and rare cord compression from osteophytes growing in a posterior direction.

The etiology of pain in cervical osteoarthritis without neurocompression is a much debated issue. The discomfort may be perceived primarily in the cervical region or may radiate distally to the shoulder or the arm if there is neural irritation. Pain resulting from stimulation of deep nerve endings found in the joints or the outer layers of the longitudinal ligaments produce interscapular pain with occasional aching in the arm or forearm and may be confused with paresthetic discomfort from direct nerve root involvement. In addition, irritation to the innervating nerves of the bone itself may cause discomfort with abnormal motions of distorted bone surfaces. On rare occasions, upper motor neuron and long tract signs may be observed if large posterior spurs compress the spinal cord. Physical examination of the neck reveals decreased range of motion in flexion-extension, lateral rotation, or lateral flexion. In addition, neurologic changes may include diminished reflexes, sensory deficits, or motor weaknesses, depending upon the variable presence of nerve root irritation and/or compression.

Surveys of musicians would suggest that neck discomfort is fairly frequent, with involvement in up to 25% of individuals. Whether the discomfort comes from soft tissue injury, early disc disease or apophyseal osteoarthritis is difficult to determine because few details are available from such studies. Lederman (59) did describe three individuals with cervical radiculopathy, but details concerning these cases are lacking. Treatment of symptomatic osteoarthritis of the cervical spine includes soft collar immobilization and use of analgesics or nonsteroidal antiinflammatory drugs. Problems suggestive of early neurocompression can be managed in a similar manner with a large percentage of patients showing improvement and return to normal function. Cervical collars should be properly fitted and are most effective when used with the neck in 15° flexion. The narrow part of the collar anteriorly facilitates this forward flexion of the cervical spine. On occasion, cervical traction may be indicated, but it should be managed through a knowledgeable physical therapist. If the pain becomes disabling or if muscle weakness occurs, suggesting continued compression of cervical roots, a neurosurgical consultation should be requested.

Neck discomfort seems to affect string players to a greater extent than other musicians. Physical examination of the neck while the musician is playing may reveal abnormal neck postures, inappropriate use of muscles not essential to playing, or an ill-fitting shoulder rest. Each of these factors, though not leading to osteoarthritis, may exacerbate underlying discomfort. In addition, a musician should bring a music stand to the examination so as to determine the posture of the entire spine as it relates to the height of the stand. Correcting simple postural problems will oftentimes relieve musculoskeletal tension across diseased apophyseal joints or discs.

Just as low back pain is a common and potentially serious problem in the general population, lumbago may affect any musician, leading to discomfort while playing. Surveys of musicians would suggest that low back discomfort is not uncommon, especially among cello and bass players. Again, as in the case of cervical discomfort, there is little information in surveys concerning the etiology of back discomfort, be it soft tissue injury, osteoarthritis, or disc disease. As in the case of cervical spine disease, therapy is conservative with use of physical therapy, nonsteroidal antiinflammatory drugs, and neurosurgical consultation if nerve root compression is suggested by the history and physical examination. A full evaluation of the musician's discomfort should include an examination while playing so as to assess the posture of the lower lumbar spine during the standing and sitting positions. The height of the cellist's chair, position of the buttocks over the seat of the chair, and posture of the posterior spine should be carefully evaluated while playing. Modifications of posture should be undertaken with the help of knowledgeable teachers.

In addition to the four anatomic sites mentioned above, musicians may experience osteoarthritic discomfort in the temporomandibular joints. Violinists and violists, woodwind players, and brass instrumentalists may be especially prone to this disorder. Further discussion of this condition is found in Chapter 4.

Other Rheumatologic Conditions

Epidemiologic studies have suggested that up to 10% of individuals in our population may at one time or another be affected by rheumatologic conditions. Common arthritic disorders may often lead to partial disability, loss of normal day-to-day function, and severely impair an individual within the work force. Such disorders spare no particular socioeconomic, racial, or educational group, including musicians. It is not possible to cover the entire scope of rheumatologic conditions as they may affect musicians—instead, we have chosen to briefly review three common disorders often observed in the clinical setting.

Juvenile rheumatoid arthritis is the most common chronic arthritic disorder found in children. Estimates vary as to its prevalence, but between 200,000 and 500,000 children are affected in the United States alone. Children may present with one of three well-described clinical subtypes: pauciarticular arthritis, polyarticular arthritis, or a systemic illness also known as Still's disease. Pauciarticular arthritis most often occurs in the preschool age group, is more common in girls than boys, and often presents with a chronic monarticular arthritis involving the knee, ankle, or wrist. Though pain may be minimal in these children, stiffness and decreased function may lead to day-to-day impairment. Physical findings include synovial hypertrophy, loss of range of motion, and muscular atrophy surrounding the affected joint. Laboratory studies may reveal an elevated antinuclear antibody, elevated sedimentation rate, and x-rays may show periarticular osteoporosis, and periostosis with soft tissue swelling. Most children respond quite well to nonsteroidal antiinflammatory therapy and an occupational therapy–physical therapy program. Children with polyarticular arthritis usually present during elementary school years with

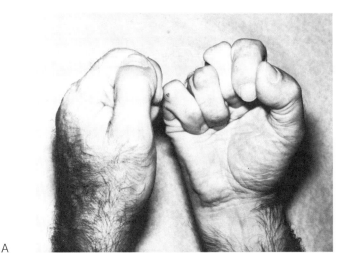

A

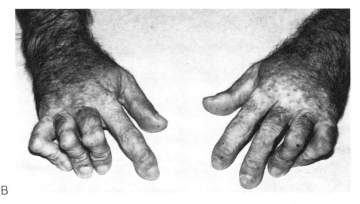

B

FIG. 3.12. Musicians may adapt to chronic arthritic changes.

a symmetrical arthritis involving the distal interphalangeal joints, proximal interphalangeal joints, metacarpophalangeal joints, wrists, elbows, shoulders, cervical
spine, temporomandibular joints, hips, knees, ankles, and toes. Physical examination reveals synovial bogginess of the affected joints, effusions, decreased range of
motion, and pain with motion and localized pressure in the affected areas. Functional impairment is usually more severe than in children with pauciarticular juvenile rheumatoid arthritis, but aggressive occupational therapy and physical therapy
with use of splinting can lead to return of normal function on a day-to-day basis.
Unlike children with monarticular involvement, the older age group may require use
of second-line agents such as gold, hydroxychloroquine, penicillamine, prednisone,
or methotrexate to control their arthritis. Up to 25% of children with polyarticular
juvenile rheumatoid arthritis may suffer severe joint destruction from their disease,
with need for future joint replacement and/or continued adaptive devices throughout

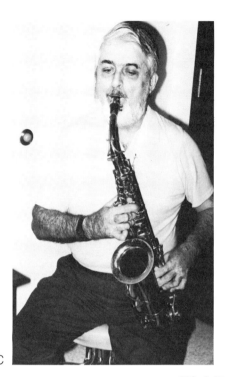
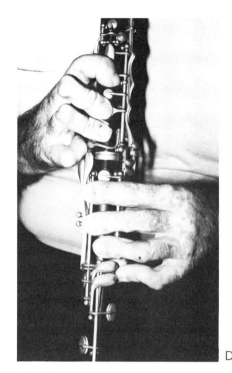

C

D

FIG. 3.12. *Continued.*

life. Children with systemic juvenile rheumatoid arthritis usually show minimal joint involvement unless the disease course changes toward that of polyarticular juvenile rheumatoid arthritis.

An overall treatment goal for all three types of juvenile rheumatoid arthritis is a "mainstreaming" of the child through the developmental years. Children are encouraged to participate in extracurricular activities at school, both in the classroom setting and in physical education classes. If children with juvenile rheumatoid arthritis show interest in musical studies, they should not be discouraged from participating and often can function as well if not better than children with no impairments, as in the case of a 52-year-old white man who developed polyarticular juvenile rheumatoid arthritis at the age of three. His disease course was characterized by severe joint involvement and destruction of the small joints of his hands, wrists, neck, hips, and knees, but a strong desire for a musical career lead to his initial study of the trombone. When severe contractures developed in his elbows and he was unable to extend a trombone slide to its fullest extent, he changed to the clarinet and saxophone in high school and graduated with a major in music from a large state university. Throughout his life, he has continued to have problems with morning discomfort and pain secondary to his polyarthritis but has learned to adapt with his medical therapy, limited to nonsteroidal antiinflammatory drugs. To this day, he continues to perform in two local orchestras on a regular basis (Fig. 3.12).

In a similar manner, rheumatoid arthritis may affect musicians just as it does the general population. Though it may present in several ways, rheumatoid arthritis is most often a slowly progressive disease, characterized by morning stiffness and pain in the metacarpophalangeal, proximal interphalangeal, and wrist joints with additional discomfort in the elbows, knees, ankles, and toes. Though physical findings may be limited to joint tenderness and loss of strength of the intrinsic muscles of the hands early in the course of the disease, as time progresses, polyarthritis reveals itself with joint swelling, synovial hypertrophy, effusions, and rheumatoid nodules in a minority of patients. Laboratory studies include elevated sedimentation rate and positive rheumatoid factor. X-ray changes may show soft tissue swelling, periarticular osteoporosis, joint space narrowing, and erosive disease. Though a diagnosis of rheumatoid arthritis may strike fear in the heart of the musician, just as in the case of children with juvenile rheumatoid arthritis, clinicians must be optimistically supportive and maximize their patient's ability to teach or perform. Education as to the nature of the disease is paramount in early stages since most laypeople have great misconceptions regarding the general long-term outcome of rheumatoid arthritis. Treatment modalities may oftentimes bring about partial or complete remission of disease symptoms, allowing return to nearly normal day-to-day functions. Therapeutic programs designed specifically for musicians include practice sessions or teaching sessions in afternoon and evening hours after "morning stiffness" has lessened. A close working relationship with an occupational therapist may improve hand function through joint protection, education, and use of splints to decrease excessive motion across joints when the musician is not practicing or performing. Medications can be tailored to the stage of the disease and the individual needs of the patient, but must take into account side effects such as tinnitus, drying of the mucosal membranes, or other side effects which may impair music performance. Attitudes toward corticosteroids have varied over the past 30 years, but most recent studies suggest that dosages of 7.5 mg per day of prednisone or less are certainly safe on a short-term basis, and on a long-term basis have markedly fewer side effects compared to dosages in the range of 20 to 30 mg per day. Though nearly all rheumatologists would agree that they would prefer not to use corticosteroids for rheumatoid arthritis, nearly all do so in some patients so as to optimize their day-to-day performance, maximize their work activities, and allow patients to remain gainfully employed. In a similar vein, physicians must realize the importance of teaching and playing as a source of income for musicians, and tailor use of medications to benefit the patient as much as possible.

Over the past 20 years, fibromyalgia syndrome or fibrositis has become recognized as a leading cause of rheumatologic discomfort. Though first described in the 1800s, only recently have diagnostic criteria been proposed and the syndrome accepted as a separate rheumatologic entity. Though no comprehensive epidemiologic studies have been performed, it is estimated that between 3 and 6 million patients in the United States suffer from this condition. The exact etiology and pathophysiology of this syndrome are not well understood; though the condition has also been called fibrositis, there has been no indication of an inflammatory component to the illness. Patients complain of generalized aches and pains about the neck, shoulders, arms, lower back, and upper legs. Although individuals may describe muscle weakness, objective changes on physical examination and laboratory studies reveal no significant muscle disease. Patients may also report a subjective feeling of swelling or tightness in the hands and feet, but physical examination will reveal no changes. In addition, patients may complain of paresthetic-like discomfort or numbness and tingling of the forearms, hands, and lower legs but, again, the neurologic examination is unremarkable. Historical data often includes a disturbed sleep pattern, generalized fatigue, chronic headaches, irritable bowel syndrome, and the only consistent findings on physical examination have been multiple trigger points at characteristic locations (Fig. 3.13). A complete evaluation of the patients suspected of having fibrositis should include a thyroid panel to rule out occult thyroid disorders, and in older patients a sedimentation rate, complete blood count, and rheumatoid factor to rule out early systemic disease. Treatment of fibromyalgia consists of reassurance as to the relatively benign nature of the illness, education about the condition, and instruction in a generalized exercise program to increase cardiovascular reserve and muscle tone. In addition, medications such as amitriptyline and cyclobenzaprine have been shown to decrease symptomatology, perhaps by reversing the α-wave

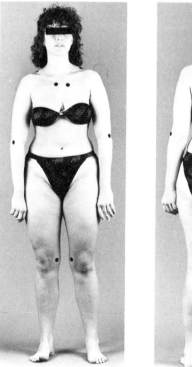 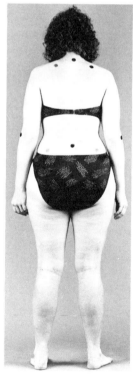

A B

FIG. 3.13. Classic trigger points (filled circles) in fibrositis.

intrusion of Δ-sleep found in studies by Moldofsky et al. (60). Though he and his coworkers were able to induce fibromyalgia symptoms in healthy volunteers through depriving individuals of Δ-sleep, the α-wave intrusion into Δ-sleep is not specific, since it may occur in rheumatoid arthritis, depression, or after trauma such as an automobile accident. Nonsteroidal medication may improve symptomatology but not with the same frequency and dependability as found in inflammatory conditions.

Though there are few, if any, descriptions of fibrositis in performing artists, in light of the frequency of the condition, one would suspect that musicians have problems similar to the remainder of the population. In reviewing the health surveys of professional musicians, though many complained of musculoskeletal discomfort in various anatomic regions, it is not possible to know whether some individuals suffered from fibrositis. Fibrositic trigger points may present as a localized musculoskeletal problem and, unless a careful history and physical examination is performed, a diagnosis may be missed, as in the case of a 46-year-old violinist who presented with shoulder discomfort thought to be bursitis, related to increased playing time in two symphony orchestras. A careful history and physical examination revealed that she had had chronic discomfort in the cervical spine along the upper aspect and midline aspect of her trapezius muscle. In addition, she described generalized aches and pain in the morning when she would rise, feeling as if she had not slept the night through. Physical examination revealed multiple trigger points over the cervical spine, trapezius region, radial heads, and distal and proximal to the knee joint. No evidence for localized soft tissue injury could be found, suggestive of tendinitis or bursitis. Her laboratory studies were unremarkable. She was given a diagnosis of fibromyalgia syndrome, reassured as to the relatively benign nature of her condition and treated with low-dose amitriptyline. She returned three weeks later markedly improved, noting increased ease of playing in both orchestras, but more importantly described an increased sense of well-being throughout the entire day. Though the patient suffered occasional recurrences of fibrositic symptoms over the next two years, low-dose amitriptyline allowed her to function at near maximum potential.

When treating fibromyalgia syndrome, side effects of low-dose tricyclics and cyclobenzaprine must be tailored to the individual and the musical instrument. Whereas a slight dryness to the mouth from a low-dose tricyclic may cause no discomfort in the string player, such a side effect may cause a significant problem for a woodwind or brass instrumentalist. Cyclobenzaprine may also cause dryness of mucosal membranes; in our experience, this side effect has occurred more commonly than with low-dose tricyclics. Studies are in progress at this time to determine the effects of alprazolam and fluoxetine on fibromyalgia. Though no controlled studies have been completed, anecdotal reports would suggest that these medications may be effective in fibromyalgia syndrome. Perhaps, more important than a pharmacologic approach to fibrositis, musicians should be instructed in an exercise program with aerobic conditioning. Such programs must be initiated slowly, increased gradually, and tailored to the musician's teaching, practice, and performance schedule. Exercise programs such as swimming, bicycle riding, or race walking have all been shown to be successful therapeutic regimens. In addition, the education of the musician about the condition will often lead to an acceptance of chronic, mild, low-grade pain.

Although a number of musculoskeletal problems in musicians have been reviewed, it should be emphasized that the majority of injuries, if identified early, can be treated with minimal intervention and excellent results. Those musicians in whom the diagnosis is delayed may take longer to recover, but the prognosis is still quite good. Those with chronic problems such as osteoarthritis, even though they may continue to have minor problems, can anticipate some degree of improvement in their symptoms and continued performing. It is hoped that musicians will be healthier and their careers will be longer as a result of the partnership being formed among musicians, music educators, and health care providers. The ultimate goal of prevention of injuries now seems more likely as a result of this partnership as well.

REFERENCES

1. Fry HJH. Incidence of overuse syndrome in the symphony orchestra. *Med Probl Perform Art* 1986; 1:51–55.
2. Fry HJH. Prevalence of overuse (injury) syndrome in Australian music schools. *Br J Ind Med* 1987; 44:35–40.
3. Caldron PH, Calabrese LH, Clough JD, et al. A survey of musculoskeletal problems encountered in high level musicians. *Med Probl Perform Art* 1986; 1:136–139.
4. Lockwood AH. Medical problems in secondary school–aged musicians. *Med Probl Perform Art* 1988; 3:129–132.
5. Fry HJH. Overuse syndrome of the upper limb in musicians. *Med J Aust* 1986; 144:182–185.
6. Fishbein M, Middlestadt SE, Ottatic V, et al. Medical problems among ICSOM musicians: Overview of a national survey. *Med Probl Perform Art* 1988; 3:1–8.
7. Brandfonbrener AG. The medical problems of musicians. *American Music Teacher* 1988; 37:11–25.
8. Ziporyn T. Pianist's cramp to stage fright: The medical side of music-making. *JAMA* 1984; 252:985–989.
9. Browne CD, Nolan BM, Faithfull DK. Occupational repetition strain injuries: Guidelines for diagnosis and management. *Med J Aust* 1984; 140:329–332.
10. Dawson WJ. Hand and upper extremity problems in musicians: Epidemiology and diagnosis. *Med Probl Perform Art* 1988; 3:19–22.
11. Newmark J, Lederman R. Practice doesn't necessarily make perfect: Incidence of overuse syndromes in amateur instrumentalists. *Med Probl Perform Art* 1987; 2:142–144.
12. Fry HJH. Overuse syndrome in musicians: Prevention and management. *Lancet* 1986; 1:728–731.
13. Spaulding C. Before pathology: Prevention for performing artists. *Med Probl Perform Art* 1988; 3: 135–139.
14. Poore GV. Clinical lecture on certain conditions of the hand and arm which interfere with the performance of professional arts, especially piano playing. *Br Med J* 1897; 1:441–444.
15. Harding DC, Brandt KD, Hillberry BM. Minimization of finger joint forces and tendon tensions in pianists. *Med Probl Perform Art* 1989; 4:103–108.
16. Bejjani FJ, Fenara L, and Pavlidis L. A comparative electromyographic and acoustic analysis of violin vibrato in healthy professional violinists. *Med Probl Perform Art* 1989; 4:168–175.
17. Bejjani FJ, Ferrara L, Xu N, et al. Comparison of three piano techniques as an implementation of a proposed experimental design. *Med Probl Perform Art* 1989; 4:109–113.
18. Salmon P, Newmark J. Clinical applications of MIDI technology. *Med Probl Perform Art* 1989; 4:25–31.

19. Hochberg FH, Lavin P, Portney R, et al. Topical therapy of localized inflammation in musicians: A clinical evaluation of Aspercreme versus placebo. *Med Probl Perform Art* 1988; 3:9–14.
20. Goodman G, Staz S. Occupational therapy for musicians with upper extremity overuse syndrome: Patient perceptions regarding effectiveness of treatment. *Med Probl Perform Art* 1989; 4.9–14.
21. Levine WR, Irvine JK. In vivo EMG biofeedback in violin and viola pedagogy. *Biofeedback Self Regulation* 1984; 9:161–165.
22. Spire M. The Feldenkrais method: An interview with Anat Baniel. *Med Probl Perform Art* 1989; 4:159–162.
23. Rosenthal E. The Alexander technique—What it is and how it works. *Med Probl Perform Art* 1987; 2:53–57.
24. Lederman RJ, Calabrese LH. Overuse syndromes in instrumentalists. *Med Probl Perform Art* 1986; 1:7–11.
25. Hoppmann RA, Patrone NA. A review of musculoskeletal problems in instrumental musicians. *Seminars Arth Rheum* 1989; 19:117–126.
26. Fry HJH. Physical signs in the hand and wrist in the overuse (injury) syndrome. *Aust NZ J Surg* 1986; 56:47–49.
27. Fry HJH. Overuse syndrome—alias tenosynovitis—tendinitis—the terminological hoax. *Plast Reconstr Surg* 1986; 78:414–417.
28. Fry HJH. Overuse syndrome in musicians. *Med J Aust* 1987; 146:390.
29. Lederman RJ. Overuse syndrome in musicians. *Med J Aust* 1987; 146:390.
30. Dennett X and Fry HJH. Overuse syndrome: A muscle biopsy study. *Lancet* 1988; i:905–908.
31. Huddelston CB, Pratt SM. Cymbal-player's shoulder. Letter *N Engl J Med* 1983; 309 (23):1462.
32. Nolan WB, Eaton RG. Thumb problems of professional musicians. *Med Probl Perform Art* 1989; 4:20–24.
33. Beighton P, Grahame R, Bird H. *Hypermobility of joints*. Springer-Verlag, Berlin, Heidelberg, New York, 1983.
34. Finkelstein H. Joint hyponatremia. *NY Med J* 1916; 104:942–943.
35. Key JA. Hypermobility of joints as a sex linked hereditary characteristic. *JAMA* 1927; 88:1710–1712.
36. Sutro J. Hypermobility of knees due to over lengthened capsular and ligamentous tissues. *Surgery* 1947; 21:67–76.
37. Kirk J, Ansell B, and Bywaters E. The hypermobility syndrome. *Ann Rheum Dis* 1967; 26:419–425.
38. Carter C, Wilkinson J. Persistent joint laxity and congenital dislocation of the hip. *J Bone Joint Surg* 1964; 46B:40–45.
39. Arroyo I, Brewer E and Giannini E. Arthritis/arthralgia and hypermobility of joints in school children. *J Rheum* 1988; 15:978–980.
40. Biro F, Gewanter H, and Baum J. The hypermobility syndrome. *Pediatrics* 1983; 72:701.
41. Larsson L-G, Baum J, Mudholkar GS. Hypermobility: Features and differential incidence between the sexes. *Arthritis Rheum* 1987; 30:1426–1430.
42. Bejjani FJ, Stuchin S, Winchester R. Effect of joint laxity on musician's occupational disorders. *Clin Research* 1984; 32:660A.
43. Graham R and Jenkins J. Joint hypermobility—Asset or liability. *Ann Rheum Dis* 1972; 31:109–111.
44. Nicholas J. Injuries to knee ligaments. *JAMA* 1970; 212:2236–2239.
45. Klemp P, Stevens J, and Isaacs S. A hypermobility study in ballet dancers. *J Rheum* 1984; 11:692–696.
46. Brandfonbrener A. Personal communication.
47. Beighton P, Solomon L, Soskolne C. Articular mobility in an African population. *Ann Rheum Dis* 1973; 32:413–418.
48. Silman A, Haskard D, Day S. Distribution of joint mobility in a normal population: Results of the use of fixed torque measuring devices. *Ann Rheum Dis* 1986; 45:27–30.
49. Silverman S, Constine L, Harvey W and Grahame R. Survey of joint mobility and *in vivo* skin elasticity in London school children. *Ann Rheum Dis* 1975; 34:177–180.
50. Shah J, Jayson M, and Hanson N. Low tension studies of collagen fibres from ligaments of the human spine. *Ann Rheum Dis* 1977; 36:139–145.
51. Handler C, Child A, Light N. Mitral valve prolapse, aortic compliance and skin collagen in joint hypermobility syndrome. *Br Heart J* 1985; 54:501–508.

52. Bird HA, Wright V. Traumatic synovitis in a classical guitarist: A study of joint laxity. *Ann Rheum Dis* 1981; 40:161–163.
53. Wilson J. A dental appliance for a clarinetist experiencing temporomandibular joint pain. *Med Probl Perform Art* 1989; 4:118–121.
54. Patrone N, Hoppmann R, Whaley J and Schmidt R. Digital nerve compression in a violinist with benign hypermobility. *Med Probl Perform Art* 1989; 4:91–94.
55. Patrone NA, Hoppmann RA, Whaley J, et al. Benign hypermobility in a flutist. *Med Probl Perform Art* 1988; 3:158–161.
56. Scott D, Bird H, and Wright V. Joint laxity leading to osteoarthritis. *Rheum Rehab* 1979; 18:167–169.
57. Hadler N, Gillings D, Imbus H et al. Hand structure and function in the industrial setting. *Arthritis Rheum* 1978; 21:210–220.
58. Bard CC, Sylvestre JJ, Dussault RG. Hand osteoarthropathy in pianists. *J Can Assoc Radiol* 1984; 35:154–158.
59. Lederman R. Nerve entrapment syndrome in instrumentalist musicians. *Med Probl Perform Art* 1986; 1:45–48.
60. Moldofsky H, Scarisbrick P, England B et al. Musculoskeletal symptoms in non-REM sleep disturbances in patients with "fibrositis syndrome" and healthy subjects. *Psychosom Med* 1975; 37:341–351.

Textbook of Performing Arts Medicine, edited by R. T. Sataloff, A. Brandfonbrener, and R. Lederman. Raven Press, Ltd., New York © 1991.

4

Temporomandibular Joint Disorders, Facial Pain, and Dental Problems in Performing Artists

James A. Howard

Department of Orthodontics, University of Washington, Dental Division, Children's Hospital, Seattle, Washington 98105

An evolutionary transgressor strategically suspended in limbo between medicine and dentistry, the temporomandibular joint (TMJ) is often misaligned by nature, misused by man, maligned by the medical profession, and misunderstood by most. This paired joint, perhaps the synovial magna cum laude, has not yet joined the other articulations in orthopedics, and has been turned a deaf ear by otolaryngology and neglected by neurology.

The oral cavity serves as the junction of creativity for speech, poetry and song. The jaws serve as the scaffolding upon which the wind instrumentalists support the tools of their careers, vocalists extend to their fullest limit, and violinists thrust into their performance. Man's outlet for emotions expressed both verbally and nonverbally, the jaw is set in determination, grimaces in pain, and gnashes in anger. For any performing artist voicing a complaint of headache or facial pain, the orofacial structures and the function of the temporomandibular joints should be evaluated.

Masquerading as multiple other medical maladies, temporomandibular joint disorders (TMD) are increasingly invoked as the diagnosis for a variety of symptoms including headache, facial pain, neck pain, and otologic complaints. In 1934, Costen (1) described a syndrome of dizziness, tinnitus, earache, stuffiness of the ear, dry mouth, burning in the tongue and throat, sinus pain, and headache. He attributed this myriad of symptoms to overclosure of the bite resulting in direct compression of the chorda tympani and auriculotemporal nerves by posterior displacement of the mandibular condyle. Subsequent anatomic dissections (2) disproved Costen's theory of pressure on the nerves by the mandibular condyle. However, the medical profession continued to assign the diagnosis of Costen's syndrome, based upon the erroneous belief that overclosure of the bite caused the symptoms, for over forty years. Some dentists still provide a variety of bite-raising dental procedures for symptoms thought to be related to condylar malposition.

When a performing artist presents with facial pain that could be related to a TMJ disorder, the clinician is often unfamiliar with the examination procedure for TMJ problems and is confused by the numerous and conflicting concepts of etiology. Because of the clinician's diagnostic uncertainty, TMD patients are sometimes subjected to costly and unnecessary diagnostic procedures such as electromyographic evaluation, mandibular movement studies, and sophisticated imaging studies. While these techniques have limited application for complex TMJ problems, their routine use cannot be justified (3,4). If the diagnosis of TMD is established, the clinician may be reluctant to recommend therapy since clear criteria have not been established for selection of the diverse treatments advocated for TMJ dysfunction (5). A study of 145 TMD patients randomly referred to two clinics revealed that despite the markedly different diagnostic and treatment methods employed, there were no important differences in treatment outcomes at 1-year follow-up (6). This variability in clinical methods for treating TMD, especially the use of irreversible and surgical therapies, is not a benign phenomenon. The search for a cure for TMD can be an expensive and risky undertaking that often results in more harm than benefit. Iatrogenic adventurism can interrupt the performing artist's career, especially if the clinician does not understand the significant impact that TMJ problems can have on vocalists, wind musicians, violinists, and violists.

EPIDEMIOLOGY

A study of Group Health Cooperative (GHC) patients, a Seattle-based health maintenance organization of over 360,000 enrollees, revealed that the mean age of 3,428 patients referred for evaluation of TMJ related disorders was 33.8 years for females and 34.2 years for males. Of those seeking treatment, 85% were female (Fig. 4.1). Patients under the age of 15 years accounted for 4.3% of the referrals. Those 15 to 29 years old accounted for 38% and those between 30 and 44 years old accounted for 38.8% of the referrals. Only 12.3% were between 45 and 59 years old, and only 6% were 60 years of age or older. Approximately 2 out of every 1,000 Group Health enrollees (0.2%) are referred each year by their primary care physician for evaluation of TMD.

TMJ EMBRYOLOGY

In the evolution from reptiles to mammals the reptilian jaw joint, the articular-quadrate joint, migrates posteriorly and evolves into the mammalian middle ear ossicles, the malleus and incus. In the human embryo the mandibular condyle and adjacent temporal bone develop between the seventh and thirteenth weeks. As these

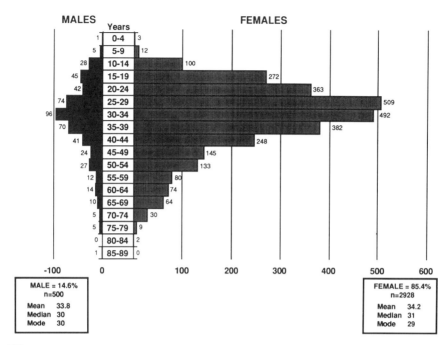

FIG. 4.1. Age and sex distribution of 3,428 TMD patients presenting with temporomandibular joint disorders.

structures approximate, rhythmic movement of the mandible results in clefts of the adjacent mesenchyme that develop into superior and inferior joint cavities (7). Closely related trigeminal motor pathways with interconnected synaptic patterns are established in the brainstem at an early period in development, with the jaw joint and ear ossicles moving in synchrony during eleven weeks of prenatal life (8). The articular disc develops from a mesenchymal layer and from the tendon of the lateral pterygoid muscle that passes through the Glaserian fissure to attach to the malleus (9). The disc maintains this attachment to the malleus until fetal joint development is completed. A persistent connection between the posterior aspect of the TMJ capsule and the malleus is found in some adult TMJ cadaver specimens. This remnant of the lateral pterygoid tendon, extending through the lateral aspect of the petrotympanic fissure, is known as the discomallear ligament (10). Using a dissecting microscope, a distinct discomallear ligament was found in 15 of 52 adult cadavers. However, when tension was applied to the ligament, there was no movement of the malleus in any specimen (11).

The trigeminal nerve innervates the TMJ, the muscles of mastication, as well as the tensor tympani (TT) and the tensor veli palatini (TVP) muscles. The TT arises from the cartilaginous portion of the eustachian tube (ET) and inserts onto the malleus. Both the tension on the tympanic membrane (TM), through the attachment of the TT to the neck of the malleus, and the maintenance of equalized air pressure on the TM, by the action of the TVP on the ET, are controlled by the motor root of the trigeminal nerve, a nerve that subserves mastication.

It has been suggested that the ET can be opened by protrusion of the lower jaw or through contraction of the pterygoid muscles. Anatomically, the levator veli palatini and medial pterygoid muscles both appear to have the potential to constrict the ET (12). However, Rich (13) demonstrated in dogs that neither changes in jaw position nor contraction of the medial pterygoid muscle have any effect upon the ET. The TVP is the only muscle that can actively dilate the lumen of the ET. The TVP arises from the sphenoid bone and wall of the ET, and inserts onto the aponeurosis of the soft palate. Casselbrant et al. (14) injected botulinum into the TVP of eight rhesus monkeys and observed a resultant lack of constriction as well as a lack of normal dilatation of the ET. The authors concluded that both constrictions and dilatations of the ET are caused by the activity of a single paratubal muscle, the TVP. The embryologic relationships and the common innervation by the trigeminal nerve help explain the frequent and varied otologic complaints reported in association with TMD. The concurrence of TMD and ET dysfunction can have special significance to those performing artists whose skills are intimately related to the perception of tone, since hearing may be impaired when pressure equilibrium is not established through the ET.

TMJ ANATOMY

The TMJ is enveloped by a well-innervated and vascularized fibrous capsule that blends with the periosteum on the neck of the condyle except on the anterior boundary, where the capsule blends with the attachment of the lateral pterygoid muscle. The capsule plays an important role in mandibular proprioception, with the anterior capsule innervated by the masseteric nerve and the posterolateral aspect by the auriculotemporal nerve, both branches of the mandibular division of the trigeminal nerve. During function, the medial aspect of the capsule is not under a strain and is neither strong nor thick. Laterally the capsule is very dense and is reinforced by the lateral ligament, a fibrous thickening attached to the zygomatic process of the temporal bone and to the condylar neck. The lateral ligament stabilizes the TMJ during translatory or sliding movements and becomes taut upon wide opening, preventing condylar dislocation.

The blood supply of the TMJ is derived primarily from branches of the internal maxillary, transverse facial, and superficial temporal arteries (15). The vascular supply to the lateral pterygoid muscle also supplies the anterior aspect of the joint. The load-bearing surfaces of the joint are avascular, while the non-load-bearing posterior attachment and medial capsular wall are highly vascularized. Because of its unique embryologic origin, the articular surfaces of the TMJ are covered by fibrous connective tissue and lack the hyaline articular cartilage typical of other synovial joints. The synovial membrane extends just to the margins of the stress-bearing joint surfaces. The synovial fluid provides lubrication, nutrition, and immunological capacity, and the fluid contains macrophages capable of removing tissue debris caused by the normal wear of articular surfaces.

During fetal life the entire disc is vascularized, but the central portion becomes avascular because of its compression between the condyle and the articular tubercle. The biconcave shape of the disc is determined by functional requirements, with the steepness of the eminence, the depth of the glenoid fossa, and the morphology of the condyle all influencing disc shape. The periphery of the disc remains vascular and innervated, and this less dense tissue merges with the surrounding capsule to sub-divide this synovial joint into non-communicating superior and inferior bursal spaces.

TMJ BIOMECHANICS

The interposed disc functions as a shock absorber and serves as a congruous surface between the incongruous condyle and articular tubercle. The complex hinge and sliding movements of the compound TMJ are facilitated by the independent rotation and translation of the disc over the condylar head. This shifting position of the disc is necessary to maintain contact between the articular components during chewing.

When the mouth is opened, the condylar head initially rotates around the inferior surface of the stationary disc. As the degree of opening increases, the disc rotates posteriorly about the condyle, and the disc-condyle complex translates forward and downward, guided by contact of the upper surface of the disc against the inclined articular tubercle. With wide opening, the condyle and disc translate smoothly together to the edge of or beyond the articular tubercle (Fig. 4.2) (16).

Mandibular opening occurs as the result of contraction of the suprahyoid, digastric, and lateral pterygoid muscles. The lateral pterygoid is also active in protrusive movements (17) and is subject to fatigue from the repetitive or prolonged protrusion of the mandible required when playing certain wind instruments. The paired temporalis, medial pterygoid and masseter muscles are the primary jaw closers. The superior head of the lateral pterygoid stablizes the joint during closure by varying the disc position to provide a moving wedge that maintains near continuous contact between the disc-condyle complex and the articular tubercle.

An internal derangement is any intracapsular mechanical alteration that interferes with the smooth action of a joint. In the early stage of a TMJ internal derangement, there is usually a normal mandibular range of motion (ROM) with deviation and clicking. The disc displaces anteromedially toward the pterygoid plates, the origin of the lateral pterygoid muscle. Upon opening, the condyle travels over the posterior band of the disc, and the clicking sound occurs as the condyle impacts against the temporal bone through the thin central portion of the disc (Fig. 4.3). Partial disc

NORMAL

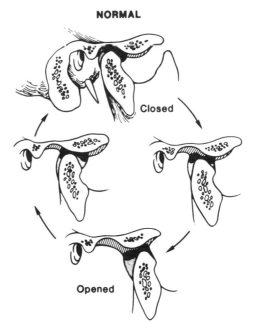

FIG. 4.2. Normal relationship of the disc and condyle during the mouth opening and closing cycle. Translation of the disc and condyle beyond the height of the tubercle is a normal finding.

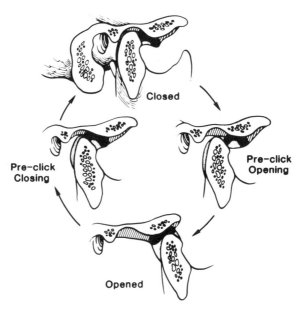

FIG. 4.3. Anteromedial disc displacement with reduction upon opening. The click occurs from the impact of the condyle against the articular tubercle through the thin central portion of the disc.

displacement occasionally occurs, with the lateral aspect of the disc displaced an- terolaterally. Posterior disc displacements are uncommon and initially result in the inability to bring the teeth into full contact on the affected side.

The displacement of the disc is accompanied by elongation or stretching of the disc attachments to the capsule. Degeneration and deformation of the disc often precede displacement, and the roughened articular surfaces alter the smooth gliding movements of the joint. The resulting hesitation and catching places additional strain on the disc attachments and can lead to disc displacement. During the initial stage of an internal derangement, the TMJ will usually click consistently on open- ing, closing, and in translation. Following displacement, continued deformation of the disc can change the character, position, and intensity of joint sounds. If the posterior band of the displaced disc becomes thinner over time, the clicking could resolve. However, if the posterior band becomes thicker, and if the attachments of the disc become further stretched, episodes of catching and locking can occur. If there is progressive thinning of the posterior attachment, crepitus is usually de- tected. If the disc bunches up in front of the condyle (Fig 4.4), the condylar transla- tion and mandibular ROM will be limited. With progression to a nonreducing disc there is often an increase in joint pain because of the additional strain placed on the highly vascularized and innervated retrodiscal tissue. The impact of joint motion

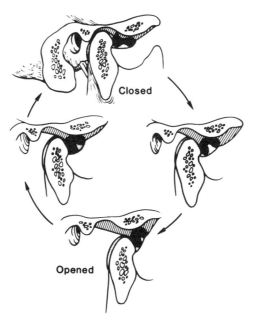

FIG. 4.4. Anteromedial disc displacement without reduction. The condyle engages the poste- rior aspect of the disc upon opening, folding the disc and blocking the translation of the con- dyle.

will no longer be evenly distributed over the articular surfaces and can result in a perforation, increasing the likelihood of osteoarthrosis. Nonreducing displacements are often accompanied by alterations in condylar morphology and position and can result in discernible changes in the bite.

In the hypermobile joint with capsular laxity the joint noise occurs from incoordinated movement of the condyle and disc as they translate over the height of the tubercle. In some instances the condyle travels onto or beyond the anterior band of the disc (Fig. 4.5). This can result in episodes of painful locking in an open position. The range of motion typically exceeds 55 mm, and the opening click usually occurs at greater than 30 mm of opening. The closing click is often louder and more painful than the opening click.

HISTORY OF THE CHIEF COMPLAINT

For many individuals, TMJ disorders are recurrent but self-limiting. Approximately 5% of the population seeks treatment for painful TMJ conditions at some time (18). The preponderance of young females and the relationship this might have to psychosocial stressors should not be overlooked when evaluating TMD patients. The ratio of females to males with signs of TMD in the general population is 1.8:1,

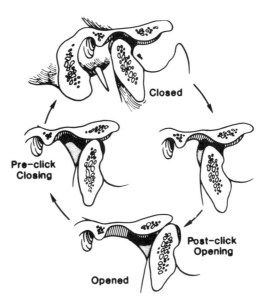

FIG. 4.5. Condylar hypermobility asociated with joint laxity. Clicking occurs with wide opening as the condyle translates beyond the height of the tubercle and travels onto or beyond the anterior band of the disc. A closing click can also occur as the disc re-centers over the condyle during mouth closure.

yet the ratio of females to males seeking treatment for these disorders is 7:1. A variety of explanations have been offered, the most common being that in response to stress, females are more likely to exhibit musculoskeletal pain, particularly in the head and neck region, whereas men are more likely to be cardiovascular responders. Stress is undeniably one of the primary factors in the timing of patients seeking treatment for facial pain. This observation is consistent with the high prevalence of TMD in the second and third decades of life, a period of significant psychosocial stressors.

An age-stratified sample of 1,265 enrollees of GHC between 18 and 75 years of age received a survey questionnaire on 5 common pain conditions: back pain, headache, abdominal pain, chest pain, and TMD pain. The screening questionnaire included identical batteries of items for each pain condition. The severity and duration of the pain were assessed as well as the degree of psychological distress, as measured by the depression, anxiety, and somatization scales of the symptom checklist 90 (SCL 90-R). Of the 1,016 respondents to the survey (80.3% response rate), 123 cases had experienced TMD pain during the previous 6 months, a prevalence of 12.1%. TMD-related pain was reported with about the same prevalence as chest pain (12%), but was less common than abdominal pain (17%), headache (26%), and back pain (41%) (19).

The 123 community cases with TMD plus 246 randomly-selected community controls who did not report TMD pain were interviewed and examined for TMD problems. These data were compared with the records of 261 consecutive patients seeking treatment for TMD. Subjects from all three groups completed identical questionnaires and received the same interview and clinical examination. While referred to as temporomandibular joint disorders, the majority of TMD patients report both muscular and articular involvement. Pain in response to palpation of the masseter muscle was reported by 58% of the TMD patients, as compared to only 14% of the community controls. Anterior temporalis pain in response to palpation was reported by 32% of the clinic cases but by only 6% of the controls. Pain in response to palpation of the lateral aspect of the TMJ was reported by 57% of the clinic cases but by only 10% of the controls. TMJ noises were detected in 57% of those seeking treatment versus 36% of the controls. However, joint noise is seldom the chief complaint, with 97% of the clinic cases seeking treatment for pain and only 3% for noise or other problems as the chief complaint. Grating sounds, suggestive of osteoarthrosis, were detected in 7% of the clinic cases but in less than 1% of the controls. There was an average of 5.2 mm reduced maximum passive mouth opening for clinic cases as compared to controls, or about a 10% reduction in mandibular range of motion (ROM) (20).

A history of clicking sounds was reported by 39% of male and 49% of female college students responding to a questionnaire. Episodes of locking had been experienced by 7% of males and 13% of females, but only 4% of males and 7% of females reported impaired function associated with the clicking. Fatigue of the jaw muscles was reported by 15% of males and 25% of females (21).

The masticatory system is adaptive and TMJ internal derangements can be, but are not necessarily progressive. Some patients will remain indefinitely in an early, nonpainful stage of clicking. Others will have short duration in an early stage with rapid transition into a more dysfunctional and painful stage, including catching and locking. Muscle splinting often occurs to protect the painful or deranged TMJ with resulting masticatory myalgia and temporal headaches. When the disc becomes displaced, the posterior attachment of the disc often undergoes metaplastic conversion from a vascular, loose connective tissue to a dense, avascular fibrous cushion that resembles the disc proper. Most TMD patients who progress to a nonreducing disc displacement and limited ROM will, with or without treatment, have gradual return to near normal opening with pain free function. Crepitus or grating sounds can develop and are usually a sign of osteoarthrosis. Rasmussen (22) followed 119 patients with advanced TMJ arthropathy (more than half of whom received no treatment), and nearly all had returned to pain-free function within three years. Displacement of the disc was found at autopsy in 64% of randomly-selected specimens from elderly individuals. In most cases osteoarthrosis was seen in association with disc displacement (23), suggesting that these findings may represent the natural aging process for the TMJ. Many individuals advance through all of the stages of internal derangement and develop osteoarthrosis, yet never experience any TMJ pain.

TMJ CLINICAL SCREENING EXAMINATION

A screening examination for facial pain and TMJ disorders requires only a few minutes. The range of mandibular motion, joint noise, and the response to muscle and joint palpation are evaluated. An intraoral examination, a routine head and neck examination, and a cranial nerve examination should all be completed. An excellent guideline for the examination and diagnosis of TMD has been presented by Clark et al. (24).

Range of Motion

The normal range of mouth opening was measured for 1,160 individuals between 18 and 70 years of age with no history of TMJ involvement. The mean mandibular opening, as measured between the incisal edges with no compensation for dental overbite, was 52.85 mm (SD 7.41 mm) for the 500 men and 48.34 mm (SD 5.64 mm) for the 660 women (25). For both sexes the mean opening diminished slightly with age. The ability to place three fingers in a handshake position vertically between the incisor teeth, the "three-finger test," usually indicates a normal range of mandibular opening of 40 mm to 50 mm. Thus, the clinician's first three fingers can be used clinically to verify a normal ROM. If it is not possible to get even two fingers between the patient's incisal edges, then the reason for the limited opening should be investigated. If four fingers fit between the patient's incisal edges, then there could be capsular laxity and hypermobility. Mandibular movement to each side is normally 8 mm to 12 mm. The width of a maxillary central incisor is 8 mm to 9 mm, so if the patient can move the lower jaw sideways the width of the upper central incisor, this should be considered normal. Any mandibular deviation, catching, locking, or pain associated with these ROM measurements should be noted.

Provocation of TMJ Pain

The lateral aspect of the capsule is examined bilaterally by having the patient open halfway and placing the clinician's index fingers firmly in the depressions created behind each condyle, just in front of the tragus of either ear. The patient is instructed to open and close their mouth slowly, and the presence of discomfort is noted. TMJ palpation not only reveals the level of discomfort, but also allows the clinician to feel asynchronous movements and clicking or crepitation. A functional test for TMJ discomfort is to place a folded-over cotton roll or gauze between the second molars on one side and have the patient repeatedly bite up and down. This squeezing action will torque the joint on the opposite side and can cause the clicking and joint or muscle pain experienced by the patient when eating.

DIFFERENTIATION OF TMJ SOUNDS

Temporomandibular joint noises are categorized as either clicking (including popping and snapping), soft-tissue crepitus, or hard-tissue grating. The irregularities in movement that accompany these sounds can be felt by placing a finger over the lateral aspect of the joint. The use of a stethoscope applied lightly over the joint is helpful in categorizing the nature and severity of the sounds. If the clinician is having difficulty detecting the TMJ sounds reported by the patient, applying upward pressure at the angle of the mandible will usually increase the intensity of the sound. The most common cause of TMJ noise is internal derangements; but altered synovial lubrication, deviations in shape of the disc, condyle, or tubercle, and incoordination between the disc and condyle during movement can all cause TMJ sounds. Not all TMJ internal derangements are progressive and clicking need not change in character over time and can actually diminish. However, the lack of joint sounds does not always equate with the absence of pathology. When a displaced disc becomes nonreducing, also known as a mandibular closed lock, there is usually a concurrent limited ROM, joint pain, deviation to the affected side, and a cessation of joint sounds, because the condyle no longer translates onto the displaced disc.

Provocation of Muscle Pain

The muscles most consistently tender and easiest to palpate in association with TMD are the temporalis and the masseter. Firm bilateral finger pressure should be applied over these muscles as the patient's teeth are clenched. Note the degree of discomfort and whether the pain is unilateral or bilateral. There can be referral patterns to other structures in the head, including the teeth, eyes, sinuses, and ears. Masseter muscle hypertrophy is often present in cases of chronic bruxism.

Palpation of the cervical musculature should also be part of this examination as mandibular posture is closely related to cervical posture. The masticatory muscles and the suprahyoid muscles, also known as the accessory muscles of mastication, constantly readjust the position of the mandible and work in conjunction with the cervical musculature to stabilize head posture and maintain the airway. The degree of cervical discomfort often correlates with stress levels and unfavorable occupational postures, especially common in musicians. Identifying and altering those factors that perpetuate myofascial pain are critical in the management of chronic head and neck pain (26).

Intraoral Examination

A quick scan of the dentition will reveal obvious sources of dental pain. The absence of posterior teeth or presence of ill-fitting dentures can trigger jaw muscle fatigue and compromise a wind musician's performance. The functional relationship of the teeth and the presence of significant mandibular dental or skeletal malocclusion should be noted. Tooth abrasion can help identify a teeth-grinding habit, and pronounced ridging of the cheeks can be a sign of teeth clenching. The health of the oral mucosa, the appearance of the tongue, and alteration of salivary flow can be clues of systemic diseases. The salivary glands should be examined for enlargement or tenderness, and the nasopharynx should be inspected for deviation or mass.

Head and Neck Evaluation

Presence or absence of tender lymph nodes, skin changes, swellings, masses, and other deviations from the norm should be noted. Facial asymmetry and chin scars can be evidence of a traumatic etiology of a TMJ problem and should be discussed with the patient. The thyroid gland should be carefully palpated. Gentle compression of the facial and temporal arteries when considering giant cell arteritis (GCA), and of the carotid arteries to evaluate for carotodynia, can be revealing for some patients. A cranial nerve examination should be completed and an otoscope should be used to rule out obvious otologic problems. Appropriate hearing tests should be requested if recent hearing loss is suspected. A neurologic consultation is indicated if there are cranial nerve sensory deficits, muscle weakness, or areas of unexplained facial numbness or paresthesia.

Imaging

Much of the confusion about the diagnosis of TMD stems from the reality that these disorders have multiple etiologies, and the signs and symptoms are variable in their expression. In an attempt to overcome this diagnostic uncertainty, the clinician often resorts to other "diagnostic methods" such as joint imaging. Relying on imaging to decrease diagnostic uncertainty or establish an etiology for TMD is fallacious in many instances. Imaging studies are often superfluous and seldom provide additional information about TMD etiology. A screening panoramic or circular tomogram is often adequate for TMJ evaluation. Axially corrected tomography is the most commonly used technique when a panoramic film is unavailable or is not adequate. The combination of lateral and frontal thin-section tomography provides excellent visualization of bony defects, can be used to locate mandibular fractures, and can establish the condylar position in the fossa. Tomography is indicated when there is a history of recent mandibular trauma, if the patient has painful episodes of locking, or if advanced degenerative joint disease is suspected (4).

Computerized tomography (CT) is superior to any other technique for the detection of maxillofacial bony fractures (27) and should be requested when there is a clinical suspicion of a fracture or tumor. The shape and position of the disc are not accurately portrayed because of soft tissue inhomogeneities, and CT is not recommended for the evaluation of TMJ internal derangements.

Arthrography has rapidly advanced the understanding of TMJ internal derangements because of the ability to visualize the location and morphology of the disc as well as its dynamic relationship with the condyle and articular tubercule during mandibular movements. While this information can be useful, this imaging method is typically reserved for use as a presurgical diagnostic aid. At present, because of the ability to visualize perforations and adhesions, arthrography is superior to magnetic resonance imaging (MRI) and, when combined with videofluoroscopy, arthrography is the only technique permitting dynamic evaluation of TMJ function. This relatively inexpensive technique is invasive, but the diagnostic yield is high and the morbidity is minimal when performed by a technically competent clinician (28).

MRI will in the future play an important role in TMJ diagnosis when the scan time and expense are reduced and the reliability and accuracy improve. New dynamic MRI techniques to illustrate joint movement also show promise. MRI is strongly recommended for the assessment of trigeminal neuropathy because the clinical presentation of symptoms is inaccurate for lesion localization, and MRI, especially with contrast enhancement, is superior to CT in displaying the extent of trigeminal tumors and their relationships to other cranial structures (29).

Scintigraphy is a very sensitive technique for detecting inflammation or change within the joint but is nonspecific and plays no practical role in the diagnosis or management of TMJ disorders, other than for assessment of suspected condylar or mandibular hyperplasia in nongrowing individuals.

Electronic thermography to assess thermal asymmetry in the orofacial region is a very technique-sensitive method that requires additional research prior to its acceptance for nonresearch clinical application in the diagnosis of facial pain, TMD, headache, and atypical odontalgia (30,31).

Historically, sialography has been the most widely used diagnostic method for salivary gland disorders. Sialography is primarily indicated for nonneoplastic conditions such as Sjögren's syndrome or granulomatous disease in which the bilateral inflammation results in alteration of the ductile system. It is unsatisfactory for tumor diagnosis because lesions less than 1 cm are usually not detected and space-occupying lesions are only indirectly visualized when they displace or disrupt the ductile system (32). Differentiating between an intrinsic or extrinsic location and predicting the benign or malignant nature of tumors are more accurately accomplished with CT and MRI. The radiosensitivity of the parotid gland is added justification for the use of MRI over CT.

Electronic Diagnostic Devices

There has been an increasing tendency by dentists to rely on technological devices for the diagnosis and treatment of TMD, despite the lack of scientific evidence to support their use. The questionable clinical relevance of, and the associated fees for, these "diagnostic tests" has engendered considerable controversy in the dental profession (5). A thorough review of the literature relating to adjunctive diagnostic tests and treatment devices for TMD, including electromyography, electrical stimulation devices, mandibular tracking devices, and sonography for the evaluation of joint sounds, has been presented by Widmer et al. (3). The authors concluded that at present there is not sufficient evidence to support routine use of any of these electronic devices for diagnosis and treatment of temporomandibular joint disorders. This excellent review is recommended for any clinician involved in the management of a TMD patient for whom these unproven modalities are being recommended by the treating dentist.

Psychological Testing

The initial examination for headaches and facial pain should include questions to evaluate behavioral, social, emotional, and cognitive factors that can relate to the patient's pain condition. Comprehensive psychological inventories such as the Minnesota Multiphasic Personality Inventory (MMPI) are not necessary for routine screening. Less involved testing such as the Beck Depression Inventory (33) or the SCL-90-R (34) can be helpful for patients with chronic facial pain or headache (35).

Thirty women referred to a multidisciplinary pain center because of failure to respond to typical muscular or vascular headache treatment regimens were questioned about sexual and physical abuse. All patients were administered the MMPI and were examined by a physician, a psychologist, and a physical therapist. Repeated abuse was reported by 66% of this group of nonresponders. Physical abuse was experienced by 61%, sexual abuse by 11%, and 28% had both sexual and physical abuse. A major difference between the two groups was the age of onset, with 86% of the nonabused women developing headache problems before the age of 20 years while 75% of abused women developed their headache pain after the age of 20 years. The women in this sample were not abused as children, but rather after the age of 20 years. The MMPI revealed significant elevations of the hypochondriasis, depression, and hysteria scales for the abused headache patients as compared to the nonabused headache patients (36).

ETIOLOGY

Additional study is needed to delineate the predisposing, initiating, and perpetuating factors for TMD. It is important not only to identify what could have initially caused the pain and dysfunction, but also to identify and minimize etiologic factors that perpetuate the patient's symptoms. There is often undue focus on correcting suspected initiating factors such as dental malocclusion, or modifying structural alterations of the joint with surgery, when simple elimination of perpetuating factors such as pain-provoking habits or activities might have provided relief. Evaluation of 3,428 patients by the author during the past 8 years has revealed the contributing factors discussed below for facial pain and temporomandibular joint disorders.

Oral Habits

Bruxism is defined as rhythmic or spasmodic clenching and grinding of the teeth. The mandible is the vehicle for bruxism, driven by the trigeminal motor nucleus and fueled by heightened levels of anxiety, excessive use of caffeine and psychosocial stressors. Bruxism is a common predisposing and perpetuating etiology for facial pain and over 20 years ago was purported to be the major etiology for myofascial pain and dysfunction (37). However, bruxism occurs in nearly equal prevalence in both sexes and most individuals who brux do not develop painful TMD. Bruxism has a cortical origin, with a central nervous system "rhythm generator" that is modulated by various oral reflexes that can be switched on by activity in higher centers and by sensory stimuli in the oral region. Jaw reflexes are influenced by interneurons in descending pathways from the cerebral cortex to the trigeminal motor neurons and can be influenced by emotions through the limbic system. Electromyographic studies have shown that anxiety and muscle tension are interrelated phenomena (38). Performing artists frequently report teeth clenching as one of the physiologic reactions associated with performance anxiety. Voluntary or conscious habits such as teeth tapping to music, setting the jaw during intense concentration, and teeth clenching in association with physical exertion are also classified as oral parafunction or bruxism.

Teeth grinding episodes occur in all stages of sleep, although they predominate in transition from sleep to wakefulness. Bruxism associated with rapid eye movement sleep is of short duration. More prolonged episodes of bruxism occur in stage I and stage II sleep and are accompanied by tachycardia and peripheral vasoconstriction. Episodes of bruxism can be induced by giving arousal stimuli to sleeping subjects, and the stage of sleep following a bruxism event is never a deeper stage than before the bruxism (39).

Administration of dopamine precursors such as L-dopa, commonly used in the treatment of Parkinson's disease, can provoke oral dyskinesia that can include deleterious bruxism and jaw dislocation (40). Phenothiazine medications can trigger bruxism, and with prolonged use the resultant receptor stimulation in the extrapyramidal system can precipitate oral dyskinesia, including severe bruxism (41) and TMJ subluxation (42). Bruxism following cortical injury, occurring with coma (43), and associated with cerebellar hemorrhage (44) have all been reported.

A written survey of 2,290 college students between the ages of 16 and 36 years revealed 5.1% were aware of current bruxism episodes, with no significant difference between men and women (45). The same question posed to the parents of 1,157 children between 3 and 17 years of age revealed 5.5% had a current bruxism habit. In this group there was an age-related decline: from 14.4% in those aged 3 to 7 years, to 6.6% in the children 8 to 12 years of age, to 1.2% in the 13- to 17-year age group. Although the use of a questionnaire and self-report to determine bruxism might not be valid, it is interesting to note that there was an age-related decline on the parental report, and that there was no difference in frequency of occurrence between the sexes. The age-related decline could be an artifact of the parents checking on their children during sleep less often as the children get older. Other studies report the awareness of bruxism in the adult population as high as 19% (46). Nevertheless, patient history denying bruxism may not be a reliable indicator of its presence, as some people are unaware that they have the habit.

Bruxism is a risk factor in developing TMD, but for most patients it is not the sole etiologic factor. Teeth grinding can cause muscle fatigue with associated temporal headaches and facial pain. The repetitive movements and the excessive loading of the TMJ can gradually stretch the disc attachments, and increased friction between the articular surfaces can lead to disc displacement. However, bruxism occurs in many individuals who experience no headaches, facial pain, or TMJ disorders, and there are many patients with TMJ disorders who do not grind their teeth. No strong correlation exists between the severity of tooth wear associated with bruxism and the presence of TMD (47). Bruxism should not be considered a pathologic condition and by itself is not an indicator of psychopathology. Unless the bruxism is causing headaches, facial pain, TMJ instability, severe tooth attrition, or tooth mobility, it does not require treatment.

Fingernail biting is a surprisingly common habit, and examination of the fingernails and cuticles should be included in a TMJ screening examination. A questionnaire completed by 2,905 subjects revealed a declining prevalence of fingernail biting with age. Of students 15 to 19 years of age, 28% were nail biters. Of college students 21 to 26 years of age, 21% were nail biters. In nonstudent adults between 19 and 66 years of age (mean age 32 years), 19% were nail biters (48). In a study of 1,077 college students, 29.3% of males and 19.3% of females were active nail biters (49). Social disapproval of nail biting could have more impact on women, accounting for the sex difference. Compared to controls, nail biters have higher anxiety scores (50). Experimental studies have shown that repetitive jaw protrusion

(51) necessary for nail biting creates preauricular pain, probably from lateral pterygoid muscle fatigue. The TMJ is loaded more heavily when biting between the incisors, as in fingernail biting, than when biting an object between the molar teeth (52). A simple and effective treatment for nail biting is to have the patient place a small adhesive bandage over the fingernail on one finger the first week, over two fingernails the second week, over three fingernails the third week, and continue to increase the number of fingernails covered by bandages each week. Given motivation from the knowledge that this habit is contributing to facial pain, this simple behavior modifier often enables the patient to stop nail biting within a few weeks.

Object biting, including lip, cheek, and tongue biting can be noted by careful observation while taking the history or by looking at the intraoral soft tissues for mucosal ridging. The patient should be asked about habitual biting of pens, pencils, paper clips, hairpins, split ends of hair, and other objects.

Oral sex can also cause TMJ sprain, pain, and clicking. The patient often first seeks treatment because of an episode of painful jaw locking in a wide-open position.

Occupational Activities and Hobbies

Scuba diving and snorkeling require gripping a regulator between the teeth. Because the bitewings or tabs of the mouthpiece do not extend to the back of the mouth, the open space between the molars creates a fulcrum that unfavorably loads the temporomandibular joints. A custom mouthpiece that extends over the molars can be fabricated by a dentist.

Frequent swimming has been reported as an aggravating or perpetuating factor for TMJ internal derangements by several teenagers. If breathing techniques are proper it is unlikely that swimming would cause the onset of a TMJ problem. However, if there is preexisting TMJ pain and dysfunction, then swimming can increase the symptoms, especially if the mandible is thrust excessively to breathe.

Wind instrumentalists, including flute and brass players, repetitively protrude the mandible while playing. Any alterations in the normal smooth gliding mechanism of the TMJ or fatigue of the masticatory muscles will be more noticeable to these wind musicians. Whereas playing a wind instrument is seldom the primary etiologic factor in precipitating a TMJ problem, once jaw pain has developed, playing a wind instrument can be an aggravating or perpetuating factor for TMD.

Singing often extends the jaw beyond the normal ROM. Vocalists seeking treatment for TMD nearly always exhibit a greater range of mandibular opening than do nonvocalists with TMD. Painful catching or locking of the TMJ in a wide open-mouthed position interferes with singing and is often associated with temporal headaches. The widest opening encountered in a sample of 3,428 TMD patients was the 77 mm active opening of the lead singer for a heavy metal rock band. This man's jaw frequently stuck open during performances without the audience becoming aware that there was a problem. Without interrupting the music, the singer would kneel with his back to the audience, in front of the percussionist, who would reduce the open lock.

A peculiar problem associated with singing was presented by a 15-year-old female with bilateral TMJ clicking, pain, excessive range of motion, and temporal headaches, all of recent onset. The clinical examination and history did not clarify the etiology. Close examination of the hands revealed calluses on the knuckles of the right hand. Despite the lack of related findings, bulimia was suspected. Upon further questioning, the patient admitted to and demonstrated placement of her hand, to a position beyond the knuckles, in her mouth. She had been doing this before falling asleep for about four months. The mother, who accompanied the patient to the examination, had not detected this unusual behavior. The patient was in a youth choir and the choral director had advised an exercise to increase mouth opening and improve the dynamic range. This girl had decided that rather than do the exercise, she would just sleep with her hand in her mouth and in this way stretch the opening, which she had managed to increase to 61 mm. The facial pain and TMJ dysfunction resolved when she stopped this jaw "exercise" performed during sleep.

Violinists and violists apply an upward and backward force against the right TMJ that can result in right TMJ pain and dysfunction, as well as condylar remodeling and facial asymmetry. A group of 51 professional violists and 15 violinists, as well as a control group of 115 subjects who had never played a violin or viola were examined for mandibular ROM, deviation on opening, joint sounds, and joint pain (53). TMJ pain was present in 73% of the violinists, 78% of the violists, and 3% of the controls. TMJ clicking was evident in 93% of the violinists, 92% of the violists, and 28% of the controls. There was a significant difference in the mean ROM of 43 mm for the violinists, 48 mm for the violists, and 55 mm for the controls. Deviation of more than 3 mm to the right upon opening occurred in 88% of these string players, as compared to 28% of the controls. TMJ pain and the degree of mandibular deviation upon opening were significantly greater in violists than in violinists. The age and number of hours the instrument was played was comparable for the two groups, and this difference could relate to the greater weight and size of the viola. Mandibular asymmetry to the right side and advanced degenerative joint disease of the right TMJ has been reported in young violinists (54,55).

Balancing the instrument between the chin and shoulder can also cause cervical strain. A survey by the author of 543 professional violin and viola players revealed that 40% experienced neck pain. Of those with neck pain, 43% reported that playing the violin or viola accentuated the neck pain. These figures for musicians are much higher than the 12% of the adult female and the 9% of the adult male population that experience current neck pain (56). The prevalence of ongoing neck pain in musicians is even higher than the 35% of the population that recalls any past episode of neck pain. Unlike the 70% of cervical pain patients who visit their doctor and are well or improved within one month (57), the musician's cervical pain is more likely to persist because of repetitive overuse or misuse.

Trauma

Trauma is a common etiology of TMJ sprain and disc displacement, with over 38% of TMJ patients reporting that general trauma and motor vehicular accidents contributed to the onset of their problem (58). A study by the author of 455 patients with painful TMJ internal derangements revealed that 164 (36%) reported facial trauma related to the onset of their TMJ dysfunction. Chin scars from a fall or direct blow to the mandible were exhibited by 13%, and an additional 4% of the patients had chin scars but could not recall any mandibular trauma.

Falls onto the chin (12.3%) resulting in a chin scar and the onset of TMD, were reported by 56 individuals. Falls occur more often in the younger age group, with bicycle accidents being the most common cause of this type of injury. This finding is consistent with the report of 8,814 head injury patients (59), 21.6% of whom were under the age of 14 years. Falls and bicycle accidents combined were a more common cause of head injury than motor vehicular accidents under the age of 14 years. Motor vehicular accidents were the predominant form of head injury in all other age groups until the age of 65 years, when falls again become the primary cause of head injury.

Physical abuse by nonfamily members (8.4%), including being struck by a fist or other object, was the cause of the TMJ problem for 38 individuals. This category of trauma occurred more frequently in men.

Physical abuse by a spouse or parent (3.5%) involving a blow to the mandible, precipitated the TMJ dysfunction and pain for 16 individuals. This category of trauma occurred more frequently in women.

Motor vehicular accidents (5.7%) involving striking the chin or side of the face, with subsequent onset of TMD, were reported by 26 individuals. In addition to direct blows to the jaw, hyperextension injuries of the TMJ with no direct blow to the mandible do occur, and can result in painful TMJ capsular sprain. A history of whiplash injury, not necessarily related to the onset of the TMJ problem, was reported by 20.4% of the 455 internal derangement patients. As with any other joint sprain, the onset of TMJ pain should occur soon after the hyperextension injury if the TMJ problem is related to a whiplash. This is an area of great uncertainty, with much misinformation about cause-and-effect relationships being provided by clinicians to attorneys and patients.

Sports-related injuries (4.4%), including glancing or direct blows from contact sports, were an initiating factor for TMJ problems for 20 individuals, most often in the age range of 15 to 30 years. Injuries from boxing, football, hockey, soccer, basketball, volleyball, gymnastics, water polo, water skiing, snow skiing, golf, and karate were all reported.

Iatrogenic trauma (1.8%), including routine dental procedures, was reported by 8 individuals as the cause of their TMJ disorder. Traumatic extraction of teeth, cementation of crowns and bridges, and deep cleaning on the lower dental arch were reported by 6 patients, and oral intubation for general anesthesia was reported by 2 patients as the initiating factor for TMD. In a patient with significant TMD, nasal intubation should be considered. Fibrous adhesions of the temporalis muscle to the temporal bone following craniotomy can result in extreme limitation of mandibular movement and deviation to the affected side. This complication of neurosurgery can usually be prevented by aggressive jaw exercise following craniotomy to maintain the range of motion. Milwaukee braces and cervical traction devices have also been implicated as causing TMJ problems or exacerbating existing TMD.

Dental Malocclusions

Historically, the dental profession has viewed malocclusion as the primary etiology for TMJ disorders, but there is little scientific evidence to support this point of view. An intraoral exam and a brief dental history should be completed in an attempt to identify possible occlusal factors. An extremely deep overbite or retroinclination of the upper incisors can contribute to TMD. Precise guidance of the mandible in the closing phase of mastication is necessary to avoid interference of the incisors, and with deep overbites this guidance is obtained by strong retrusive action of the posterior temporalis muscles upon closure (60). The loss of posterior molar support or the presence of ill-fitting dentures can also contribute to TMD, and visual inspection of the oral cavity for these conditions is advised for all facial pain patients. The loss of posterior tooth support can cause TMJ internal derangements, and this group is the most likely to have progression to degenerative joint disease (61).

DIFFERENTIAL DIAGNOSIS

The signature of a TMJ disorder is pain provoked by jaw function (62). Resting pain that is unrelated to jaw function is much less common and should alert the clinician to an alternative diagnosis (63). Differential diagnosis of facial pain is difficult because of the overlapping and complex innervation of the cranial nerves with interconnecting pathways, resulting in confusing patterns of referred pain. Pain of the masticatory muscles commonly refers to other facial structures. Temporalis pain is frequently interpreted by the patient as ophthalmologic pain or as frontal sinus pain. The masseter refers pain along the entire length of the zygoma and is often interpreted as maxillary sinus pain or as tooth pain. The lateral pterygoid will refer pain to the TMJ, the ear, and the nasal region; and the medial pterygoid to the submandibular region. A sustained clench during muscle palpation can elicit these referral patterns.

For patients presenting with facial pain, serious pathology can be overlooked if a careful history and examination are not completed. For example, otalgia is often associated with TMD, but otalgia can also be caused by intrinsic ear disease, referred pain from a dental abscess, giant cell (temporal) arteritis, auriculotemporal or glossopharyngeal neuralgia, carotodynia, atypical odontalgia, nasopharyngeal tumor, laryngeal tumor, acoustic neuroma, sinus disease, and obstruction or tumor of the parotid gland.

Congenital and Developmental Conditions

Connective tissue disorders that affect other articulations can involve the TMJ, with juvenile rheumatoid arthritis (JRA) being the most common. Ronning et al. (64) observed radiographic lesions of the TMJ in 28.9% of 249 children with JRA who were under the age of 15 years. Clinical symptoms including TMJ pain, limited range of motion, severe retrognathia and anterior open-bite malocclusion were present in 40% of the children with radiographic changes.

Condylar hyperplasia is uncommon, more frequent in males, and usually unilateral. The bony remodeling is a progressive but self-limiting growth disturbance that causes facial asymmetry and altered occlusion. This benign process can cause muscle or TMJ pain secondary to the skeletal asymmetry and often results in TMJ clicking on the contralateral side.

Malignancies in the region of the TMJ are exceedingly rare, with only seven occurring in the TMJ out of over 3,200 head and neck tumors treated over a 20-year period (65). Synovial chondromatosis of the TMJ has been reported to extend intracranially, resulting in facial nerve paralysis (66).

Idiopathic condylolysis is an uncommon phenomenon of sudden onset that is not yet understood. It occurs primarily in young females and causes unexplained severe bilateral resorption of the condylar heads. There is an associated sudden change in the dental occlusion with progressive development of an anterior open bite. Only 14 cases, all young females, have been detected in a sample of 3,428 TMD patients. Rabey (67) reported on four bilateral cases and recommended the use of the term be reserved for cases which demonstrate normal mandibular growth until the occurrence of a lytic event that is not caused by infection and does not result in ankylosis.

Elongated styloid processes of the temporal bone can result in facial pain, painful swallowing, and the sensation of a lump in the throat. Stylohyoid or Eagle's syndrome (68) can cause carotodynia from compression of the external or internal carotid arteries by an elogated styloid process. This vascular compression can result in periorbital, retro-ocular, TMJ, and otologic pain—all regions that receive their blood supply from branches of the external carotid artery.

Embryologically the styloid process and the attached stylohyoid ligament derive from the second branchial cartilage that divides into four cartilaginous fragments. When only the tympanohyal segment is ossified, a short styloid process exists. When the adjacent stylohyal ossifies, then a longer styloid process exists. The ceratohyal cartilaginous fragment usually degenerates in intrauterine life, becoming the stylohyoid ligament, but on rare occasion it also ossifies (69).

A macroscopic inspection of 404 styloid processes from macerated skulls revealed that 24% of the specimens had a length less than 20 mm, with 29% over 30 mm length (70). The mean length was 26 mm, with the maximum length 53 mm. There was no variability by sex or age, suggesting that elongation does not occur with advancing age.

The styloid process is easily visualized on a panoramic radiograph and historically has been judged to be elongated and capable of inducing symptoms when over 30 mm in length (71). Correll et al. (72) evaluated 1,771 panoramic views and found the incidence of elongation to be 18.2%, with 93% exhibiting bilateral elongation. Only eight patients had symptoms, nearly all unilateral, that might be related to the elongation. The high anatomic occurrence of long stylohyoids is in contrast with the low clinical manifestation of symptoms. The length of the process alone is not as pathognomonic as the shape of the process; its incurvation and whether or not the adjacent calcified segments are joined as a solid structure are factors in compression of the carotid artery. In a sample of 3,428 TMD patients, only 2 exhibited symptoms confirmed to be caused by stylohyoid compression of the carotid artery. Schmidt (73) reported on a 27-year-old male opera singer experiencing difficulty sustaining his vocal register because of fatigue of his throat muscles and lumps in his throat. Bilateral surgical removal of the distal end of the calcified stylohyoid ligaments resolved his complaints. Sataloff and Price (74) reported a case of styloid pain syndrome caused by stretching of the stylomandibular ligament following mandibular osteotomy. The 26-year-old female had immediate improvement in pain and a return to normal mandibular excursion following excision of the styloid tip and division of the stylomandibular ligament. The authors pointed out that not only the stylohyoid attachment, but also the stylomandibular ligament can cause facial pain and limited mandibular ROM.

Systemic ligament laxity should be considered in the diagnosis of TMD, especially in a population such as wind musicians and vocalists who subject their temporomandibular joints to repetitive, prolonged, or excessive movements. At any age, in a normal population, females have greater peripheral joint mobility than males (75). The degree of joint laxity diminishes rapidly throughout childhood, continuing to fall at a slower rate in adult life (76). Women have a smaller maximum jaw opening than men; however, this sex difference is not evident in children. Females with hypermobility of peripheral joints show significantly higher prevalence of TMJ dysfunction than do females without hypermobility (77). A highly significant correlation exists between wrist and elbow laxity and internal derangements of the TMJ for females (78). A study of 40 TMJ patients (79), 37 of whom had failed conservative therapy and were scheduled for TMJ surgery, revealed that 52.5% had systemic joint hypermobility based on the Beighton (76) scoring system. Joint laxity can predispose for TMD in individuals who receive mandibular trauma or who grind their teeth. TMJ hypermobility can predispose wind musicians and vocalists to experience articular complaints and should be suspected as a contributing factor to facial pain if systemic hypermobility is evident.

Neurologic Conditions

Trigeminal neuralgia or tic douloureux is a recurrent, excruciating, lancinating pain that radiates along the maxilla or mandible. Seldom occurring in the ophthalmologic division of the trigeminal nerve, it is almost always unilateral and typically occurs in elderly patients, with a 2:1 predominance in women and a 3:2 predominance on the right side. Trigger zones are exquisitely sensitive locations on the face that provoke instantaneous severe pain when stimulated by pressure or touch. This condition occurs in 2% to 4% of patients with multiple sclerosis.

Glossopharyngeal neuralgia, also known as vagoglossopharyngeal neuralgia, is a rare condition that occurs most often in males over the age of 50 years. The onset is usually abrupt, with severe, paroxysmal, lancinating pain radiating to the throat, teeth, ear, and tongue. The pain is unilateral 98% of the time and is accompanied by trigeminal neuralgia 10% of the time. Trigeminal neuralgia is 70 times more common than glossopharyngeal neuralgia (80). The tic-like pain can be triggered by movement of the tonsillar region, such as occurs with swallowing or coughing. Branches of the glossopharyngeal nerve include the tympanic nerve, a somatic afferent, the lingual branch, a special afferent that supplies taste receptors in the posterior third of the tongue, and visceral efferents that join with the auriculotemporal nerve to supply secretomotor fibers to the parotid gland. The carotid branches are visceral afferents to the carotid body and sinus that can trigger reflex responses to alter respiration, blood pressure, and cardiac output. Because glossopharyngeal neuralgia is closely associated with the trigeminal, vagus, and accessory nerves, its symptoms, in particular the cardiac changes, are often misdiagnosed due to other symptoms including altered parotid salivary flow, neck pain and syncope (81).

Postherpetic trigeminal neuralgia typically precedes or occurs in conjunction with an acute vesicular eruption, usually in the ophthalmologic branch or first division of the trigeminal nerve. The postherpetic neuralgia has a characteristic burning character with intolerable pain that can last for months or years.

Auriculotemporal syndrome is also referred to as Frey's syndrome and involves preauricular sweating and flushing associated with salivation. The sweating is caused by aberrant reinnervation following a blow (82), injection trauma, or surgical injury to the auriculotemporal nerve, with a high incidence following total parotidectomy (83). The sweat glands on the affected side become reinnervated by parasympathetic fibers of the glossopharyngeal nerve that travel in juxtaposition to the auriculotemporal nerve to innervate the parotid gland (84). Thermal sweating is reduced or abolished in the affected areas. This crossover innervation results in gustatory sweating that can be a social embarrassment, requiring repeated wiping of the zygomatic region during eating. For the performing artist affected by Frey's syndrome, the gustatory sweating can be controlled with scopolamine, 3% to 5% in a topical cream (85). A possible complication is blurring of vision, should the drug inadvertently come in contact with the eyes.

Cluster headache is uncommon, with a calculated prevlaence of 0.4% in males and .08% in females, and is the only type of headache that predominates in males

(86). The pain is unilateral, almost always around the eye, and frequently radiates to the teeth, gingiva, face, ear, nose, and neck. The duration is short, being minutes to hours, and characteristically builds to a maximum intensity over a short period of time, plateaus as a severe, lancinating pain and remits over a short period of time. These headaches appear in bouts, or clusters, with unexplained remissions. Lacrimation, stuffy nose, facial flushing, and photophobia are common. A hallmark of the headache is agitation, with the patient restless and pacing the room or moving other parts of the body. To date, there is no one hypothesis that explains the pathophysiology of cluster, but the symptoms appear to relate to changes in the carotid artery proximal to its bifurcation.

Facial migraine, also referred to as lower half headache or atypical facial pain, is of vascular origin and presents as a recurrent, unilateral throbbing headache with pain in the retro-orbital, frontal, and ear regions. The facial pain persists for several hours and is relieved by vasoconstrictor drugs.

Idiopathic toothache is less correctly referred to as atypical odontalgia, and is a poorly understood phenomenon characterized by persistent pain arising from the teeth and their supporting structures without any apparent cause. The pain is almost continuous and throbbing, and often spreads across the midline. Unlike pain from pulpal pathology, the pain is not relieved by somatosensory anesthetic block (87). These patients have often been unsuccessfully treated for this pain with root canal therapy and tooth extraction. The diagnosis is complicated by spontaneous remissions. An overwhelming majority of patients are female with history of migraine and depression and often respond to tricyclic antidepressants (88). Atypical odontalgia has also been described as a "dental migraine" that responds to vasoconstrictors (89) but a vascular mechanism seems unlikely, given the continuous, steady pain.

Atypical facial pain is a group of disorders that do not fit into major neurologic classifications and show no definable dental, neurologic, vascular, or medical condition that can account for the persistent, often vague complaints of these patients. The pain is often nonanatomic and nondermatomal in geography and has been suggested to be a psychiatric condition. A study of 121 patients referred to a pain center for treatment of atypical facial pain revealed that 29% had previously undiagnosed medical and dental pathology (90). The diagnosis was deferred for 9% of patients, and 62% met the American Psychiatric Association DSM-III criteria for psychiatric disorders. Depression was the diagnosis for 26% and somatoform disorders, including hysterical conversion, was the diagnosis for 24% of the patients with psychiatric illness. The mean age of the sample was 52.4 years, and 82.6% were female.

Glossodynia is often a somatic manifestation of a psychiatric disorder, more common in women over the age of 40 (91). Glossodynia can be disabling for the wind musician, and it is important that the clinician not overinterpret a musician's understandably anxious behavior. It is essential that nutritional deficiencies be ruled out as an etiology. The tongue's rich vascularity, rapid cellular turnover rate, and intimate contact with a broad spectrum of microorganisms make it an early indicator of many nutritional deficiencies (92). Burning or soreness of the tongue is common in iron deficiency anemia, with the tongue exhibiting a smooth surface and papillary atrophy. Changes in the appearance of the tongue and glossodynia nearly always occur with folic acid deficiency and vitamin B_{12} deficiency. Laboratory confirmation should be followed by replacement therapy. Xerostomia can also induce glossodynia as the saliva plays an important antibacterial and lubrication role. A wide variety of pharmacologic agents found in prescription and over-the-counter medications have anticholinergic effects. Of the 20 medications most frequently prescribed in 1986, 11 have xerostomic side effects (93). Xerostomia can occur as part of several chronic diseases, including diabetes mellitus and autoimmune disorders such as scleroderma, systemic lupus erythematosus, and Sjögren's syndrome (94). Radiation therapy for head and neck cancer usually results in xerostomia.

Systemic Diseases

Giant cell arteritis has an incidence of 9.3 cases per 100,000 individuals, with the rate twice as high for females (12.4) as for males (6.1). GCA has an age-specific incidence with an increase from 6.6 cases per 100,000 in the sixth decade to 73.1 cases in the ninth decade (95). GCA can be mistaken for TMD because of the temporal headaches and the jaw claudication when chewing, however, careful examination reveals the tenderness to be related to the temporal arteries in GCA, not the temporalis muscle, as is seen with TMD. Placing a patient in the reclined position will usually cause engorgement of the cranial arteries, including the facial artery as it crosses under the lower border of the mandible. In addition to symptoms referable to the temporal artery, visual changes, polymyalgia rheumatica, weight loss, and malaise in elderly individuals are important diagnostic clues (96). Neurologic findings and symptoms in biopsy proven GCA occurred in 31% of 166 patients, including tongue numbness and otalgia (97). Appreciation of mild or systemic manifestations can lead to early recognition of GCA and prevent morbidity, preserve vision, and prolong life.

Sjögren's syndrome can be mistaken for TMD because of swelling of the parotid gland that is misinterpreted as pain or swelling of the adjacent masseter muscle. Facial pain and neurologic findings can be present, including trigeminal neuropathy (98). Reduced salivary flow along with dryness of the eyes are common findings. Lesions of the TMJ and of the modified synovial joints between the ear ossicles (99) may occur, and hearing loss may be evident (100).

Bulimia, a cycle of food binges followed by purging, has an estimated incidence of 2.1% in young females (101). Bulimia is easily detected when there is erosion of the lingual surfaces of the upper teeth caused by the regurgitation of stomach acids (102). A diminished gag reflex requires that the patient put his or her hand or other object further down the throat to induce the vomiting, and at times a callus on the knuckles is evident. The repetitive vomiting can result in temporomandibular joint hyperextension and sprain. Headaches can occur as a result of the poor nutritional status and from the strain imposed on the temporalis muscles from TMJ hypermobility. Esophageal inflammation and benign, painless bilateral parotid gland enlargement are often seen in association with chronic bulimia (103).

Fibromyalgia is a form of nonarticular rheumatism with diffuse musculoskeletal aches and stiffness and exaggerated tenderness at multiple known anatomical sites. Also described as fibrositis (see Chapter 3), this is a less exact term that refers to pain and tenderness of muscles to palpation, regardless of anatomic site, a condition known as myofascial pain syndrome (104). As is the case with facial pain associated with bruxism, this condition affects predominately women between the ages of 20 and 50 years, and is associated with nonrestorative sleep, muscle stiffness, and chronic headaches. Pain thresholds of the tender points located in the temporalis and trapezius muscles are significantly lower than normal in fibromyalgia patients (105). Recommended treatment includes lifestyle changes to reduce stress, biofeedback and relaxation training programs, improved sleep habits, physical fitness training, heat, cyclobenzaprine or tricyclic antidepressants, and nonsteroidal antiinflammatory medications (106).

TMJ AND DENTAL PROBLEMS OF WIND INSTRUMENTALISTS

Expression of a musical composition as a woodwind or brass melody requires precise neuromuscular control of the orofacial complex. The mouth and associated musculature are the crucial links between the wind instrument and the instrumentalist. For some musicians the musical melody becomes medical malady through trauma, overuse, or misuse of the orofacial structures.

The individual variability of these structures and their adaptability throughout life should be considered when a musician initially chooses a wind instrument (107). The embouchure, the manner or method of applying the lips and tongue to the mouthpiece of a wind instrument to produce a tone, requires integrated action and positioning of the lips, tongue, and teeth. The word *embouchure* is French in origin and means "opening into." Each different wind instrument mouthpiece requires a specific muscular force pattern to form the embouchure, and a quality performance requires precise lip control. The ease of positioning the instrument relative to the anterior teeth contributes to forming the embouchure, and some dental and facial patterns facilitate (whereas other patterns complicate) the adaptation of the mouth to the mouthpiece. Ignoring the physical requirements of forming a correct embouchure can result in the selection of an instrument that is not suited to his or her morphology, which may limit the musician's ability to play to full potential. Poor lip control, muscle fatigue, sores on the lips, or pain of the temporomandibular joints can all compromise the embouchure.

The Embouchure

Neuromuscular control, as evidenced by the skillful and repetitious coordination between the mouth and the mouthpiece, reaches its acme in woodwind and brass performances (108). The lip muscles form the embouchure and act as a flexible washer to prevent the escape of air, with the mouth serving as a funnel to deliver the flow of pressurized air from the lungs. The intrinsic and extrinsic tongue muscles act as a valve to control the flow of air (109). The tongue is to the wind instrument what the bow is to the stringed instrument, with individual notes determined by each stroke of the tongue. The tonal quality is determined by tongue position in coordination with the muscles of respiration and soft palate in controlling the column of exhaled air. Depending upon the position of the anterior teeth, the form of the palate, and the size and position of the tongue, a reed wind musician will raise or lower the instrument to facilitate the embouchure and improve sound production.

The temporomandibular joints and the associated muscles of mastication, including the suprahyoid musculature, determine the position of the lower jaw when playing a wind instrument. The cervical musculature is highly active and important in stabilizing head posture and in maintaining the airway. Changes in head posture result in compensatory changes in the position of the mandible, changes in the pharyngeal airway, and an increase or decrease in lip pressure, all of which can alter tonal quality. When playing the trumpet, the tone and pitch are varied by the three pistons of the instrument and by alteration of the size of the lip aperture, change in the tension of the embouchure musculature, and changes in mandibular position. The body posture of 16 virtuoso trumpeters was evaluated during performance of musical tasks while standing (110). Photographic coordinates for the teeth, head, neck, sacrum, knee, and heel were digitized and a vector sum of body segment angles was computed for a neutral standing position and position while playing three different notes. The postural changes observed can be explained in large part by the respiratory process. There was a significant correlation between the angle of the horn and degree of the overbite. The greater the overbite when playing, the less horizontal the horn position. The overbite ratio is varied by changing the position of the mandible, which results in a compensatory change in the angle at which the trumpet is held.

The buccinator muscle (in Latin, buccinator means "trumpeter"), is the facial muscle most active when playing a wind instrument. This circumoral muscle is described as a purse string for the mouth that draws the corners of the mouth laterally, pulling the lips backward against the teeth. The buccinator actively compresses the cheeks when blowing and also aids in swallowing by helping to form a lip seal. It is composed of three groups of fibers or bands with the upper band and lower band each separate and continuous from side to side without decussation. The fibers of the middle band decussate and join the fibers of the orbicularis oris, thus permitting independent or coordinated control of the upper and lower lip (Fig. 4.6).

Blanton et al. (111) studied the activity of the buccinator using fine wire electrodes in 32 individuals with normal occlusion and found the muscle is involved in nearly all oral activities, including swallowing. Working in concert with the orbicularis oris muscle, the buccinator was most active in blowing and in pulling the lips back against the teeth, both of which are actions required in maintaining the embouchure. Williams et al. (112) studied the bilabial compression forces and found a significant difference in performance with and without the teeth clenched.

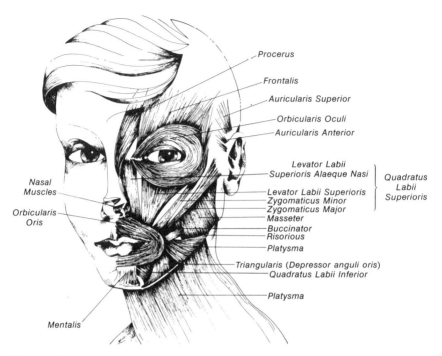

FIG. 4.6. Orofacial musculature. The muscles of facial expression are very superficial and all of them attach to the skin, at least at their insertion. Some attach to the skin at both the origin and insertion. These muscles give character and diversity to the human face. They also perform many other important functions such as closing of the eyes, moving the cheeks and lips during mastication and speech, and revealing some psychological activities. All of the muscles of facial expression receive innervation via the seventh cranial nerve. (From Fried LA: Anatomy of the Head, Neck, Face and Jaws. Philadelphia, Lea & Febiger, 1976, with permission.)

Bilabial compression force is essential in maintaining a lip seal when playing brass instruments. For all subjects, the maximum bilabial compression force they could exert against with their teeth lightly clenched was less (mean 411 g) than the force they could sustain with their teeth not in contact (568 g). It appears that by posturing the mandible such that the molar teeth do not contact, the subjects used bracing action of the jaw elevator muscles to gain additional bilabial compressive force that could not be obtained by lip muscle function alone.

White and Basmajian (113) used fine wire electrodes to compare the muscle activity of nine advanced and nine beginning trumpeters. The advanced trumpeters demonstrated no difference in the level of EMG activity of the upper lip versus the lower lip when playing, but the beginning trumpeters demonstrated more EMG activity of the upper lip. As was expected, the EMG activity was greater when playing the higher registers than when playing low registers. Complete and abrupt cessation of all lip muscle activity occurred precisely with the end of the tone in 17 of the 18 trumpeters. This very precise control over the tension and movement of the lips occurs because the tongue serves as a valve-like mechanism to immediately stop the tone, resulting in a sudden increase of intraoral air pressure that is quickly reacted to by the circumoral musculature.

Classification of Wind Instruments

Strayer (114) classified the woodwind and brass instruments into four groups by the configuration of each mouthpiece (Fig. 4.7). He indicated those instruments he thought were most appropriate for each type of dental occlusion; however, no data were presented to support his observations.

Class A instruments have cup-shaped mouthpieces made of metal that vary in size and in the depth and width of the brim. These include the trumpet, cornet, bugle, French horn, trombone, tuba, euphonium, and the alto, baritone, bass, and flügelhorn. To form a proper embouchure, the upper and lower incisors are aligned in a vertical plane and the mouthpiece is applied with backward pressure, compressing the lips against the upper and lower incisors. In playing brass instruments the borders of the lips are positioned inside the mouthpiece and vibrate, behaving as a biologic double reed. Precise lip control is required as the borders must vibrate at a

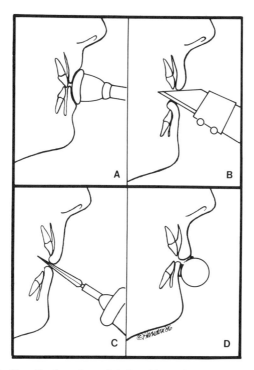

FIG. 4.7. Classification of woodwind and brass instruments by Strayer.

different frequency for each note played. The vibration is somewhat analogous to the phonation of the vocal cords as they vibrate when an exhaled stream of air passes between them. With the larger mouthpieces, more of the border of the upper lip is positioned inside the mouthpiece than for the lower lip. The lip musculature is more tensed for higher tones than for lower tones.

Class B instruments have wedge-shaped mouthpieces with a single reed clamped over a rectangular, smooth, and flat opening on the undersurface. This group includes the saxophones and clarinets. Although the saxophone is constructed mainly of metal, it is considered a woodwind because the sound is produced by vibration of the reed. The upper incisors rest against the hard, sloping top surface of the mouthpiece. The lower lip is curled over the edge of the lower incisors, forming a cushion for the reed, known as the "lay." Some single-reed musicians use a double-lip embouchure by also curling the upper lip over the upper incisal edges. Sound is produced by vibration of the tip of the reed over the rectangular opening as wind is applied.

Class C instruments have a double-reed mouthpiece and include the English horn, oboe, oboe d'amore, sarrusophone, bassoon and contra bassoon. The double reed, with its buttonhole-shaped aperture, is inserted between the upper and lower lips, which are curled backward over the incisors, forming a double-lip embouchure. Sound is produced by the two flexible, almost parallel reeds vibrating against the lips, and the pitch is raised by pushing the reeds further into the mouth and by pressing the lips more firmly together. Excessive lip pressure results in failure of the reeds to vibrate properly. Some musicians place the reed in the mouth at a slant to prevent excessive lip pressure and to allow them to maintain a more normal head posture.

Class D instruments have an aperture in the head of the instrument that serves as the mouthpiece. This group includes the flute and piccolo. The aperture rests against the lower lip, which is rolled along the side of the instrument and is active in stabilizing the position of the instrument. The upper lip is stretched and drawn downward over the upper incisors to provide a narrow opening between the lips, permitting a controlled stream of exhaled air to flow into and across the aperture. For low notes the upper lip is more tensed than for high notes.

Classification of Dental Occlusion

In an ideal dental occlusion there is no dental crowding, and the mandible or lower jaw bone and its teeth are in a correct relationship to the maxilla, or upper jaw bone, and its teeth. Dental relationships, including irregularity or tipping of the incisor teeth, can be important in selecting a wind instrument. Positioning of the mouthpiece is in part determined by the overjet, the horizontal distance between the upper and lower incisors, and overbite, which is the vertical overlap of the upper incisors over the lower incisors (Fig. 4.8).

Malocclusions were classifed by Angle (115), based upon the relationship of the

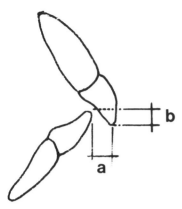

FIG. 4.8. Overjet (*a*) is the horizontal distance between the incisors. Overbite (*b*) is the vertical overlap of the upper over the lower incisor.

mandibular and maxillary molar and incisor teeth (Fig. 4.9). Crowding, open bites, crossbites and other dental irregularities are also considered, and in a class I malocclusion there are dental irregularities, but there is a correct anteroposterior relationship of the mandibular teeth to the maxillary teeth. In a class II malocclusion the mandible and its teeth are in a posterior or retruded relationship to the maxillary

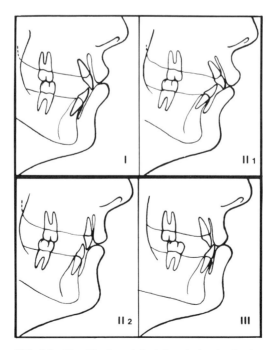

FIG. 4.9. Classification of dental occlusion by Angle.

teeth. Class II malocclusions are subdivided according to the relationship of the upper to the lower incisor teeth. In division 1 the upper anterior teeth have normal or excessive forward inclination, often with an excessive horizontal overjet. In division 2 the upper incisors are upright or inclined backward, often with an excessive overbite. In a Class III malocclusion the mandible is postured too far forward in relationship to the maxilla. The incisor teeth often have no overjet or overbite and are in an edge-to-edge relationship. In other Class III cases the anterior teeth are in crossbite with a negative horizontal overjet, resulting in the lower lip protruding ahead of and overlapping the upper lip.

Blake (116) reported the distribution of occlusal types, as classified by Angle, in the general population (Table 4.1). Class III malocclusion, with a prognathous mandible, is more prevalent in black and Japanese populations.

Wind Instrument Selection

Depending upon the type of mouthpiece, the number of hours the instrument is played, and the position of the teeth, the forces introduced by the tongue and facial muscles while playing a wind instrument can alter the equilibrium between dental and skeletal structures (117). The adaptability of the orofacial complex to these muscular forces is age-related, and maintaining the stability of this intimate relationship between the mouth and mouthpiece is essential for the career musician. Alterations in the occlusion are more likely to occur in the growing individual, especially during the period of permanent tooth eruption, and often coincide with the age at which most musicians select their initial instrument. Ignoring the individual's dental relationships and the character of the lip and facial muscles in selecting a wind instrument could compound an existing malocclusion. Proper instrument selection can enhance orofacial form and function and improve dental relationships through the repetitive application of the muscular forces associated with playing a wind instrument, and this should be considered in orthodontic treatment planning for wind musicians.

Herman (118) utilized dental casts in a prospective study of the dental changes occurring between 11 and 13 years of age in 127 wind instrumentalists. He concluded that the wind instrument that is suited to the patient's dental occlusion is a welcome aid in orthodontic treatment. He provided a guide for instrument selection for the beginning wind musician, so as to facilitate and not hinder orthodontic treatment objectives. Herman suggested that class A, or cup-shaped mouthpieces, such

TABLE 4.1. *Distribution of Angle's occlusal categories in 802 control subjects*

Class I	76%
Class II, division 1	17%
Class II, division 2	5%
Class III	2%

as brass instruments, have a tendency to reduce overjet and to decrease overbite. He stated that class B, or single-reed mouthpieces such as the clarinet or saxophone, tend to increase overjet and overbite, and that class C or double-reed mouthpieces such as the oboe and bassoon, tend to reduce overjet and increase overbite. Class D instruments with aperture mouthpieces such as the flute and piccolo were said to reduce overjet and increase overbite and were thought to be beneficial for a person with a short or weak upper lip or a protruding lower lip. While Herman's conclusions seem logical, his findings were not statistically significant.

Shimada (119) used dental casts and cephalometric radiographs for a retrospective study of dental and skeletal changes in 55 young wind instrumentalists. The mean age was 16 years and 4 months, and the mean length of musical experience was 3 years and 3 months, with a mean playing time of 2 $^1/_2$ hours per day. The data were reported by class of instrument, and there was no significant difference in the skeletal pattern between the groups. A definite difference in the inclination of the maxillary and mandibular incisors was observed in class B instrumentalists. The maxillary incisors were inclined more labially and the mandibular incisors more lingually, with a net result of an increased horizontal overjet. In class C and class D musicians there was a slight increase in the labial inclination of both the maxillary and mandibular incisors with no net increase in overjet. A tendency for the mandibular dental arch to be decreased in width and increased in length was attributed to the sustained contraction of the muscles at the corner of the mouth when playing wind instruments.

Pang (120) evaluated the effect of playing wind instruments on anterior tooth relationships of 76 seventh graders. Dental casts were obtained before the students selected their instruments and again 6 months later. This double-blind study used an equal number of controls matched for age, sex, weight, and height. The author acknowledged that the major weakness of the study was the short 6-month interval. Pang failed to correlate the number of hours each individual played with the amount of dental change observed. Playing wind instruments had no effect on the overbite. The greatest reduction in overjet occurred with class A instruments, with 16 of the 19 students showing a decrease in overjet in only 6 months. However, the average difference was less than 1 mm and was not statistically significant. A tendency toward reduction of overjet with class C and a tendency for an increase in the overjet with class D instruments was also noted. Class B instruments had little effect on dental protrusion. This conflicts with the report by Herman (118) of increased overjet in class B musicians, which he related to an increase in maxillary incisor protrusion. Pang concluded that for the growing individual the effect of playing a wind instrument on the position of the anterior teeth is unpredictable, and that only on a group basis can a class of wind instruments be theorized to alter skeletal and dental relationships.

Gualtieri (121) studied the occlusion of 150 adult professional musicians, and found that the only significant difference between the 82 wind instrumentalists and the nonwind instrumentalists was a difference in overjet. This difference existed primarily in class B musicians with single-reed mouthpieces. The increased overjet was attributed to increased lower incisor lingual inclination, found to be twice as prevalent in clarinet and saxophone players as compared to the nonwind musicians.

Seidner (122) examined 200 professional wind instrumentalists using lateral cephalometric radiographs taken while the musicians were actually blowing into the mouthpieces. The headfilms provide a graphic portrayal of the pressure against the lips, the degree of mouth opening, and the lower jaw position in forming the embouchure. He concluded that individuals with a narrow upper dental arch and a high palate, characteristic of a Class II malocclusion, were best suited to playing a clarinet. Class III malocclusions favored the adaptation of the mouth to the mouthpiece of the oboe and bassoon. His comments were directed at the tonal quality of music rather than what effect playing the wind instrument might have on the occlusion.

Lip Form and Anterior Dental Crowding

Cheney (123) examined the dental occlusion and lip form of 100 college wind instrumentalists majoring in music. His rating of dental variables was matched with each musician's own rating of the difficulty they encountered in forming the embouchure of their primary instrument. Problems adjusting to the embouchure were reported by 26% and included lip and facial muscle fatigue, difficulty posturing the lower jaw far enough forward, lip irritation, and air leakage around the mouthpiece. Difficulties were reported by 5% of the woodwind musicians, 27% of the large brass, and 47% of the small brass players. Of the small brass instrumentalists who were classified as having a Class II dental malocclusion, 79% reported difficulty. For all occlusal classifications, the deeper the overbite the greater the tendency for embouchure difficulties. Cheney noted that maxillary dental protrusion was considered a problem by all of the brass players whom he had classified as having forward tooth position. The dental protrusion was reported to interfere with lip placement and required greater forward posturing of the lower jaw to form the embouchure. This was most often reported by those playing brass instruments with small mouthpieces, which require a great deal of precision in aligning the lower incisors directly below the upper incisors to provide equal support of the mouthpiece by the upper and lower lips. Anterior dental open bites were a problem for brass players but were particularly disturbing to woodwind musicians because they experienced difficulty in preventing the escape of air from the corners of the mouth during prolonged playing. Of the 36 subjects Cheney rated as having significant maxillary anterior tooth crowding, only 5 complained that tooth irregularity caused them any difficulty. Of the 40 subjects he rated as having significant mandibular anterior dental crowding, only 3 reported this to be a source of difficulty. Anterior tooth crowding appears to be much less of a problem for wind musicians than had previously been reported. Anterior crossbites in association with incisor crowding caused lip irritation in woodwind musicians. Cheney rated lip form according to height and thickness and found that variations in lip form were not a significant factor in embouchure formation. Only two musicians, both small brass players, reported that their lip form compromised tone control.

A short upper lip is thought to contribute to protrusion of upper incisors and also represents an aesthetic concern. Some orthodontic patients are advised that playing a wind instrument will serve as a lip-strengthening exercise and improve tooth position and soft tissue profile. Ingervall and Eliasson (124) studied the effect of lip training in growing children with a short upper lip who were judged to have lip incompetency and were unable to form a lip seal. They compared 10 controls with 15 children who received specific lip-training exercises over a period of 1 year. Soft tissue and dental variables, including overjet and overbite, were evaluated using radiographs. They demonstrated that it clearly is possible to influence the morphology of the lips with exercise. A significant increase in the height of both lips and a decrease in lip separation occurred in the exercise group with no change in the controls. It should be emphasized that lip training did not affect tooth position. Lip muscle activity was compared using surface EMG, and there was no change in muscle activity when swallowing after 1 year of lip exercises.

Natural lip function in professional musicians was studied by Fuhrimann et al. (125). The morphology of the face, the lip strength, muscle activity, and lip pressure against the teeth were compared in 12 trumpeters, 12 clarinetists, and 12 nonwind instrumentalist controls. Using a water-filled transducer system and fine wire hook electrodes, the lip pressure and muscle activity were recorded with the lips at rest and during chewing. Among the three groups, there were no significant differences in lip pressure or muscle activity. When playing the trumpet the median pressure was 524 g/cm^2 for the upper lip and 188 g/cm^2 for the lower lip. The corresponding measures for clarinetists were 121 g/cm^2 for the upper and 229 g/cm^2 for the lower lip. The authors concluded that the intensive use of the lips by professional musicians does not result in increased lip strength, and that playing either type of wind instrument had no effect on tooth position as compared to the control group. These findings contradict the claims of Parker (126), who used cephalometric radiographs to evaluate instrument placement and upper incisor angulation in 84 accomplished student wind musicians. He stated that playing a wind instrument results in balanced muscle tonicity, and that playing any brass or woodwind instrument is helpful for a mouth-breather or a person with a short upper lip. No EMG activity or lip pressure recordings were made in support of his observations. Parker noted that reed musicians compensate for excessive overbite or overjet by raising or lowering the instrument to meet the individual need. He commented that a trumpet player with a Class II, division 1 malocclusion has to thrust the lower jaw excessively forward to maintain the embouchure, and he conjectured that this could result in lateral pterygoid muscle fatigue and thus TMJ symptoms.

Lamp and Epley (127) rated the musical performance aptitude of 151 students, 14 to 15 years old, by having each try out on a brass, a woodwind, and a string instrument. Their performance ability was correlated with an irregularity index of their anterior teeth. The correlation coefficient between evenness of incisor teeth and a high aptitude for playing was only 0.13 for woodwinds and 0.10 for brass instruments. The correlation for tooth evenness and string performance, an irrelevant correlation, was 0.16. It can be concluded that crowded or irregular anterior teeth are not an obstacle in the initial attempt to play wind instruments. However, it is unknown whether anterior dental crowding could limit the ultimate level of performance with certain wind instruments, and rotated and protruded teeth, dental spacing, and missing teeth could compromise proficiency.

Lip, Muscle, Tongue, and Soft Tissue Problems

Tooth position and contour are important to all wind instrumentalists but appear to be most critical to the brass musician. Wind instrumentalists with a diastema, or space between the upper central incisors, can develop severe irritation from the upper lip being drawn into the diastema when forming the embouchure. Chronic lip irritation resulting from the mouthpiece pressing against crowded, chipped, or worn teeth can be alleviated by reshaping the teeth with grinding or bonding techniques.

Newmark and Lederman (128) reported that a rapid increase in practice time, especially superimposed upon a baseline of relatively little routine practice, predisposes a musician to overuse injuries. They defined overuse as those symptoms associated with activity exceeding the biological limits of the tissue involved. They surveyed 79 participants, all but 3% of whom were amateur musicians, at a week-long music conference that included 3 $\frac{1}{2}$ hours of intensive coaching on their instruments each day. For nearly all participants, playing time and intensity were increased over their usual routine, with 54% averaging less than 1 hour per day practice during the prior year. During the week, 72% developed new playing-related medical problems, most of which the authors regarded as overuse. Of the 22 wind musicians, 4 reported soreness of the lip muscles, and 3 reported canker sores.

Lederman (129) reported on occupational cramps in 21 musicians, 7 of whom were wind players. Muscle involvement of the lips and face, affecting the embouchure, was reported by 4 of the 7, including 1 bassoonist with involvement of the jaw, tongue, and laryngeal muscles. Lederman noted that these patients had symptoms consistent with focal dystonias, and that only 4 of the 21 musicians mentioned pain as a prominent feature, making it unlikely that the occupational or "musician's cramp" is a continuum of painful muscle-tendon overuse.

Focal dystonias of the tongue are uncommon. This highly developed sensorimotor organ is closely integrated with the activity of the muscles of mastication and mandibular movement, as is evident by how seldom we bite our tongues when chewing. The jaw-tongue reflex coordination is one of the most intricate biological control systems, with interplay between the hypoglossal motor neurons and the trigeminal muscle afferents. The masticatory muscles, primarily the temporal muscle (130), and the TMJ mechanoreceptor afferents have a direct influence on tongue activity. This could explain the difficulty encountered by some wind musicians who try to play through the joint and muscle pain, not realizing that there is a reflex alteration in tongue coordination.

Krivin (131) describes the fabrication of a clear vinyl plastic lip shield, or embouchure aid, from a model of the lower teeth. The device was tested daily for over a year by two clarinetists and two saxophonists who were experiencing lip irritation. All four were able to extend their playing regimen by three more hours per day without discomfort, and the chronic lip problems were quickly eliminated without disturbing the embouchure. This flexible yet durable device can be inexpensively fabricated by a dental laboratory from a stone cast of the lower teeth. Lip shields should be resilient to cushion the lip, smooth to avoid lip abrasion, thin to minimize interference, and transparent so that they will not be noticed. Lip shields for the brass musician are of minimal value and cause lip muscle fatigue. Nixon (132) reported that those brass players with irregular or crowded upper incisors have a tendency to establish an "embouchure of comfort" by positioning the mouthpiece to one side of the midline to avoid irritation of the inner aspect of the lips.

Hellsing and L'Estrange (133) studied lip pressure in 15 adults with Class I occlusion who were not wind musicians and were not mouth-breathers. The subjects had normal overjet and overbite and lip competency. Lip pressures were recorded using strain gauge transducers attached to the incisors. Each five-second recording was repeated ten times for nasal breathing with the mandible at rest and head posture normal. Lip pressure for nasal breathing with the head in flexion and in extension was also recorded, as was lip pressure during mouth breathing. The millivolt readings were converted to grams/cm^2. The lip pressure exerted during nasal breathing with natural head position and the mandible at rest was 3.65 g/cm^2 for the upper lip and 8.32 g/cm^2 for the lower lip. During induced mouth breathing the upper and lower lip pressures decreased significantly. During head extension there was a highly significant increase in upper and lower lip pressure, thought to be related primarily to soft tissue stretching. During head flexion there was a highly significant decrease in upper lip tension. Muscle activity in the mentalis region caused by head flexion interfered with accurate recording of the lower lip pressure. Precise control of lip pressure is critical to the embouchure, and the variable lip pressure resulting from changes in head posture can have a significant impact on tone quality. Wind musicians with altered head posture caused by cervical pain from injury or from occupation- or emotion-induced cervical muscle hypertonicity can have difficulty adjusting their embouchure.

Repetitive, coordinated lip muscle activity can improve hypotonic or flabby lips. However, lip pressure associated with embouchure formation, measured to be as high as 130 mm Hg (134) as compared to normal speech pressure that rarely exceeds 6 mm Hg, can also be traumatic if sustained over long periods of time. Planas (135) described a trumpet player with ruptured fibers of the orbicularis oris muscle in the lower lip. A fibrous band of scar tissue within the muscle was surgically removed and the trumpeter was able to continue his career.

The extremely high intraoral air pressure must be directed to the mouthpiece without any leakage of air around the lips. A palatal seal is required to prevent air leakage through the nasal passages. Tonsillectomy and adenoidectomy can result in velopharyngeal insufficiency, and the altered muscle tonicity can compromise sound production because the desired intraoral pressure cannot be sustained (136). Wind musicians should be discouraged from playing for at least 2 weeks following tooth extraction, particularly for extractions in the maxillary arch where the high intraoral pressure could cause a rupture of the mucosa into the maxillary sinus (137). The double-reed instruments such as the oboe and bassoon require the highest sustained intraoral pressure to maintain the necessary airflow through the narrow aperture between the reeds. The large brass instruments such as the tuba and trombone require large volumes of air but require less intraoral pressure and are more dependent upon precise shaping of the lips and tongue for tone control. The smaller brass instruments, including the coronet, trumpet, and French horn, require the greatest variability in intraoral pressure, reaching exceedingly high pressure with sustained, loud, or high-pitched notes. Single-reed instruments such as the clarinet and saxophone require moderate intraoral pressure, whereas the flute and piccolo require the least air pressure (138).

High intraoral pressure can force saliva retrograde into the parotid salivary gland (139) through Stensen's duct, located in the cheek adjacent to the upper molars. This retrograde flow occasionally results in bacterial infection, with blockage of the duct and painful swelling. This condition can be treated with antibiotics, but its prevention is difficult. Viral parotitis also occurs. Blowing a saliva spray into the mouthpiece must be avoided, as it is incompatible with producing a pure tone and will cause a loss of volume.

The concern over shared mouthpieces in school bands has typically focused on the spread of respiratory infections (140). Calabrese (141) addressed the impact of AIDS on performing artists. There is no evidence that saliva transmits the AIDS virus, but it has been isolated from the saliva in about 5% of infected individuals. Despite repeated exposure to saliva, there are no known cases of transfer of the virus to dentists in the absence of contact with blood. The AIDS virus does not appear to be highly contagious, and intimate and usually repeated sexual contact is the primary source of disease transmission. Shared use of eating utensils, toothbrushes, or combs has not resulted in known transmission (142). However, even in the absence of salivary transmission of AIDS, the known transfer of hepatitis and other viral disease through saliva dictates that sharing a mouthpiece without adequate sterilization is no longer acceptable.

Drooling of saliva or formation of beads of perspiration under the lower lip, most often experienced by clarinetists, can result in "clarinetist's cheilitis" of the border of the lower lip. Contact dermatitis of the lips also occurs from prolonged contact with a metal alloy mouthpiece, in particular from sensitivity to nickel or chromium. A dermatologist can determine such sensitivities, and the skin patch test is an important diagnostic tool in differentiating allergic from contact dermatitis (143). Acne mechanica or localized acneiform eruptions of the lips can occur as a result of repetitive mechanical pressure, friction, or rubbing. "Flutist's chin" is a variation of acne mechanica, which also occurs on the neck of violists and violinists, known as "fiddler's neck" (144).

Tooth-Related Problems of Wind Instrumentalists

Engelman (117) used an intraoral pressure transducer to measure perioral forces applied against the teeth when playing various wind instruments. He found that only class A, or brass instruments with cup-shaped mouthpieces, produce a significant backward pressure against the dentition. He recorded a mean of 500 g of backward force against the incisors for class A, compared to 270 g for the classes B and C, and 211 g for the class D instruments. Proffit (145) reported that the optimal force for orthodontic movement of incisor teeth is 100 g, and only 50 g is required for tipping, rotation, or extrusion of anterior teeth. However, it is estimated that force at these levels must be sustained for at least 6 hours per day to bring about tooth movement.

Barbenel et al. (146) designed a transducer to measure the forces of the lip against the mouthpiece during trumpet playing under normal conditions. Thirty male subjects who were full-time, very proficient, professional trumpeters were compared with 30 male subjects of intermediate skills, all of whom had played the trumpet for at least 6 years. The limit of the force which the players could apply to the mouthpiece while keeping a note at a constant loudness and when playing an ascending scale was determined. Mouthpiece force increased dramatically with ascending pitch, and to a marked, but lesser extent, with increased loudness. The proficient group could maintain a mean maximum force of 77.6 Newtons (n), significantly greater than the mean of 45 n by the intermediate players. The magnitude of the mouthpiece forces were extremely high for the upper registers, with forces greater than 100 n being recorded.

Cremmel and Frank (147) reported changes in the pulp chambers of anterior teeth as a result of the repetitive force application in professional wind musicians. They observed on radiographs diffuse calcification, elongated dense calcifications, and root canal shrinkage. The localization of these changes was directly related to the diameter of the embouchure. The interposition of the lower lip in clarinetists and saxophonists did not prevent the development of changes within the pulp chambers. In clarinetists the upper incisor pulp chambers were narrowed with calcifications, and the same changes were noted in the middle and lower third of the root canal in saxophonists. Flutists showed elongated calcifications in the middle third of the lower incisor root canals. These pulpal changes are thought to be the result of modest and transient forces applied to the teeth when playing, resulting in compression of the periodontal ligament space. This compression restricts the blood flow to the pulp and results in a transient inflammatory response that can trigger abnormal calcification within the pulp chamber (148).

Periodontal disease and the associated loss of supporting bone around the teeth result in tooth mobility and is now a more common cause of tooth loss than is decay.

Playing a wind instrument has been purported to cause anterior tooth mobility, but Herman (118) and Gualtieri (121) examined wind musicians and found no evidence of increased anterior tooth mobility. Bergstrom and Eliasson (149) compared dental radiographs of 242 professional musicians between the ages of 21 and 65 years, 100 of whom were wind instrumentalists. The alveolar bone height, a reliable measure of periodontal disease, was recorded from radiographs of the molars and the mandibular incisors. There was no significant difference in bone height between the wind instrumentalists and the nonwind musicians and there were no significant differences between the brass and woodwind players. Previous studies reporting that playing a wind instrument contributes to periodontal disease did not use radiographic measures and lacked suitable controls. Bergstrom and Eliasson concluded that in the presense of good oral hygiene, playing a wind instrument does not increase the risk of alveolar bone loss or periodontal disease.

Loosening and shifting of the anterior teeth of the wind musician with periodontal disease can pose a serious problem. Mobile teeth can be treated with a removable splint for use when playing, or an unobtrusive orthodontic retainer can be bonded to the lingual aspect of the incisors to control tooth mobility. Lovius and Huggins (150) studied 20 professional wind musicians utilizing a cephalometric radiograph, dental casts, and a clinical examination. Above average oral hygiene without periodontal involvement was noted, as was a normal overjet relationship and angulation of the incisors. They stressed the importance of an intact dentition and stated that the fear of losing teeth plays a greater part in the lives of professional wind musicians than for any other group. It behooves all professional wind musicians to have dental models taken as a permanent record in case of accidental injury to the front teeth so that a dentist could accurately restore the desired tooth contours.

The wind musician in need of orthodontic therapy may want to request treatment with removable orthodontic appliances rather than the traditional bands and brackets attached to the teeth. While removable appliances can be very effective in growing individuals, it is usually necessary to place bands and brackets on the teeth near the end of treatment to achieve an ideal result. The use of removable appliances in the adult or nongrowing patient has definite limitations. Traditional orthodontic appliances can cause lip trauma and interfere with formation of the embouchure, especially for flute and single-reed instrumentalist. A lip shield can reduce irritation and protect the anterior teeth from the backward pressure. Crawford (151) reported on a 12-year-old flutist who improvised a lip shield by using an orange peel to cover the braces on her lower teeth so that she could play in comfort. Following orthodontic therapy, the wind instrumentalist, especially the class B musician, should wear a retainer for as long as possible to prevent tooth crowding and backward inclination of the lower incisors (152).

Dentures pose special problems for wind instrumentalists, especially single-reed and brass musicians. The high intraoral air pressure and the mechanical forces applied by the mouthpiece to dentures reduce retention and stability and can cause pressure sores under the dentures. These problems can be eliminated by using osse-ointegrated implants to support the denture (these now have a 95% long-term success rate). Mechanical denture aids fabricated from a soft, compressible acrylic can be positioned over a denture to create an opening compatible with playing a wind instrument (153). The compressibility of the material permits change in the position of the mandible while playing. This personalized embouchure aid stabilizes the dentures, minimizing the cheek and tongue pressure otherwise required to hold the dentures in place. Special embouchure dentures (154), worn only when playing, can be fabricated with interlocking inclined planes to improve denture stability when the mouthpiece is positioned.

Temporomandibular Joint Problems

Gualtieri (121) noted TMJ clicking or crepitus upon clinical examination in 12% of the controls, 5% of clarinet and saxophone players, and 11% of trumpet and horn players. However, 31% of the trombone and tuba players exhibited TMJ noises. Cephalometric radiographs taken with the mandible at rest were compared with radiographs taken with the mouthpiece in position. For the trombone and tuba players, the group with the highest frequency of TMJ noise, the mandible moved up and back from the rest position when the embouchure was formed. One etiology of TMJ clicking and pain is repetitive upward and backward force against the mandible, resulting in distal condylar displacement. The mandibular position noted in the radiographs for the trombone and tuba players could explain the much higher prevalence of TMJ sounds. The mandible moved either down and forward or down and back for the other instruments. Gualtieri reported subjective muscle discomfort in 28% of the trumpet and horn players, 25% of the trombone and tuba players, and only 10% of the clarinet and saxophone players.

In a written survey of 200 flutists, Koskinen-Moffett (155) found the prevalence of TMJ symptoms to be comparable to that in the general population. The mean age of the flutists was 34 years; 80% were female. Clicking was reported by 32%, and episodes of locking occurred in 12%. Instantaneous pain with the clicking was reported by 6%, with 11% experiencing TMJ pain from playing the flute. Subjective awareness of bruxism or teeth grinding and clenching was reported by 44% of the flutists as compared to 19% of the general population (46). The author surmised that the increased awareness of bruxism might be related to stress or performance anxiety.

Electromyographic (EMG) biofeedback training and stress management can effectively reduce daytime bruxism as well as reduce cervical muscle tension related to performance anxiety. Biofeedback may be an effective behavioral control technique for reducing excess muscle tension in musicians without compromising performance. The lowered EMG levels are maintained for an extended period of time without the aid of ongoing feedback training sessions (156). Levee et al. (157) reported the successful treatment of a woodwind musician with biofeedback. The musician had been unable to continue his career because of tightness of his jaw muscles and constriction of his throat that was accentuated in stressful, anxietyproking situations. EMG biofeedback is advocated as an adjunct to psychotherapeutic intervention for the performing artist with stress-related disorders.

Survey of Orthodontists

A 1977 survey by the U.S. Public Health Service of 12- to 17-year-old whites revealed that 11% of males and 13% of females receive orthodontic therapy (158). Published reports on the relationship of wind instruments to orofacial structures provide conflicting advice, often based upon conjecture rather than data. To develop an appreciation for the magnitude of these problems, and for the level of interest and knowledge, the 160 orthodontists in Washington state were mailed questionnaires about how frequently they were consulted by wind musicians with orofacial problems (159). Orthodontists were selected because the age range of their patient population overlaps the age range of the beginning wind instrumentalist and because orthodontic training includes in-depth study of the anatomy and physiology of the orofacial region.

The response rate was 57%, and the mean years of clinical experience of the 92 respondents was 14, with a range of 1 to 33 years. A surprising 48% of the orthodontists had played a wind instrument, suggesting a strong selection bias in completing the questionnaire. Only 14% use a written questionnaire as part of the initial history to inquire if new patients are currently playing or are considering playing a wind instrument. An additional 9% inquire during the patient interview. Only one orthodontist made available to patients any written or visual information about the relationship of wind instruments to orofacial structures. The orthodontists estimated that 7% of their patients play wind instruments and 28% of the orthodontists indicated that these musician-patients report lip irritation and sores more often than do their other patients. An understanding of the relationship between wind instrument mouthpieces and dental and skeletal structures was deemed inadequate by 78% of the respondents. When questioned specifically about the relationship of each class of mouthpiece to different malocclusions, 34% of the respondents stated that they would not be sure how to advise a patient. Only 23% of the orthodontists could remember a patient ever having sought orthodontic therapy because they thought it might improve their comfort or ability when playing a wind instrument.

Orthodontic tooth movement is the result of gentle but persistent forces. While the magnitude of the forces applied to the incisors when playing some wind instruments is great, the majority of the respondents doubted that the duration of these forces was adequate to bring about dental or skeletal changes in amateur wind musicians. Responses to questions about the effect of different instruments (Table 4.2) on the occlusion of growing individuals is of interest but should be viewed as opinion based upon clinical experience. These survey results do not provide a scientific basis for making recommendations. Playing a class B instrument such as a clarinet was rated harmful for a class II, division 1 malocclusion by 47% of the orthodontists. Playing a class A instrument such as a trumpet was rated as helpful for a

TABLE 4.2. *Opinion of orthodontists about the effect of playing wind instruments on dental and skeletal structures*

Is playing the *trumpet*, an instrument with a cup-shaped mouthpiece (Class A), likely to be helpful, harmful, or have no effect on the occlusion of a growing individual with the malocclusion listed below?

	Class I	Class II Div 1	Class II Div 2	Class III
Helpful	4	47	4	2
Harmful	5	0	35	5
No effect	77	40	46	59
Not sure	14	13	15	34
	100%	100%	100%	100%

Is playing the *clarinet*, an instrument with a single-reed mouthpiece (Class B), likely to be helpful, harmful, or have no effect on the occlusion of a growing individual with the malocclusion listed below?

	Class I	Class II Div 1	Class II Div 2	Class III
Helpful	0	0	18	23
Harmful	8	55	17	0
No effect	73	32	48	52
Not sure	19	13	17	25
	100%	100%	100%	100%

Is playing the *oboe*, an instrument with a double-reed mouthpiece (Class C), likely to be helpful, harmful, or have no effect on the occlusion of a growing individual with the malocclusion listed below?

	Class I	Class II Div 1	Class II Div 2	Class III
Helpful	0	14	11	12
Harmful	7	18	12	0
No effect	73	52	57	59
Not sure	20	16	20	29
	100%	100%	100%	100%

Is playing the *flute*, an instrument with an aperture mouthpiece (Class D), likely to be helpful, harmful, or have no effect on the occlusion of a growing individual with the malocclusion listed below?

	Class I	Class II Div 1	Class II Div 2	Class III
Helpful	2	22	6	13
Harmful	4	19	28	4
No effect	76	43	50	62
Not sure	18	16	16	21
	100%	100%	100%	100%

From Howard and Lovrorich, ref. 159.

patient with a Class II, division 1 malocclusion by 55% of the orthodontists. The double-reed or class C instruments were thought to have the least effect on dental occlusion. Class I malocclusions were rated as the least likely to be affected by playing a wind instrument, and Class II division 1 as the most likely to be affected. The greatest uncertainty was the effect of playing wind instruments on Class III malocclusions.

Survey of Wind Instrumentalists

   To gain insight into the frequency and severity of head and neck problems, a self-completion questionnaire was distributed to be completed by 135 amateur wind instrumentalists (159), each averaging less than 10 hours per week playing time during the last year. The response rate was 53%, and of the 72 respondents, 42% were female. The mean age was 37 years with a range of 15 to 69 years. The mean duration of playing was 21 years with a range of 4 to 60 years and a standard deviation of 13 years. Several musicians played more than one wind instrument but were asked to respond about their primary instrument. Class A (cup-shaped mouthpieces) accounted for 47% of the musicians; class B (single-reed) for 29%, class C (double-reed) for 13%, and class D (aperture mouthpiece) for 11 % of the musicians.
   The mean age at which the musician began playing a wind instrument was 11 years with a range of 5 to 37 years of age. Orthodontic treatment had been completed for 24% of respondents with 93% undergoing treatment between the age of 11 to 16 years—the same age period in which 94% of the musicians began playing their first wind instrument. The coincident age of orthodontic therapy and instrument selection reinforces the importance of increasing orthodontists' awareness of the interplay between wind instruments and the dental occlusion. Only 35% of the musicians surveyed had ever discussed with a health care provider the dental implications of playing a wind instrument. One brass player responded that she was reluctant to seek dental care because her dentist was insensitive to the condition of her lips and the inside of her mouth during dental procedures.
   The most common problem experienced by wind musicians was lip discomfort caused by sharp teeth. This was reported as a problem by 36% of the musicians. However, 81% of the single-reed musicians reported this as a problem, as did 77% of the double-reed musicians. The offending sharp teeth had been smoothed by a dentist for 14% of the musicians. Lip shields had been tried by 38% of the single-reed players but only 10% routinely used a lip shield. Most musicians had made their own shield from tape, cigarette paper, pieces of rubber glove, or commercially available denture reline material.
   The prevalence of TMJ pain and dysfunction in wind musicians is comparable to that in the general population. Subjective awareness of a restricted mouth opening was reported by 13%. The three-finger test could not be accomplished by 6% of the respondents and was possible, but with pain, for 22%. TMJ sounds were reported by 35%, but only 7% heard the noise on a daily basis and considered it a problem. A

history of catching and locking was reported by 13%. Stiff or sore jaws upon awakening were present in 14% of the sample, and 22% reported morning headaches. Temporomandibular joint pain was reported by 21% of the wind musicians, with 30% reporting that playing accentuated their joint pain.

Teeth clenching during the day was reported by 21%, and 24% were aware of night grinding. Nightguards for bruxism had been worn by 13% of the wind musicians. Treatment specifically for a TMJ problem had been received by 6%, which is the same percentage of the general population that seeks treatment for TMJ-related disorders (18). Neck pain was experienced by 43% of these musicians; 39% of those with pain reported that playing accentuated the neck pain. Surprisingly, only 32% of those with neck pain had sought treatment for this problem.

A history of frequent ringing in the ears, or tinnitus, was reported by 10% of the respondents as compared to 9% in a comparable age group in the general population (159a). The term *tinnitus* describes a sensation, not a mechanism. It is not a disease itself, but a symptom that occurs in conjunction with several disorders, and in most cases the etiology is uncertain. Steffan (160) advises that when musicians first experience tinnitus, hearing protection should be utilized to help prevent progression. This is appropriate especially if the musician is exposed to excessive noise, as discussed in Chapter 9 on hearing loss in musicians. Foam earplugs offer up to 35 decibels of sound reduction across most of the musical frequency spectrum, while still allowing the musician to hear what is being played.

There was no significant difference in reporting of signs and symptoms between males and females. The small size of the sample precludes statistical analysis between the different instrument groups or correlation of the number of years played and the age of the musician with the reported problems. All of these could be important variables and should be examined in future studies. This preliminary report of amateur instrumentalists reveals the need for a larger survey of professional wind musicians early in their careers, as well as those with many years of experience, to determine if professional wind musicians develop an increase in orofacial problems over time.

Despite a variety of symptoms associated with playing wind instruments, only 15% of the amateur musicians in this study had ever sought treatment for these problems from a physician. Even so, this could represent a significant number of medical consultations as a 1978 Gallup Poll survey of 15,000 families estimated that there were 10,863,000 amateur wind instrumentalists in the United States (161).

Further study is needed to delineate the full range of TMJ-related and orofacial problems experienced by musicians and vocalists. Only when the interplay between the orofacial complex and musical instruments is understood by the music teacher and the clinician can the beginning instrumentalist be properly guided in instrument selection and technique of playing. For the wind musician, improper selection as it relates to tooth position, skeletal pattern, and lip morphology can limit the musician's success, resulting in mediocre performance because of the inability to form and maintain a correct embouchure. Instrument selection should be based upon the student's preference, the ease of forming and maintaining an embouchure, and physical characteristics such as adequate respiratory function, hand size, and arm length.

DISCUSSION

The suspected high prevalence of medical problems in musicians was confirmed by the self-completion questionnaire returned by 2,212 of the 4,025 professional musicians of the 48 affiliate orchestras of the International Conference of Symphony and Opera Musicians (ICSOM) (162). Medical problems were reported by 82% of all musicians with 76% listing at least one problem as severe in terms of its effects on their performance. Of the 55% responding, 353 were class A wind musicians, 83 were class B, 168 were class C, and 95 were class D musicians. The sample was slightly disproportionate with respect to gender, instrument group, and type of orchestra as compared to the total ICSOM population. The data were statistically weighted to project the occurrence in the total ICSOM population, 33% of whom are women, with a mean age of 40 years for females and 43 years for males. It is interesting to note that for brass players only 10% are female, for flute and piccolo 53% are female, and for the reed instruments 22% are female musicians. For string players, which comprise 62% of the musicians, 41% are female. The average age at which the ICSOM musician began playing the orchestral instrument was 10 years. The authors pointed out that the reported prevalence of medical problems in this population might underestimate the actual risk, because those with severe problems might no longer be able to perform and could have dropped out of the population. The medical problems were divided into musculoskeletal and non-musculoskeletal groups. Orofacial and TMJ problems, incorrectly grouped as non-musculoskeletal, were reported by 11% of all musicians. No specific data were given for wind instrumentalists, but of all respondents, 3% indicated an acquired dental malocclusion, 2% a loss of lip control, 1% a loss of lip seal, and 3% mouth lesions.

Harman (163) divided the diverse occupational diseases reported by instrumentalists into six categories: dermatitis, nerve compression syndromes, occupational cramps, intraoral pressure problems, cardiac abnormalities, and miscellaneous ailments. An excellent article by Hoppmann and Patrone (164) reviews the incidence and prevalence of musculoskeletal problems in instrumental musicians. The authors identified the three most common classes of performance-related problems in musicians in order of their occurrence as: musculotendinous overuse, nerve entrapment/thoracic outlet syndrome, and motor dysfunction. Lederman (165) evaluated 226 instrumentalists seeking treatment for playing-related symptoms, 29% of whom were diagnosed as having peripheral nerve disorders. Musculoskeletal problems were diagnosed for 62%, generally involving the upper extremities, and especially prevalent were left-sided arm problems for violinists and violists.

Wind instrumentalists report medical problems in each of these categories, yet only a small percentage seek professional medical advice (159). Perhaps this reluctance to seek treatment is because of a perceived lack of interest or knowledge on the part of health care providers about the problems encountered by wind musicians. The ICSOM survey (162) revealed that for hand problems, rest was helpful for 84%, physical therapy helpful for 82%, seeing a neurologist helpful for 13%, and seeing a general practitioner was rated as helpful by only 6% of the musicians.

Usually the musician perceives that something is wrong with the body that prevents proper playing. All too often it is something wrong with the style of playing that is the cause of the medical condition, and solving the problem involves changing the technique of playing. Musicians are encouraged to tell their health care providers about their musical activities and, when possible, to demonstrate by bringing their instrument to the provider's office. Observing the patient play the instrument can be the key to diagnosis and will help guide appropriate therapy.

INITIAL TMJ THERAPY

Therapy for musculoskeletal problems is familiar to all and can be applied to the muscles of the head and neck region. Treatment should focus on directing the patient to control his or her own musculoskeletal symptoms. Aggravating factors should be identified and avoided. A caring, reassuring attitude that TMJ/facial pain disorders have a favorable prognosis and that the physician has a clear understanding of the nature of the patient's problem will have therapeutic value. In many cases the primary care physician can provide the initial therapy and no referral will be necessary other than perhaps to physical therapy and counseling, if appropriate.

Patients with painful TMJ derangements will usually benefit from referral to a dentist for treatment with an intraoral appliance. For those patients who do not have derangements but present with evidence of a severe bruxism habit, the physician will need to decide if the patient would benefit more from an appliance or by stress management, including cognitive awareness training and progressive muscle relaxation. The following is a brief guide to the management of TMJ/facial pain disorders.

Home Use of Physical Therapy

The patient is advised to apply moist heat over the areas of discomfort and to vigorously massage the muscles following the application of heat. Gentle, passive range-of-motion exercises are indicated if a limited mandibular range of motion persists. Cervical and facial muscle soreness can usually be reduced by focusing on habitual postures that contribute to the pain and implementing exercises to improve muscle tone and increase resistance to fatigue.

Pharmacotherapy

Nonsteroidal antiinflammatory drugs (NSAIDS) are usually helpful in controlling the muscle and joint inflammation and as analgesics. The dose should be tailored, as for any other orthopedic condition, to the patient's current level of symptoms. Gastrointestinal tract side effects occur in 20% to 30% of patients who take NSAIDS in therapeutic doses (166), and these medications should not be used long-term without clinical supervision. It should be recognized that elderly individuals are subject to cognitive dysfunction and mood alterations as a common side effect of NSAIDS (167). The decreased attention span and the loss of short-term memory are side effects that would not be tolerated by the elderly, active performing artist.

"Muscle relaxants" are thought to be effective because of their sedative effect, and at the common doses prescribed do not elicit actual muscle relaxation (168). These medications play a role in the short-term management of acute muscle discomfort and headaches but are not a realistic treatment option for the chronic facial pain or headache patient. Whenever such medications are used there should be a paralleling effort to alter the patient's stress levels and activities that produce the muscle pain.

Phenothiazine medications should be avoided whenever possible as they can have an adverse effect on these patients by increasing bruxism or even triggering extrapyramidal reactions resulting in facial, neck, jaw, and tongue muscle spasms (41,42).

Antianxiety and antidepressant medication to improve poor sleeping patterns can significantly reduce bruxism and therefore decrease facial pain and headaches upon awakening. Amitriptyline has been shown to have analgesic properties independent of an antidepressant action and can be effective in dosages as low as 10 mg to 30 mg in the treatment of muscle contraction headache and facial pain (169).

Narcotic analgesics play little role in the management of these patients other than for episodic and severe muscle contraction headache. Caffeine intake through beverages should be considered a self-prescribed drug, and the patient should be informed of its potential to contribute to caffeine withdrawal headaches, alter sleep patterns, and increase bruxism.

Modification of Chewing

The patient should be advised to avoid hard or sticky foods for several months. Incisal biting or tearing of foods with the front teeth increases the loading of the joint and should be avoided indefinitely. Foods that are normally bitten off with the front teeth should be cut up into small pieces and chewed in the back of the mouth. The mouth should not be opened more than the width of two fingers when eating. The clinician should have the patient chew on a folded-over cotton roll to determine if there is a side on which the patient can chew with less joint noise and discomfort. If so, the patient should make every effort to chew only on that side. Gum chewing is not necessarily harmful but large pieces of gum or bubble gum should be avoided. The gentle rhythmic action of gum chewing serves as a muscle exercise and relieves muscle tension for some patients. Unshelled sunflower seeds, beef jerky, licorice, caramels, and taffy are not to be eaten. The patient should obey the rule: "If it hurts to chew it, then don't do it."

Modification of Hobbies and Habits

Laying on the floor with the chin propped on one hand while reading or watching television or when seated at a desk can stress the jaw joints and should be avoided. The mouthpiece used for scuba diving and snorkeling torque the TMJ and can aggravate an asymptomatic TMJ condition. Holding the telephone between the shoulder and the mandible and talking out of the side of the mouth for extended periods of time can also exacerbate TMJ and cervical problems.

Awareness of Clenching and Grinding

Patients should make every effort to not clench or grind their teeth. They should think about the times they would be most likely to grind their teeth, including with physical exertion, freeway driving, waiting in lines or at doctor's offices, and at other times of high stress. When aware of clenching their teeth they should remember the phrase "lips together/teeth apart." By forming a seal with their lips and gently puffing air, the masseter becomes relaxed, the teeth separate, and the clenching cycle is interrupted. When the patient has the urge to clench the teeth, the tip of the tongue should be placed in the vault of the palate and upward tongue pressure should be applied, allowing only partial mouth opening.

Behavioral Medicine

Increasing the awareness of the relationship between stress and physical symptoms, changing maladaptive habits and behaviors, and improving coping skills are important parts of the overall treatment program for TMD and headache patients. Enrolling in stress management classes, cognitive awareness training, and EMG and thermal biofeedback training should be encouraged in selected cases. These approaches allow identification and control of the stressors that lead to the muscle tension that is causing the musculoskeletal pain. The clinician should assist the patient in verbalizing stress management goals and should monitor progress with follow-up visits. If individual psychotherapy is needed, psychological care should be coordinated and integrated with the other treatments. This referral should be made as soon as the need is identified, not after the patient fails to respond to the other therapies.

Trigger Point Injections

Selective injection of anesthetic, with or without cortisone, can be a valuable adjunct for the patient with isolated areas of persistent cervical and facial muscle pain and identifiable trigger zones.

Temporomandibular Joint Injections

Diagnostic injections of the auriculotemporal nerve or into the TMJ can introduce infection, and sterile technique including skin preparation is essential. The injection of steroids into the TMJ is controversial and should not be done unless there is persistent pain that is not responsive to other therapies. Intra-articular steroids can provide temporary benefit in the treatment of osteoarthrosis, but they have a short duration of action (170). The articular surface of the TMJ is fibrous connective tissue, not hyaline cartilage, and the reaction to cortisone injections could be different from other joints.

Referral for Physical Therapy

The patient with generalized neck and facial muscle soreness will usually benefit from a referral to physical therapy. The therapist will focus on habitual postures that can contribute to the pain and teach the patient exercises to improve muscle tone and resistance to fatigue. The use of heat, ice, diathermy, or ultrasound in combination with passive stretch and deep tissue massage is appropriate for both cervical and facial pain. Cervical problems and TMJ/facial pain are closely related for some patients, and simple alterations of sleeping postures, the use of a cervical pillow or neck roll, and neck-strengthening exercises can indirectly improve a jaw problem. Caution is advised if cervical traction is to be used, as this can apply excessive loads directly to the temporomandibular joints.

Intraoral Appliance Therapy

Referred to as splints, braces, nightguards, orthotics, and repositioning appliances, these interocclusal appliances have been used with success for managing facial pain (171) for over 100 years. These removable acrylic devices are always worn at night and for a variable number of hours during the day, depending upon the nature of the problem. For some violinists and violists it is helpful to wear the appliance when playing. It is not usually necessary to wear the appliance when eating. There are several designs of appliances, and it usually makes little difference if it is worn over the top or bottom teeth. Clear, hard acrylic, 2 mm to 3 mm thick between the molar teeth is the design used most often. Some clinicians provide soft vinyl splints that are easier to fit to the teeth but can trigger increased clenching in some patients and can aggravate an existing jaw derangement. Wearing a splint increases the patient's awareness of jaw habits and trains the patient to rest the jaw in a more open position. The splints are in effect a behavior modification tool, and EMG monitoring of the masseter muscle has shown that the level of bruxism activity is decreased when the appliance is worn. It does not, however, provide a cure, and the bruxism returns to the pretreatment level when appliance therapy is terminated. People with severe bruxism should continue to wear a splint at night in the long term to prevent abrasion, fractures, and mobility of the teeth.

In addition to their use for control of bruxism, splints can also provide templates or occlusal supports for stabilization of TMJ derangements and with full-time wear these appliances can negate many significant occlusal problems. The splint alters the loading of the joints and can reduce the amount of muscle activity. Most TMJ derangements are not progressive disorders, and in conjunction with rest, the patient might need to use the appliance for only a short time to control symptoms and promote the natural healing capacity of this joint. Although these appliances seldom resolve TMJ noises, they almost always control the painful locking episodes that are often the chief complaint (172). The appliance protects the teeth from abrasion caused by bruxism, and for this reason it is often recommended by dentists for habit control, even when there is no evidence of TMD.

Temporary Mandibular Immobilization

A careful history can reveal the cause of the joint laxity and hypermobility. Aggravating factors include bulimia, cheerleading, frequent singing, and oral sex. The patient with an excessive ROM with clicking on wide opening and painful episodes of locking can easily be treated with a combination of jaw exercise, habit modification and the use of elastic bands to restrain mouth opening. This inexpensive treatment involves attaching an orthodontic bracket on the facial surface of the canine teeth and then having the patient wear an interarch elastic band on each side of the mouth. Usually the translation over the tubercle, which is what causes the clicking and episodes of locking, occurs beyond 30 mm of opening. The length of the rubber band can be set to allow for 25 mm of opening, therefore preventing the subluxation but still permitting enough freedom of mandibular movement for normal speech and eating. The use of this temporary restraint will control unexpected yawns, excessive translation of the jaw caused by laying on the side of the face during sleep, and will promote cautious eating habits. The rubber bands do not cause eruption of the canine teeth and are not uncomfortable to wear. This simple treatment controls temporal headaches and locking episodes and decreases the posttreatment ROM in nearly all TMJ hypermobility patients. Interocclusal appliance therapy is sometimes used in conjunction with the elastic immobilization if there is evidence of bruxism.

Temporomandibular Joint Surgery

The increased emphasis on TMJ internal derangements has resulted in increased diagnostic imaging to identify disc position and morphology and has resulted in more frequent surgical intervention. Patients who have been diagnosed as having a TMD and are concerned that it might require surgery should be reassured that the probability of needing surgery is about 1%. Before recommending surgical intervention, the clinician and the patient should clearly understand the natural course of internal derangements (173).

Arthroscopy of the superior compartment of the TMJ has been reported as a successful technique for painful nonreducing disc displacements and for limited mandibular mobility associated with arthrosis (174). The favorable response is probably in large part related to the flushing-out of this synovial joint and also the manipulation through a wide range of motion while under general anesthesia. Puncture of the inferior joint compartment with the arthroscope increase the risk of tissue damage and provides very limited access of the bursal spaces, and typically is not done (175).

SUMMARY

The temporomandibular joints are subject to the same misuse, overuse, trauma, aging, and systemic diseases as are the other synovial articulations. The muscles of mastication, subservient to this joint and sharing its innervation, are the most common source of facial pain. The majority of TMJ-related disorders will respond to the same physical therapy and anti-inflammatory medication that would be used for cervical myalgia, a problem that often coexists with TMD in the performing artist. Irreversible and expensive changes in the dental occlusion to resolve TMJ disorders are usually unnecessary, and surgical treatment is seldom warranted. Reversible methods including removable interocclusal orthotic appliances (otherwise known as splints, biteplates, or nightguards) can be very effective in managing both joint and muscle pain. In addition to their role in providing orthopedic stabilization, these appliances are also effective in reducing nocturnal bruxism and the associated facial pain and temporal headaches.

If the initial examination reveals that the patient has a painful TMJ derangement, it is usually beneficial to immediately refer the patient to a dentist for treatment with an intraoral appliance. Stress management can be effective for daytime bruxism habits such as clenching and tooth tapping. Pain control and behavior modification through the use of cognitive therapy, EMG biofeedback training, and relaxation skills are effective. However, this training does not necessarily carry over to sleeping hours, and for control of nocturnal teeth grinding with evidence of severe bruxism facets and masticatory muscle pain, a bruxism appliance is usually beneficial.

TMJ/facial pain disorders have a favorable prognosis. The physician can provide initial therapy for nearly all patients presenting with TMD. The therapy should focus on directing the patient to prevent and control his or her own musculoskeletal symptoms. Aggravating factors should be identified and avoided and when appropriate, technique of playing an instrument or singing should be modified. A caring, reassuring attitude that addresses both the physical and emotional component of the problem is necessary. Psychosocial stressors as an etiologic factor must always be considered, and close follow-up is important.

CONCLUSIONS

Physicians and dentists are encouraged to take an active role in documenting and reporting their own experiences in the prevention, detection, and management of the medical and dental problems encountered in performing artists presenting as patients. Medical injuries related to music making are an important problem that is likely to have implications during even the early phases of musical training (176), making early detection by the primary care physician essential. The interested clinician needs to coordinate care with physical therapists, occupational therapists and mental health providers knowledgeable about the special problems encountered by performing artists, and with musicians and their teachers. For career instrumentalists or vocalists, the adverse affects of their art can transform musical melody to medical malady. The providers of music medicine must recognize the role of the instrument in causing or perpetuating the symptoms, search for effective methods of prevention and treatment, and avoid recommending that the performer give up music. Our current knowledge is insufficient, and we have the opportunity to learn from every performing artist we see and from each new problem we encounter; but our current information allows us to help preserve a healthy performing career in almost all cases.

REFERENCES

1. Costen JB. Syndrome of ear and sinus symptoms dependent upon disturbed function of temporomandibular joint. *Ann Otol Rhin Laryngol* 1934; 43:1–15.
2. Sicher H. Temporomandibular articulation in mandibular closure. *J Am Dent Assoc* 1948;36:131–139.
3. Widmer CG, Lund JP, Feine JS. Evaluation of diagnostic tests for TMD. *Calif Dent Assoc J* 1990; 18(3):53–60.
4. Howard JA. Imaging techniques for the diagnosis and prognosis of TMD. *Calif Dent Assoc J* 1990; 18(3):61–71.
5. Greene CS. Can technology enhance TM disorder diagnosis? *Calif Dent Assoc J* 1990; 18(3):21–24.
6. Von Korff MR, Howard JA, Truelove EL, Sommers E, Wagner EH, Dworkin S. Temporomandibular disorders: variations in clinical practice. *Med Care* 1988; 26:307–314.
7. Moffett BC. The morphogenesis of the temporomandibular joint. *Am J Orthod* 1966; 52:401–407.
8. Du Brul EL. Origin and adaptations of the hominid jaw joint. In: Sarnat BG and Laskin DM, eds. *The temporormandibular joint*. Springfield: Charles C. Thomas Publishers, 1980.
9. Moffett BC. The prenatal development of the human temporomandibular joint. In: *Carnegie Institution of Washington: Contributions to Embryology* 1957; (Publication 611)36:19–28.
10. Rees LA. The structure and function of the mandibular joint. *Br Dent J* 1954; 96:125–133.

11. Loughner BA, Larkin LH, Mahan PA. Discomalleolar and anterior malleolar ligaments: possible causes of middle ear damage during temporomandibular joint surgery. *Oral Surg Oral Med Oral Path* 1989; 68:14–22.
12. Cantekin EL, Doyle WJ, Reichert TJ, Phillips DC, Bluestone CD. Dilation of the eustachian tube by electrical stimulation of the mandibular nerve. *Ann Otol Rhinol Laryngol* 1980; 89(Suppl 68):47–53.
13. Rich AR. A physiologic study of the eustachian tube and its related muscles. *Bull Johns Hopkins Hosp* 1920; 31:206–214.
14. Casselbrant ML, Cantekin EI, Dirkmaat DC, Doyle WJ, Bluestone CD. Experimental paralysis of tensor veli palatini muscle. *Acta Otolaryngol* 1988; (Stockh) 106:178–185.
15. Stingl J. Blood supply of the temporomandibular joint in man. *Folia Morphol* 1964; 13:20–24.
16. Kofler TJ, Howard JA. Temporomandibular joint arthrography. *Curr Probl Diagn Radiol* 1985; 14(1):1–54.
17. Carlsöö S. An electromyographic study of the activity, and an anatomic analysis of the mechanics of the lateral pterygoid muscle. *Acta Anat* 1956; 26:339–351.
18. Rugh JD, Solberg WK. Oral health status in the United States: temporomandibular disorders. *J Dent Educ* 1985; 49:398–405.
19. Von Korff M, Dworkin SF, LeResche L, Kruger A. An epidemiologic comparison of pain complaints. *Pain* 1988; 32:173–183.
20. Dworkin SF, Huggins K, LeResche L, Von Korff M, Howard J, Truelove E, Sommers E. Epidemiology of signs and symptoms in temporomandibular disorders: clinical signs in cases and controls. *J Am Dent Assoc* 1990; 120:273–281.
21. Pullinger AG, Monterio AA. Functional impairment in TMJ patient and nonpatient groups according to disability index and symptom profile. *J Craniomandib Practice* 1988; 6:156–164.
22. Rasmussen CO. Clinical findings during the course of temporomandibular arthropathy. *Scand J Dent Res* 1981; 89:283–288.
23. De Bont L, Boering G, Liem R, Havinga P. Osteoarthrosis of the temporomandibular joint. A light microscopic and scanning electron microscopy study of the articular cartilage of the mandibular condyle. *J Oral Maxillofac Surg* 1985; 43:481–488.
24. Clark GT, Seligman DA, Solberg WK, Pullinger AG. Guidelines for the examination and diagnosis of temporomandibular disorders. *J Craniomandib Disord Facial Oral Pain* 1989; 3:7–14.
25. Mezitis M, Rallia G, Zachariades N. The normal range of mouth opening. *J Oral Maxillofac Surg* 1989; 47:1028–1029.
26. Graff-Radford SB, Reeves, JL, Jaeger B. Management of headache: effectiveness of altering factors perpetuating myofascial pain. *Headache* 1988; 27:186–190.
27. DeMarino DP, Steiner E, Poster RB. Three-dimensional computed tomography in maxillofacial trauma. *Arch Otolaryngol Head Surg* 1986; 112:146–150.
28. Kaplan PA, Tu HK, Sleder PR, Lydiatt DD, Laney TJ. Inferior joint space arthrography of the temporomandibular joints: reassessment of diagnostic criteria. *Radiology* 1986; 159:585–589.
29. Hutchins LG, Harnsberger HR, Hardin CW, Dillon WP, Smoker WR, Osborn CA. The radiologic assessment of trigeminal neuropathy. *Am J Radiol* 1989; 153:1275–1282.
30. Gratt BM, Pullinger A, Sickles EA, Lee JJ. Electronic thermography of normal facial structures: a pilot study. *Oral Surg Oral Med Oral Path* 1989; 68:346–351.
31. Finney JW, Holt CR, Pearce KB. Thermographic diagnosis of temporomandibular joint disease and associated muscular disorders. *Postgrad Med* March (Special Issue): 1986; 93–95.
32. van den Akker HP. Diagnostic imaging in salivary gland disease. *Oral Surg Oral Med Oral Path* 1988;66:625–637.
33. Beck AT, Ward CH, Mendelson M, Erbaugh J. An inventory for measuring depression. *Arch Gen Psychiat* 1961; 4:564–571.
34. Lee YO, Lee SW. A study of the emotional characteristics of temporomandibular disorder patients using SCL-90-R. *J Craniomandib Disord Facial Oral Pain* 1989; 3:25–34.
35. Speculand B, Goss AN. Psychological factors in temporomandibular joint dysfunction pain. *Int J Oral Surg* 1985; 14:131–137.
36. Domino JV, Haber JD. Prior physical and sexual abuse in women with chronic headache: clinical correlates. *Headache* 1987; 27:310–314.
37. Laskin DM. Etiology of the pain dysfunction syndrome. *J Am Dent Assoc* 1969; 9:147–153.
38. Sainsbury P, Gibson JG. Symptoms of anxiety and tension and the accompanying physiological changes in the muscular system. *J Neurol Neurosurg Psychiat* 1954; 17:216–224.

39. Satoh T, Harada Y. Electrophysiological study on tooth grinding during sleep. *Electroencephalo Clin Neurophysio* 1973; 35:267–275.
40. Magee KR. Bruxism related to levodopa therapy. *J Am Med Assoc* 1970; 214:147–150.
41. O'Hara VS. Extrapyramidal reactions in patients receiving prochlorperazine. *New Engl J Med* 1958; 259:826–828.
42. Ryan M, LaDow C. Subluxation of the temporomandibular joint after administration of prochlorperazine: report of two cases. *J Oral Surg* 1968; 26:646–648.
43. Pratap-Chand R, Gourie-Devi M. Bruxism: its significance in coma. *Neurol Neurosurg* 1985; 87:113–117.
44. Pollack IA, Cwik V. Bruxism following cerebellar hemorrhage. *Neurol* 1989; 39:1262.
45. Reding GR, Rubright WC, Zimmerman SO. Incidence of bruxism. *J Dent Res* 1966; 45:1198–1204.
46. Gross AJ, Rivera-Morales WC, Gale EN. A prevalence study of symptoms associated with TM disorders. *J Craniomandib Disord Facial Oral Pain* 1988; 2:191–195.
47. Seligman DA, Pullinger AG, Solberg WK. The prevalence of dental attrition and its association with factors of age, gender, occlusion and TMD symptomatology. *J Dent Res* 1988; 67:1323–1333.
48. Kleinrok M, Meilnik-Hus J, Zysko-Wozniak D, Szkutnik J, Kaczmarek A, Doraczynska E, Pyc K. Investigations on prevalence and treatment of fingernail biting. *J Craniomand Practice* 1990; 8:47–50.
49. Westling L. Fingernail biting: a literature review and case reports. *J Craniomandib Practice* 1988; 6:182–187.
50. Coleman JC, McCalley JE. Nail-biting among college students. *J Abnorm Soc Psychol* 1948; 43:517–525.
51. Scott DS, Lundeen TF. Myofascial pain involving the masticatory muscles: an experimental model. *Pain* 1980; 8:207–215.
52. Ito T, Gibbs CH, Bonnet RM, Lupkiewicz SM, Young HM, Lundeen HC, Mahan PE. Loading on the temporomandibular joints with five occlusal conditions. *J Prosthet Dent* 1986; 56:478–484.
53. Hirsch JA, McCall WD, Bishop B. Jaw dysfunction in viola and violin players. *J Am Dent Assoc* 1982; 1044:838–843.
54. Kovero O. Degenerative temporomandibular joint disease in a young violinist. *Dentomaxillofac Radiol* 1989; 18:133–135.
55. Reider CE. Possible premature degenerative temporomandibular joint disease in violinists. *J Prosthet Dent* 1976; 35:662–664.
56. Lawrence JS. Disc degeneration. Its frequency and relationship to symptoms. *Ann Rheum Diseases* 1969; 28:121–127.
57. British Association of Physical Medicine. Pain in the neck and arm. A multicentere trial of the effects of physical therapy. *Brit Med J* 1963; 2:1607–1616.
58. Pullinger AG, Seligman DA. Association of TMJ subgroups with general trauma and MVA. *J Dent Res* 1988; 67:403.
59. Luerssen TG, Klauber MR, Marshall LF. Outcome from head injury related to patient's age. *J Neurosurg* 1988; 68:409–416.
60. Möller E. Action of the muscles of mastication. In Kawamura Y, ed. *Frontiers in Oral Physiology*, vol 1. Basel: Karger, 1974; 121–158.
61. Christensen LV, Zeibert GJ. Effects of experimental loss of teeth on the temporomandibular joints. *J Oral Rehabil* 1986; 13:587–598.
62. Solberg WK. Temporomandibular disorders: background and the clinical problem. *Br Dent J* 1986; 160:157–161.
63. Bell WE. *Temporomandibular disorders. Classification, diagnosis, management*, 3rd ed. Chicago: Year Book Medical Publishers, 1990.
64. Ronning O, Valiaho ML. The involvement of the temporomandibular joint in juvenile rheumatoid arthritis. *Scand J Rheumatol* 1974; 3:89–96.
65. Nwoku AL, Koch H. The temporomandibular joint: a rare localization for bone tumors. *J Maxillofac Surg* 1974; 2:113–119.
66. Daspit PC, Spetzler RF. Synovial chondromatosis of the temporomandibular joint with intracranial extension. *J Neurosurg* 1989; 70:121–123.
67. Rabey GP. Bilateral mandibular condylysis: a morphoanalytic diagnosis. *Br J Oral Surg* 1977; 15:121–134.

68. Eagle W. Elongated styloid process: further observations and new syndrome. *Arch Otolarlyngol Head Neck Surg* 1948; 47:630–640.
69. Steinmann E. A new light on the pathogenesis of the styloid syndrome. *Arch Otolaryngol Head Neck Surg* 1970; 91:171–174.
70. Lengele BG, Dhem AJ. Length of the styloid process of the temporal bone. *Arch Otolaryngol Head Neck Surg* 1988; 114:1003–1006.
71. Sivers JE, Johnson GK. Diagnosis of Eagle's syndrome. *Oral Surg Oral Med Oral Path* 1985; 59:575–577.
72. Correll RW, Jensen JL, Taylor JB, Rhyne RR. Mineralization of the stylohyoid-stylomandibular ligament complex. *Oral Surg Oral Med Oral Path* 1979; 48:286–291.
73. Schmidt OV. Elongated styloid process which interfered with function of a singer's voice. *Arch Otolaryngol* 1950; 54:417–421.
74. Sataloff RT, Price DB. Mandibular osteotomy complicated by styloid pain. *Oral Surg Oral Med Oral Path* 1983; 56:25–27.
75. Wright V, Johns RJ. Quantitative and qualitative analysis of joint stiffness in normal subjects and in patients with connective tissue diseases. *Ann Rheum Diseases* 1961; 20:36–45.
76. Beighton PH, Solomon L, Soskolne CL. Articular mobility in an African population. *Ann Rheum Disease* 1973; 32:413–417.
77. Westling L. Craniomandibular disorders and general joint mobility. *Acta Odont Scand* 1989; 47:293–299.
78. Bates RE, Stewart CM, Atkinson WB. The relationship between internal derangements of the temporomandibular joint and systemic joint laxity. *J Am Dent Assoc* 1984; 109:446–447.
79. Harinstein D, Buckingham RB, Braun T, Oral K, Bauman DH, Killian PJ, Bidula LP. Systemic joint laxity (the hypermobile joint syndrome) is associated with TMJ dysfunction. *Arthritis Rheum* 1988; 31:1259–1264.
80. Rushton JG, Stevens JC, Miller RH. Glossopharyngeal (vagoglossopharyngeal) neuralgia: a study of 217 cases. *Arch Neurol* 1981; 38:201–205.
81. Kjellin K, Müller R, Widen L. Glossopharyngeal neuralgia associated with cardiac arrest and hypersecretion from the ipsilateral parotid gland. *Neurol* 1959; 9:527–532.
82. Olson RE, Walters CL, Powell WJ. Gustatory sweating caused by blunt trauma. *J Oral Surg* 1977; 35:306–308.
83. Laage-Hellman JE. Gustatory sweating and flushing: etiologic implications of latent periods and mode of development after parotidectomy. *Acta Otolaryngol* (Stockh) 1958; 49:306–314.
84. Daly RF. New observations regarding the auriculotemporal syndrome. *Neurol* 1967; 17:1159–1168.
85. Laage-Hellman JE. Treatment of gustatory sweating and flushing. *Acta Otolaryngol* 1958; 49:132–143.
86. Couch JR. Cluster headache: characteristics and treatment. *Semin Neurol* 1982; 2:30–40.
87. Solberg WK, Graff-Radford SB. Orodental considerations in facial pain. *Semin Neurol* 1988; 8:318–323.
88. Kreisberg MK. Atypical odontalgia: differential diagnosis and treatment. *J Am Dent Assoc* 1982; 104:852–854.
89. Rees RT, Harris M. Atypical odontalgia. *Br J Oral Surg* 1978; 16:212–218.
90. Remick RA, Blasberg B. Psychiatric aspects of atypical facial pain. *J Canad Dent Assoc* 1985; 12:913–916.
91. Sullivan PD. The diagnosis and treatment of psychogenic glossodynia. *Ear Nose Throat J* 1989; 68:795–798.
92. Dreizen S. Systemic significance of glossitis. *Postgrad Med* 1984; 75:207–215.
93. Glass BJ. Drug-induced xerostomia as a cause of glossodynia. *Ear Nose Throat J* 1989; 68:776–781.
94. Rhodus NL. Xerostomia and glossodynia in patients with autoimmune disorders. *Ear Nose Throat J* 1989; 68:791–794.
95. Bengtsson BA, Malmvall BE. Giant cell arteritis. *Acta Med Scand* 1982; (Suppl 658):1–102.
96. Healey LA, Wilske KR. *The systemic manifestations of temporal arteritis.* New York: Grune and Stratton, 1978.
97. Caselli RJ, Hunder GC, Whisnant JP. Neurologic disease in biopsy-proven giant cell (temporal) arteritis. *Neurol* 1988; 38:352–359.
98. Mellgren SI, Conn DL, Stevens JC, Dyck PJ. Peripheral neuropathy in primary Sjögren's syndrome. *Neurol* 1989; 39:390–394.

99. Gussen R. Atypical ossicle joint lesions in rheumatoid arthritis with Sicca syndrome (Sjögren's Syndrome). *Arch Otolaryngol* 1977; 103:284–286.
100. Doig JA, Whaley K, Dick WC. Otolaryngological aspects of Sjögren's syndrome. *Br Med J* 1971; 4:460–463.
101. Halmi KA, Falk JR, Schwartz E. Binge eating and vomiting: a survey of a college population. *Psychologic Med* 1981; 11:697–706.
102. Eccles JD. Erosion affecting the palatal surfaces of upper anterior teeth in young people. *Br Dent J* 1982; 152:375–378.
103. Levin PA, Falko JA, et al. Benign parotid enlargement in bulimia. *Ann Intern Med* 1980; 93:827–829.
104. Yunus MB, Kalyan-Raman UP, Kaylan-Raman K. Primary fibromyalgia syndrome and myofascial pain syndrome: clinical features and muscle pathology. *Arch Phys Med Rehab* 1988; 69:451–454.
105. Tunks E, Crook J, Norman G, Kalaher S. Tender points in fibromyalgia. *Pain* 1988; 34:11–19.
106. Buckelew SP. Fibromyalgia. A rehabilitation approach. *Am J Phys Med Rehab* 1989; 68:37–42.
107. Dunn RH. Selecting a musical wind instrument for a student with orofacial muscle problems. *Int J Orthod* 1982; 20:19–22.
108. Basmajian JV, White ER. Neuromuscular control of trumpeter's lips. *Nature* 1973; 241:170.
109. Herman E. Orthodontic aspects of musical instrument selection. *Am J Orthod* 1974; 65:519–530.
110. Bejjani FJ, Halpern N. Postural kinematics of trumpet playing. *J Biomech* 1989; 22:439–446.
111. Blanton PL, Biggs NL, Perkins RC. Electromyographic analysis of the buccinator muscle. *J Dent Res* 1970; 49:389–394.
112. Williams WN, Vaughn AO, Cornell CE. Bilabial compression force discrimination by human subjects. *J Oral Rehabil* 1988; 15:269–275.
113. White ER, Basmajian JV. Electromyography of lip muscles and their role in trumpet playing. *J Appl Physiol* 1973; 35:892–897.
114. Strayer ER. Musical instruments as an aid in the treatment of muscle defects and perversions. *Angle Orthod* 1939; 9:18–27.
115. Angle EH. *Malocclusion of the Teeth*. Philadelphia: White Dental Co., 1907.
116. Blake S. A study of the incidence of malocclusion and facial characteristics in Seattle high school students, aged fifteen to twenty years. Master thesis, Department of Orthodontics, University of Washington, 1954.
117. Engleman JA. Measurement of perioral pressures during the playing of musical wind instruments. *Am J Orthod* 1965; 51:856–864.
118. Herman E. Influence of musical instruments on tooth positions. *Am J Orthod* 1981; 80:145–155.
119. Shimada T. A morphologic study on the effect of wind instruments on the dento-oral region with reference to the growing young people. *J Nihon Univ Sch Dent* 1978; 20:23–36.
120. Pang A. Relation of musical wind instruments to malocclusion. *J Am Dent Assoc* 1976; 92:565–570.
121. Gualtieri PA. May Johnny or Janie play the clarinet? *Am J Orthod* 1979; 76:260–276.
122. Seidner S. The importance of the dental condition for players of wind instruments. *Dent Abstr* 1957; 2:68–69.
123. Cheney EA. Adaptation to embouchure as a function of dentofacial complex. *Am J Orthod* 1949; 35:440–456.
124. Ingervall B, Eliasson GB. Effect of lip training in children with short upper lip. *Angle Orthod* 1982; 52:222–233.
125. Fuhrimann S, Schupbach A, Thuer U, Ingervall B. Natural lip function in wind instrument players. *Eur J Orthod* 1987; 9:216–223.
126. Parker J. The Alameda instrumentalist study. *Am J Orthod* 1957; 43:399–415.
127. Lamp CJ, Epley FW. Relation of tooth evenness to performance on brass and woodwind musical instruments. *J Am Dent Assoc* 1935; 22:1232–1236.
128. Newmark J, Lederman RL. Practice doesn't necessarily make perfect: incidence of overuse syndromes in amateur instrumentalists. *Med Probl Perform Art* 1987; 2:142–144.
129. Lederman RJ. Occupational cramp in instrumental musicians. *Med Probl Perform Art* 1988; 3:45–51.
130. Morimoto T, Takebe H, Sakan I, Kawamura Y. Reflex activation of the extrinsic tongue muscles by jaw closing muscle proprioceptors. *Jap J Physiol* 1978; 29:461–471.
131. Krivin M. An embouchure aid for clarinet and saxophone players. *J Am Dent Assoc* 1975; 90:1277–1281.
132. Nixon G. Dental problems of the brass instrumentalist. *Br Dent J* 1963; 105:160–161.

133. Hellsing E, L'Estrange P. Changes in lip pressure following extension and flexion of the head and at changed mode of breathing. *Am J Orthod Dentofac Orthop* 1987; 91:286–294.

134. Dibbell GD, Ewanowski S, Carter WL. Successful correction of velopharyngeal stress incompetence in musicians playing wind instruments. *Plast Reconstr Surg* 1979; 65:662–664.

135. Planas J. Rupture of the orbicularis oris in trumpet players (Satchmo's syndrome). *Plast Reconstr Surg* 1982; 69:690–693.

136. Hart CW, Logermann JA. Tonsils and adenoids and the professional musician. *Med Probl Perform Art* 1986; 1:58–63.

137. Mortenson GC, Kolar LW. Understanding the procedures and risks involved in the extraction of third molars. *Med Probl Perform Art* 1988; 3:119–122.

138. Smith R, Levine H. Hypopharyngeal dilatation in musicians: etiology and treatment. *Med Probl Perform Art* 1986; 1:20–23.

139. Saunders HF. Wind parotitis. *N Engl J Med* 1973; 289:698.

140. Bryan AH. Mouthpiece hygiene: Wind instrument mouthpieces harbor countless disease germs. *Instrumentalist* 1965; 10:20–24.

141. Calabrese LH. AIDS in the performing arts. *Med Probl Perform Art* 1987; 2:113–116.

142. Friedland GH, Saltzman BR, Rogers MF, et al. Lack of transmission of HTLV-III/LAV infection to household contacts of patients with AIDS or AIDS-related complex with oral candidiasis. *N Engl J Med* 1986; 314:344–349.

143. Taylor JS. Dermatological problems of performing artists. *Symposium on medical problems of musicians and dancers.* Cleveland Clinic Foundation, 1988;74–78.

144. Dahl MC. Flautist's chin: a companion to fiddler's neck. *Br Med J* 1978; 2:1023.

145. Proffit WR. Contemporary Orthodontics. St. Louis: C.V. Mosby, 1986;228–236.

146. Barbenel JC, Kenny P, Davies JB. Mouthpiece forces produced while playing the trumpet. *J Biomech* 1988; 21:417–424.

147. Cremmel R, Frank RM. Pulp syndrome of wind instrument players. *Rev Fr Odontostomatol* 1971; 18:1027–1037.

148. Anstendig H, Kronman J. A histologic study of pulpal reaction to orthodontic tooth movement in dogs. *Angle Orthod* 1972, 42:50–55.

149. Bergstrom J, Eliasson S. Alveolar bone height in professional musicians. *Acta Odont Scand* 1986; 44:141–147.

150. Lovius B, Huggins DG. Orthodontics and the wind instrumentalist. *J Dentistry* 1973; 2:65–68.

151. Crawford PM. The flautist's shield. *Br J Orthod* 1981; 8:147–148.

152. Fine L. Dental problems in the wind instrumentalist. *Clev Clin Quart* 1986; 53:3–9.

153. Langer K. Dentures for wind instrument players. *Quintessence Int* 1973; 7:45–46.

154. Porter MM. Dental problems in wind instrument playing: single reed instruments—the embouchure denture. *Br Dent J* 1968; 124:34–36.

155. Koskinen-Moffett L. Pain behind the flute? *National Flute Association* Winter 1984.

156. Morasky RL, Creech R, Sowell LE. Generalization of lowered EMG levels during musical performance following biofeedback training. *Biofeedback Self Regul* 1983; 8:207–216.

157. Levee JR, Cohen MJ, Rickles WH. Electromyographic biofeedback for relief of tension in the facial and throat muscles of a woodwind musician. *Biofeedback Self Regul* 1976; 1:113–120.

158. Kelly J, Harvey C. An assessment of the teeth of youths 12–17 years. Washington, D.C., National Center for Health Statistics, U.S. Public Health Service 1977; DHEW Publication No. (HRA):77–1164.

159. Howard, JA, Lovrovich AT: Wind Instruments: Their interplay with orofacial structures. *Med Probl Perform Art* 1989; 4:59–72.

159a. Coles RR. Epidemiology of tinnitus. *Tinnitus: Ciba Foundation Symposium* 1981; No. 85:16–35.

160. Steffan PK. The problem of noise-induced hearing loss in musicians. *J Am Tinnitus Assoc* 1990.

161. Berg B. *American Music Conference Reports.* Chicago: American Music Conference, 1983.

162. Fishbein M, Middlestadt SE, Ottati V, Straus S, Ellis A. Medical problems among ICSOM musicians: Overview of a national survey. *Med Probl Perform* 1988; Art 3:1–8.

163. Harman SE. Occupational diseases of instrumental musicians: literature review. *Maryland State Med J* 1982; 31:39–41.

164. Hoppmann RA. Patrone NA. A review of musculoskeletal problems in instrumental musicians. *Semin Arthritis Rheum* 1989; 19:117–126.

165. Lederman RJ. Peripheral nerve disorders in instrumentalists. *Ann Neuro* 1989; 16:640–646.

166. Barrier CH, Hirschowitz BI. Controversies in the detection and management of nonsteroidal anti-

inflammatory drug-induced side effects of the upper gastrointestinal tract. *Arthritis Rheum* 1989; 32:926–932.

167. Goodwin JS, Regan M. Cognitive dysfunction associated with naproxen and ibuprofen in the elderly. *Arthritis Rheum* 1982; 25:1013–1015.

168. *American Medical Association Drug Evaluations: Drugs used to treat skeletal disorders*, 6th ed. Chicago: 1986.

169. Kreisberg MK. Tricyclic antidepressants: analgesic effect and indications in orofacial pain. *J Craniomandib Disord Facial Oral Pain* 1988; 2:171–177.

170. Stefanich RJ. Intraarticular corticosteroids in treatment of osteoarthritis. *Orthop Rev* 1986; 15:65–71.

171. Clark GT. A critical evaluation of orthopedic interocclusal appliance therapy, part I: theory, design, and overall effectiveness. *J Am Dent Assoc* 1984; 108:359–364.

172. Moloney F, Howard JA. Internal derangments of the temporomandibular joint. III. Anterior repositioning splint therapy. *Austral Dent J* 1986; 31:30–39.

173. Nickerson JW, Boering G. Natural course of osteoarthrosis as it relates to internal derangements of the temporomandibular joint. *Oral Maxillofac Surg Clin North Am* 1989; 1:27–45.

174. Sanders B, Buoncristiana R. Diagnostic and surgical arthroscopy of the temporomandibular joint: clinical experience with 137 procedures over a 2-year period. *J Craniomand Disord Facial Oral Pain* 1987; 1:202–213.

175. Holmlund A, Hellsing G, Axelsson S. The temporomandibular joint: a comparison of clinical and arthroscopic findings. *J Prosthet Dent* 1989; 6 2:61–65.

176. Lockwood AH. Medical problems of musicians. *N Engl J Med* 1989; 320:221–227.

Textbook of Performing Arts Medicine, edited
by R. T. Sataloff, A. Brandfonbrener, and
R. Lederman. Raven Press, Ltd.,
New York © 1991.

5

Neurological Problems of Performing Artists

Richard J. Lederman

*Department of Neurology and Director, Medical Center for Performing Artists,
Cleveland Clinic Foundation, Cleveland, Ohio 44195*

It is difficult to think of any activities that make greater demands on the nervous system than the performing arts. Virtually all forms of music, dance, and the dramatic arts require an extraordinary level of sensorimotor control, precision, speed, endurance, and in some cases strength. The qualities of artistic sensitivity, interpretation, and creativity must be combined with the above largely executive functions under the most stressful circumstances—performance before an audience including one's peers and critics. Every aspect of this is, of course, under the control of, and influenced by, the nervous system. It is beyond the scope of this chapter to review the complex functions of the nervous system or to analyze the various neurological and other factors that go into the making of a performing artist. Rather, this discussion presents an approach to clinical problems encountered among performing artists from the perspective of a neurologist. This will require at least some introduction to the process by which a neurologist evaluates a problem, the tools which are available to and utilized by the clinician for this analysis, and the ways in which these tools may be applied specifically to the disorders encountered in performing artists. We will confine the discussion largely to those ailments which specifically impact upon the ability to perform or sustain a performance career. Three prior reviews, reflecting somewhat different experiences and perspectives, are available (1–3).

THE NEUROLOGICAL EVALUATION

The neurologist begins by eliciting a description of the main problem for which the performer is seeking help or advice, referred to most frequently as the "chief complaint". This must be thoroughly elaborated upon and as much relevant information as possible obtained, most effectively by a combination of spontaneous exposition by the patient and directed questions by the examiner. In the case of performing artists, the information must be placed not only in the context of the general medical history but also in the setting of the artistic endeavor itself. As part of this specialized history, one needs to know how the problem relates to the performing art. Did the difficulty arise out of performance or from some unrelated activity? How does it affect performance?

It is often necessary to inquire about practice and performance schedules. In the case of the instrumentalist or vocalist, one needs to ask about duration of practice sessions, length and number of performances, and total daily or weekly time devoted to the instrument. In addition to the time spent, the "intensity" of the activity may be an important factor. This more nebulous quantity leads to a discussion of the repertoire being played or sung, the amount of repetitious activity that may be required, and the urgency with which it is being prepared. A violin student who is desperately attempting to master the fourth "Paganini Caprice," with its rapidly played double stops and tenths, spending hours a day prior to the lesson or audition repeating the relevant passages, may be subject to greater stresses than someone practicing a varied repertoire over an even longer period of time. We have noted (4,5), as have others (6,7), that sudden increases in either duration of instrumental activity or this ill-defined playing "intensity" may precipitate the development of symptoms. In the case of instrumentalists, one may need to ask about changes in the instrument itself or in various devices that are used to modify it. Violinists and violists may have recently changed chin or shoulder rests, a cellist may have begun using a different end pin, the oboist may have purchased a new instrument with different sound qualities or may have begun working with a new reed, and a flutist may have finally been able to afford a new gold flute with resultant change in weight and feel of the instrument. When evaluating students, one also inquires about recent changes in teacher or in technique. Students may begin to have problems after they change teachers; they may be told that everything they had learned previously is "wrong" and they must change the way they hold the bow or must alter their embouchure. One must further inquire about apparently unrelated activities that may impact upon the performance. A student who has taken on a job as a cashier or the young professional who has begun playing racquetball may be utilizing muscles similar to those required for instrument playing, adding to the total neuromuscular burden and precipitating the current symptoms. One also must not fail to inquire about the emotional and psychological stresses and strains under which the performer is laboring. These, of course, may have profound effect on the individual's well-being as well as on the perception of or tolerance for what might otherwise be relatively minor problems. The economic and interpersonal stresses to which the performer may be subject are often overlooked in the analysis of a somatic symptom and, not infrequently, the student or performer may not volunteer this information or recognize its relation to the problem being discussed.

The neurological examination has traditionally been subdivided along anatomical and physiological lines. A commonly used method would include sequential testing of mental status, the cranial nerves, motor systems, sensory systems, and reflexes. This, of course, is only one segment of the "complete" physical examination; the decision regarding the extent of the exam must be made by the neurologist based upon individual circumstances. Even within the neurological examination itself, certain portions may be emphasized and others performed in a more perfunctory manner, depending on the specific problem as well as upon the skills and experience of the examining physician. In this regard, the performing artist is no different from other patients and no specific guidelines need be suggested here.

The examination of the musician is supplemented whenever possible by observation while playing or singing. This is especially critical for problems which occur largely, if not exclusively, during performance. At times, this may present a number of logistical problems. The instrumentalist must be sufficiently disrobed while playing to allow the physician to examine posture and relevant portions of the anatomy; this may be accomplished using an examining gown or occasionally a swimsuit. Instrumentalists should be instructed to bring their instruments with them, if possible. Access to a piano or electronic keyboard should be arranged for the physician seeing more than an occasional musician. Videotaping of this portion of the examination may be invaluable in analyzing mechanical inefficiency and technical faults as well as allowing careful and repeated review of posture and position.

In addition to the history and examination, a variety of ancillary tools are also available to the neurologist. These are chosen as they would be in any other setting and may include blood (or other body fluid) analysis; x-ray; neuroimaging techniques such as computerized tomography (CT) scan and magnetic resonance imaging (MRI); and electrodiagnostic testing such as nerve conduction study, needle (or surface) electromyography (the two of these are generally considered parts of one test, the EMG), and evoked potentials, particularly somatosensory evoked potentials (SEP). These procedures supplement and extend the neurological examination and may provide critical information unobtainable otherwise. Techniques which are currently experimental, such as motion analysis or magnetic resonance spectroscopy, may someday prove indispensable for effective evaluation of neuromuscular problems.

DEVELOPMENTAL DISORDERS AND EFFECTS OF AGING

It seems unnecessary to state at the outset that performing artists are subject to any and all of the ailments which affect other groups. Any disease, of course, that would cause sufficient physical or mental disability at an early enough age to preclude development of musical skills, such as certain congenital or early-onset neurological disorders, may indeed never be seen in a performer. One possible exception to this might be the severely retarded or autistic child or adult who may have special musical talent (the "idiot" or "autistic savant"). Because precocious musical talent may show itself in early childhood, it is conceivable that the neurologist could encounter a neurological problem in a performer as young as 4 or 5 years of age. At the other end of the spectrum, performers, particularly instrumentalists, may continue well into their 80s or beyond. Thus the age range for neurological problems potentially may span 8 or even 9 decades. It is my experience, however, that the performer seeking neurological advice tends to be relatively young; the average age of referred performers in my practice is about 32 years, with a range from 10 to 80 years.

Aging, of course, has its effects on performers as much as, if not more than, on others. There is very little scientific data regarding this point. Certainly it is the conventional wisdom that aging takes its toll on dancers, particularly those in ballet, earlier than on any other group of performers. Instrumental musicians also may vary in their sensitivity to aging. It is generally suggested that keyboard and string instrumentalists may continue to play considerably longer than woodwind and brass players, but this may have more to do with respiratory function than neurological abnormality. The long performance life of some conductors is, of course, legendary as it is in the case of some actors and actresses. The length of performance careers in vocalists is intermediate.

In any group of performers, however, aging certainly influences performance. Many would agree that what is lost in neuromuscular function, particularly in speed and accuracy of movement, is compensated for by increasing artistry and interpretive powers. This is not always the case, of course. Famed violinist Mischa Elman may have said it best in the twilight of his career: "You know, the critics never change; I'm still getting the same notices I used to get as a child. They tell me I play very well for my age" (8).

The neuroanatomical and neurophysiological substrata for performance changes with aging are incompletely understood. Certainly a number of alterations are known to occur in the aging nervous system: there is gradual decrease in brain weight with gyral atrophy and progressive attrition of neurons; microscopic changes occur in dendritic processes and synaptic connections; a variety of chemical changes have been identified in the aging nervous system, including the activity of enzyme systems influencing neurotransmitters and the accumulation of an intraneuronal pigment called lipofuscin; changes in conduction properties of peripheral nerve are known to occur; and aging produces alteration in muscle fibers as well (9).

NEUROLOGICAL DISORDERS

Neurological disorders of performers may be divided into three basic categories. The first, which will be dealt with only briefly and very incompletely, would include those which would affect performing artists to a degree no greater or lesser than any other group. These presumably would be seen in the same proportion in performers at any given age as they would in others. The interested reader is referred to any of a number of excellent textbooks for a fuller discussion of these disorders. The second group to be considered will be those that affect performing artists with frequency equal to others, but may adversely affect performing artists more than other groups. The bulk of these disorders have specific impact on the sensorimotor systems and impair the execution of the performing art. The third and final group of disorders are those that seem preferentially to affect performing artists. Whether there is a real or only apparent increase in frequency is very difficult to say; indeed, there are no adequate statistical data to support the idea that the performing artist is in fact disproportionately affected. Nonetheless, this group of disorders accounts for a substantial percentage of performing artists who seek neurologic care for performance-related problems (4,10) and a somewhat lower proportion seeing nonneurologists, as expected (11,12). The bulk of this chapter will deal specifically with these disorders.

DISORDERS AFFECTING PERFORMERS AND NONPERFORMERS ALIKE

One would expect common neurological conditions which have neither special predilection for, nor particularly debilitating effects on, performing artists to be as common a reason for neurological consultation in this group as in any other. In this group would be such entities as the common forms of headache, including migraine or vascular headaches, muscle contraction or tension-type headaches, and others. As in the general population, these disorders are rarely debilitating but can be a cause of frequent discomfort, annoyance, and at times hours or even days of diminished productivity. The large number of medications available both for symptomatic treatment and as prophylactic regimens allows successful control in the majority of patients. A variety of nonpharmacologic approaches, such as dietary manipulation and relaxation techniques, offers satisfactory alternatives in some patients. These forms of treatment may often appeal to performing artists particularly and should be offered and supported by the sympathetic physician. Two examples of performers with headache serve to illustrate a number of features, the first of chronic tension-type (muscle contraction) headache plus occasional migraine, and the second of migraine with aura (classic or neurologic).

A 22-year-old cello student has had headaches for the past four years. These have varied from occasional severe, throbbing, largely unilateral headaches with nausea and photophobia, lasting up to 8–12 hours, to frequent nagging, bandlike headaches which might fluctuate in intensity over several days. Headaches would worsen with stress and would be aggravated by prolonged practice or playing. General and neurologic examination was normal. Physical therapy and amitriptyline were prescribed, with substantial reduction in frequency and severity of headaches.

A 25-year-old right-handed violinist was rehearsing with an ensemble when she noted spots before her eyes as if exposed to a bright flash. She then noted that the left half of a colleague's face was dark and obscured by the spots. These symptoms lasted about 15 minutes. She felt light-headed, and when she tried to write, she noted that her spelling was impaired. Twenty minutes later her right hand became cold and seemed swollen. Numbness then began in the right little finger and spread across the entire hand to the arm and then into the right lower jaw. She was unable to feel the bow as she tried to play, and her arm felt "disembodied." Over the next hour the numbness dissipated. She has a history of frequent headaches for many years but never one which could be considered severe, and there was no nausea. One of these headaches had occurred the morning of the episode, and she had another the following day as well. The patient's mother has migraine and her father a history of epilepsy. The patient smokes about one pack of cigarettes a day. She takes no medications. Neurological examination 2 days after the episode was normal. No further episodes occurred over the next 6 months, without treatment.

Another very common neurological problem which may be encountered in the performing artist is epilepsy, or seizure disorder. Symptomatic forms of epilepsy, those associated with structural or metabolic diseases affecting the nervous system, are infrequently encountered; the disability in these cases is more likely due to the underlying central nervous system disease than to the seizures which result from it. Idiopathic epilepsy, however, may occur in performing artists and tends to appear during the second and third decades particularly, although first seizures may occur well into middle and later years. Therefore, the performing artist may have a fully established career at the time of onset, and this can create a potentially devastating situation. The highly effective and relatively safe anticonvulsants which are currently available allow adequate, if not complete, control in most patients and a number of performers continue successful careers despite seizure disorders. Poor control with frequent seizures represents a very serious limitation to a successful performing arts career, as well as to many others. Details of medical as well as other forms of treatment, including surgery, for epilepsy are beyond the scope of this discussion.

This 35-year-old pianist had an episode of loss of consciousness at age 14 years, accompanied by vomiting and urinary incontinence. At age 25 there was an episode of transient unresponsiveness without loss of consciousness, lasting about 30 seconds. The patient subsequently began to experience sensations of déjà vu and perceptual distortion. One episode of repetitive speech and writing also occurred, associated with drooling and urinary incontinence. Subsequent evaluation included a normal CT scan of the head and a normal EEG, awake and asleep. Anticonvulsant medications in both single and multiple drug regimens have been only partially successful in controlling the episodes.

The special problem of so-called musicogenic epilepsy (13) deserves brief mention here. It is well recognized that certain sensory stimuli, such as flashing lights, can precipitate or trigger seizures in susceptible individuals. Less commonly, auditory input may trigger seizures, and there have been cases in which music has been the precipitating stimulus, even specific tunes or instruments. This very rare form of "reflex epilepsy" may be treated by anticonvulsant medications as well as by sensory desensitization; in a few patients, psychotherapy may be helpful. This disorder is said to occur more often in those with musical talent, although the author is not aware of a case involving a professional performer.

Another very common neurological disorder which may be expected to occur frequently in performing artists is Alzheimer's disease. As in the general population, this disorder is most likely to strike older age groups, when retirement is either imminent or already in effect, thus mitigating the impact on the performing career. This does not, however, diminish the devastation on the life of the performer or the family. Since Alzheimer's disease affects motor performance relatively later and less severely than memory and other higher cortical functions, instrumental playing may continue to be technically acceptable although the gradual impoverishment of intellect and affect or emotional expression will have deleterious effects on the creative and interpretive aspects of performance. Composer-pianist Maurice Ravel may have suffered from Alzheimer's disease or a related condition, rendering him unable to compose or play (14–16). As the number of aging performers and former performers increases along with the number of elderly in the general population, this problem will be seen with increasing frequency, but it will probably not represent a greater problem in the performing arts community than in any other.

The majority of strokes, an extremely common neurological problem in the general population, have equally damaging effects on performers and nonperformers. The severity of the residual deficit after recovery, be it in the realm of cognitive, behavioral, sensory, or motor function, will be the major factor determining the patient's ability to return to a productive performing arts career, as is the case in most other fields. Because strokes so often affect motor function, particularly of the fingers and hand (due in part to the large representation of the fingers and hand within the motor control centers of the brain), even minor residual deficits are likely to have relatively profound effects on the ability of an instrumentalist, in particular, to continue his or her career. In this case, stroke may be considered an example of the second category of neurological disease, that which would be particularly devastating to a performer. This aspect will be discussed below, along with the rare circumstance in which stroke specifically affects musical language.

A large number of other less common neurological disorders, including brain tumors, nervous system infections, and toxic or metabolic disorders, are also equally likely to interrupt and perhaps terminate the performing artist's career as any other. These will not be dealt with further here. However, an example of a central nervous system infection that may be more prevalent among performing artists than among those in other occupational groups is HIV infection (17). This prevalence is not the result of the performing arts career itself, of course, but is due to the relatively higher frequency of homosexuality among performing (and creative) artists than in the population at large. AIDS, which has already caused such devastation in the performing arts centers, particularly on the coasts of this country, commonly affects the nervous system. Primary infection of the brain by HIV, the presumed cause of AIDS encephalopathy/dementia, as well as of secondary infection with toxoplasmosis or cytomegalic inclusion disease, is being recognized in increasing numbers of AIDS patients and is now one of the most common manifestations of the disorder. Malignant brain tumors, particularly lymphoma and progressive multifocal leukoencephalopathy, are also being seen with increasing frequency. Vacuolar myelopathy and various forms of peripheral nerve and muscle disease are other neurological complications; all of these forms of neurological involvement may cause devastating effects. It can only be assumed that this will become an increasingly prevalent problem among performers as well as in the general population.

An example of selective involvement of certain performing arts groups with a toxic disorder of the nervous system would be the occurrence of drug and alcohol-related problems. Here again, it is not that the chemical substances have greater effects in performers but only that certain groups seem more prone to experiment with, and therefore become addicted to, these substances. Among the reasons cited for this are the high levels of stress in the performing arts and the relative willingness in this community to tolerate and, in some cases, encourage, wider ranges of lifestyle and behavior (18).

DISORDERS HAVING MORE PROFOUND EFFECTS ON PERFORMERS THAN ON OTHERS

A number of neurological disorders will be found to have particularly devastating effects on performing artists, despite being no more frequent among those in this group than in any other. Mostly these are disorders which in some way disrupt motor function and control. What might be a tolerable and minor motor deficit for someone in a career demanding less rigorous neuromuscular control may prove sufficient to end, or severely curtail, the career of a performing artist. A related phenomenon may at times tax the diagnostic acumen of the neurologist. The exquisite sensorimotor demands of the performing artist may bring the patient to clinical attention at such an early stage that diagnosis may be extremely difficult and routine neurological examination may well be "normal." This certainly happens in other groups as well, particularly in disorders that are characterized by fluctuations. The neurologist must avoid the temptation to reassure the performing artist that "nothing is wrong" or to conclude that the problem is "functional" or largely psychogenic. As in many other circumstances in clinical medicine, the best defense against this common error is a careful history and physical examination, serial observation, and above all, a firm commitment to "listen to the patient."

The first disorder to consider in this category is multiple sclerosis. This disease, which generally has its onset in the third and fourth decades and hence is most likely to appear in the young performing artist just establishing a career, can have effects on virtually any function of the nervous system. In its episodic form there are brief or more prolonged exacerbations or flare-ups, followed by remissions. The fleeting, and sometimes vague, disturbances of visual or sensorimotor dysfunction can sometimes present insurmountable problems in diagnosis despite recent development of highly sensitive, if not specific, diagnostic studies.

A 39-year-old right-handed French hornist had an episode of low back pain with leg weakness and incoordination 9 years previously. Because of subsequent easy fatigability, she stopped playing for 3 years. She then resumed playing the French horn but would experience episodes of severe fatigue of the facial and jaw muscles. Three years previously, a neurologist found slight pupillary asymmetry, right greater than left hyperreflexia, and bilateral Babinski responses. Because of the fatigue, an EMG was performed, including repetitive stimulation, and was normal.

She subsequently was able to play for up to an hour at a time, although fatigue of the jaw and facial muscles continued to be a problem. Our examination revealed right esotropia and slight facial asymmetry but no convincing weakness or impairment of motor control. There was slight asymmetry of speed of movement in the fingers and toes, left slower than right, and slight left hyperreflexia. Over the next 3 years, multifocal but fluctuating neurological symptoms and signs developed, further strengthening the suspicion of demyelinating disease.

In the more chronic progressive form, which may be a later phase in a patient who has begun with exacerbations and remissions, or may be the primary presentation, the question of diagnosis usually revolves around distinguishing this from other causes of progressive neurological deficit, such as degenerative diseases, tumors, and in the case of myelopathies, spinal cord compression. Here again, the array of relatively newer diagnostic studies such as MRI, evoked potentials, and sophisticated spinal fluid analysis may be of immense help in confirming the diagnosis of multiple sclerosis or in excluding other diseases.

A 46-year-old right-handed clarinetist had an episode of optic neuropathy 20 years previously. Five years later he noted difficulty with the left leg and developed paresthesias down the legs with neck flexion. He continued to play in a symphony without difficulty until 7 years previously, when he first noted difficulty with sensation and fine motor control in the right hand. The symptoms have progressed slowly, and he now has impairment in all four limbs, right worse than left, along with some difficulties with bladder control. Spinal fluid analysis showed oligoclonal bands, and MRI of the head revealed multiple periventricular areas of abnormal signal intensity. MRI of the cervical spinal cord also showed an area of abnormal signal. The patient has become progressively disabled and is no longer able to maintain his position in the orchestra.

Another ailment that can be very subtle in its earliest stages and still impair motor function significantly is Parkinson's disease. This disorder is most common in the aging population but not infrequently begins in the fifth or sixth decades, potentially at the peak of an instrumentalist's career. It is characterized by tremor most notable at rest, difficulty in initiating and sustaining repetitive movements, muscle rigidity, and impaired equilibrium. Changes in the voice are also common, leading to impairment of volume and control of articulation, both of which may be clearly evident to the performer and to the sophisticated listener but unimpressive to the musically naive. If the characteristic resting tumor is present early on, the diagnosis is relatively easy to confirm. It should be noted that this tremor is usually not a major cause of disability in performers or in others, although it can be extremely annoying and embarrassing. Because it tends to be ameliorated with voluntary action, it impairs motor function during performance only infrequently and to modest degree. In those who do not have prominent tremor, one must look for the more subtle postural changes and deficiencies in fine motor control that will likely bring the performer to the physician. Once again, serial evaluation is the most effective tool in making the diagnosis, since ancillary studies are not of significant help.

This 59-year-old right-handed double bass player began noting left shoulder and arm pain 1 1/2 years previously, along with some stiffness of the hand and fingers. Over the last 6 months he has lost facility with the left hand and is unable to play. He describes "cramping" and the need for increased effort to place his fingers on the fingerboard. He also had problems buttoning his clothes and getting his wallet out of his left rear pocket. He has noted that the left foot may scuff along the floor on occasion. When he swims, his wife has noted that his left arm makes a much smaller excursion than the right. Examination revealed asymmetric facial hypokinesia, left greater than right, and abnormal posture of the left hand and arm, which was held stiffly and moved much less than the right. There was slightly increased tone in the left arm which greatly increased during contralateral finger tapping. Repetitive finger movements on the left were difficult to sustain. There was diminished arm swing on the left with walking. A diagnosis of Parkinson's disease was made and treatment with carbidopa-levodopa, MSD (Sinemet) was instituted. This allowed him to continue most daily activities but was insufficient to allow him to play his instrument effectively. He has retired from the orchestra and is in business.

To be differentiated from the tremor of Parkinsonism is the more common and, for the performer, sometimes more debilitating problem of essential tremor. This is a tremor occurring with activity, either sustained antigravity posture or voluntary action. It tends to affect primarily the hands, the neck muscles, and, on occasion, the muscles of the face, jaw, and of vocalization. It will generally be most troublesome to the string player, in that it will interfere with bow control or vibrato; and to the wind player or vocalist, in whom it will impair embouchure or voice control, respectively. This may be a familial trait or may appear as an isolated phenomenon. It not infrequently begins in early adult life and is clearly aggravated by stress, as are most disorders of movement. The beta-blockers, such as propranolol (Inderal), are the most useful medications for controlling this tremor. Historically, alcohol has also been used frequently and is effective, but it has obvious drawbacks for the performer as well as in the general population. Primidone (Mysoline) and perhaps alprazolam (Xanax) have also been recommended; my success with these drugs has been modest.

A 34-year-old guitarist noted shaking of the left hand in certain positions and trembling of the fingers particularly when he played the guitar. This was aggravated when he was under stress. Examination revealed asymmetric but bilateral action tremor involving the upper extremities. Neurological examination was otherwise normal. The problem was ameliorated with propranolol but he remained symptomatic, although still able to play.

Motor neuron disease (amyotrophic lateral sclerosis [ALS] and other forms) may occasionally afflict a performing artist. Because of its tendency to begin asymmetrically in the distal upper extremity muscles, it may present diagnostic difficulties early in its evolution and may particularly affect instrumental performance. Although the muscular weakness, atrophy, fasciculation, and impairment of control may occasionally remain focal and only slowly progressive, it most often develops rapidly over a few years and is likely to disable the performer permanently soon after onset. There is no known cure for this ailment.

Two other types of disorders which affect motor performance more or less exclusively are the diseases of neuromuscular transmission (primarily myasthenia gravis) and the primary muscle disorders, of which the degenerative forms (dystrophies) and inflammatory types are most common. Myasthenia gravis is a rare disorder of the neuromuscular junction, usually causing fatigability and weakness which may be episodic and exercise-related. The symptoms tend to be worse as the day progresses or as a particular muscular activity continues; this history is critical in suggesting the correct diagnosis. Difficulty in supporting the instrument or in maintaining finger activity, lip control, or quality of voice may be the initial complaints (19). The diagnosis is made clinically and confirmed by electrodiagnostic studies and the presence of antibodies to a component of muscle. The disease can often be well controlled and sometimes may even be cured by appropriate medical treatment (cholinesterase inhibitors, corticosteroids, other immunosuppressant regimens) and surgical removal of the thymus gland.

Primary muscle disorders are also quite uncommon among performers. The degenerative disorders tend to be familial and of early onset; these factors tend to discourage or inhibit the development of a performing arts career. Occasionally, muscle dystrophy may initially develop later in life and these forms are more likely to afflict a performer. Inflammatory disorders of muscle, particularly polymyositis, might be more likely to occur in a performer since these tend to develop in the middle and later decades of life. Polymyositis, which may be found as an isolated disorder or in association with other systemic diseases such as the collagen-vascular disorders (systemic lupus erythematosus, rheumatoid arthritis) or cancers, usually presents with muscle weakness, fatigability, and sometimes soreness. These disorders may respond to corticosteroids or other immunosuppressant drugs but are likely to be quite disabling and tend to be career-threatening because of the need for long-term treatment or the association with debilitating systemic illnesses.

Of a variety of cranial nerve disorders, only two will be discussed in this context. The first is idiopathic facial paralysis, or Bell's palsy, which is a relatively common disorder affecting the facial muscles on one side. This is a familiar disorder to most physicians. Unilateral facial pain is often the initial manifestation, but shortly thereafter the patient notes drooping or sagging of that side of the face, with unilateral inability to wrinkle the forehead, blink, smile, or seal the lips. A sensation of numbness is not infrequent, although the sensory contribution of the facial nerve is a minor component; this symptom may reflect trigeminal involvement. The pain is usually short-lived, but the facial weakness, which may be virtually total on one side, often lasts weeks or months. It is usually self-limited, although complete recovery is not always seen. Even mild forms of this disorder are incompatible with playing a woodwind or brass instrument because of inability to effect a seal (Fig. 5.1), and singing is impaired because of the difficulty in articulating labial sounds. There is no specific predilection for performing artists of any type but, for reasons

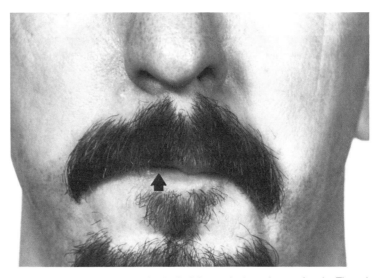

FIG. 5.1. French hornist with onset of right facial paresis 6 weeks previously. There has been substantial improvement but the slight residual lip weakness with resultant incomplete seal (*arrow*) prevents adequate formation of embouchure.

which remain unclear, I have seen this in French horn players in particular. Fortunately, all of these have returned to full capability after a number of months. Treatment with corticosteroids remains controversial; most recover more or less fully with or without treatment. Artificial tears should be used in the affected eye, especially if lacrimation is impaired, since corneal scarring is a potential complication until eyelid closure can be accomplished. Careful follow-up is mandatory, since failure to improve within a few months (or any further progression) suggests an alternative diagnosis. Further investigation, including imaging of the skull base, would be indicated at that time.

Another disorder of cranial nerves which is not rare in the general population is trigeminal neuralgia or tic douloureux. The very brief lancinating and severe pains of the face or jaw are often triggered by touching the skin or mucous membranes and by activities involving facial and jaw muscles. Hence, playing of a wind instrument, or violin and viola, may be virtually impossible. I have seen one unique case in which a clarinetist found that his episodes were almost exclusively triggered by playing. Although trigeminal neuralgia is generally controllable with medication or various surgical techniques, this patient has changed careers because of it.

It has been mentioned previously that strokes commonly affect motor function, both strength and fine motor control, and hence may be especially damaging to the instrumental musician. Levels of recovery that may be sufficient for most other activities may still preclude continuation of a career as an instrumentalist, although there are clearly many examples of musicians who have been able to return to performing careers after suffering a stroke.

A 55-year-old professional violinist was seen 2 ¹/₂ years after an episode involving apparently stepwise onset of dysarthria and left hemiparesis occurring under a situation of extreme stress. Studies at that time demonstrated a hemorrhagic right frontoparietal infarction. Six months later he developed focal seizures involving the left face and arm and subsequently had a generalized seizure, after which he was treated with anticonvulsants. His current problem is in sight reading, finding it difficult to translate the notes into finger movements. He also describes inability to execute passages which require rapid or complex finger movements. Examination revealed mildly increased tone in the left arm and leg and mild impairment of fine motor control in the left fingers. He had slight deficit on the left hand with double simultaneous touch and mildly impaired pain, light touch, and joint position sense in the left toes. Tendon reflexes were slightly hyperactive on the left and there was a Babinski response on that side. Occupational therapy seemed to help his left hand dexterity and he was able to play in a local community orchestra, but remained well below his previously attained level of accomplishment on the violin.

Rarely, a stroke may affect not the motor control but some other function intimately related to performance. In the case of music, disorders of perception or expression of musical language have been called "amusias" and may be caused by stroke or occasionally by other forms of brain injury. They are related to other more commonly recognized disorders of language (aphasias); a number of examples are available in the medical literature, some of these studied quite extensively (20,21). Because of the apparent rarity of amusias, they are of more importance to the neurologist as keys to understanding music processing within the brain than they are as clinical problems. I have not seen an example in a performer although I have had one classical-music lover who found after a right hemispheric stroke that he could not listen to orchestral music because it sounded cacophonous. By the time I saw him several weeks after the stroke, I was unable to demonstrate any perceptual abnormalities by readily available testing; he did ultimately recover his ability to enjoy music.

Generalized polyneuropathies, both the acute types such as Guillain-Barré syndrome and the more chronic forms, including diabetic and various hereditary neuropathies, may occur in instrumental musicians and other performers. The Guillain-Barré syndrome is characterized by rapid onset, usually over a period of 1 to 2 weeks, of muscle weakness of the legs, arms, trunk, and face. Details of the clinical features, as well as management, are beyond the scope of this chapter. Ultimate recovery is the rule but this may take months to years and, as with other disorders of motor function, performers may find even the slightest residual weakness debilitating. Diabetic and other polyneuropathies are generally more insidious in onset and tend to be slowly progressive, with some fluctuation not infrequent. Sensory dysfunction is often more prominent than weakness and, although involvement of the upper extremities tends to be late, again may impair instrumental performance in particular. In diabetes, it is hoped that careful medical management can retard the progression of neuropathy, but correlation between severity of the diabetes and the neuropathic complications is often imperfect.

One other entity which is common in the general population and presents a special difficulty to performing artists, particularly among dancers, warrants discussion. Back pain at all levels is a frequent symptom in performers, as it is in others. Herniated lumbar disc with resulting lumbar radiculopathy will be found in a relatively small percentage of those with lower back pain. It certainly can be seen in all types of performers but may disable the dancer more than others. Male ballet dancers may be particularly likely to develop this because of their lifting activities, although there is no evidence that the incidence is actually higher in this group. The pain pattern and the neurological signs of weakness, sensory loss, or reflex change in the lower extremity are not different in the performer and nonperformer.

The clinician often places great faith in the aggravation of pain by stretching the affected nerve root (primarily L-5 or S-1) in the straight leg raise maneuver. In dancers, this is often unreliable because of their extraordinary flexibility. The straight leg raise may often be accomplished to 90° or greater without any additional discomfort even in the face of clear disc herniation and lumbosacral root compromise. Diagnosis is usually confirmed by high resolution CT scanning or MRI. In dancers as well as in others, a period of conservative treatment is indicated unless progressive neurologic deficit is noted or pain fails to subside with bedrest, analgesics, and physical therapy.

DISORDERS WHICH SEEM PARTICULARLY PREVALENT IN PERFORMERS

The following are by far the most common neurological disorders encountered in the author's practice (24) and this experience is echoed by others who see large numbers of instrumental musicians. The two types of neurological disorders which appear to be most prevalent among musicians seeking medical help are the localized, or focal, neuropathies (24,25), often involving a single peripheral nerve or branch, and the focal dystonias or occupational cramps (26,27).

Focal Compression Neuropathies

The peripheral nervous system includes motor, sensory, and autonomic nerve fibers outside the anatomic confines of the brain and spinal cord (central nervous system). Because the functional elements of the peripheral nervous system include cell bodies of motor nerves, which are in the spinal cord or brainstem and are influenced by central connections from sensory fiber input, it is sometimes difficult to localize a clinical problem specifically to the peripheral nervous system. Nonetheless, the majority of such problems affecting performing artists are in fact compression neuropathies, hence the site of injury is usually identifiable. The terms *compression neuropathy* and *entrapment neuropathy* are often used interchangeably, although the latter designation should be reserved for those forms of compression which occur between anatomic structures within the body, differentiating them from those due to external pressure. Of course, there are other forms of localized mononeuropathy such as lacerations, local chemical injuries, and tumors, but these are uncommon in the performing artist and will not be considered in this discussion.

A brief statement about the effects of chronic compression would be helpful in understanding these disorders. Trauma from compression may injure the nerve fiber (axon) itself, the surrounding myelin sheath, the connective tissue elements of peripheral nerve, or sometimes all three components. In general, the earliest changes are seen in the myelin sheath. These cause either slowing of nerve conduction or conduction block, the inability of the nerve to transmit electrical impulses beyond the compressed segment. At times, usually with more long-lasting or severe compression, the nerve fiber itself may be damaged. Injury to the axon causes degeneration of that portion of the fiber distal to the site of injury and sometimes proximally as far as the nerve cell. While all elements of the peripheral nervous system have the capacity to regenerate and heal, damage to the nerve fiber is more likely to lead to permanent functional impairment, particularly if the surrounding connective tissue elements are also damaged. Since this is generally a result of more prolonged or severe compression, there are obvious reasons for recognizing compressive neuropathies early in their evolution. The role of ischemia, or circulatory insufficiency, in chronic compression neuropathy is uncertain but it may be a factor at least in some cases.

A number of factors may contribute to the susceptibility of nerve to compression. Nerve fibers which are located closer to the surface of the peripheral nerve trunk are more sensitive than those situated in the deeper portions of the nerve. Larger diameter fibers are more likely to be injured than thinner ones. Finally, a variety of metabolic or systemic illnesses may render the nerves more susceptible to injury, including poor nutrition, such as that which may be associated with alcoholism or eating disorders, diabetes, and kidney failure. A controversial concept suggests that sensitivity to compression at one site along a peripheral nerve may be enhanced by more proximal compression, the so-called double crush hypothesis. An example might be the greater likelihood of median nerve sensory fibers being injured at the wrist if those same fibers are simultaneously being compressed at the level of the cervical root through which they pass. This question does arise in the performing artist, but at the present time no definitive answer is available.

The clinical features of nerve compression will, of course, vary depending on the site of the injury, as well as the duration and severity. Most compression neuropathies are characterized by pain and by some sensory disturbance such as numbness, tingling, burning, or "pins and needles." The sensory symptoms are usually in the territory served by the nerve, although pain may well be more widely distributed both distally and proximally. Motor disturbances, including weakness and atrophy, may also be seen, particularly in longstanding compression. Impairment of motor function or control in peripheral nerve injuries is usually proportional to the amount of weakness or sensory loss. This differs from some disorders of the central nervous system, in which control may be impaired more than would be expected from the amount of weakness or demonstrable sensory loss. Tendon or stretch reflexes are often diminished, even with early or mild compression. Abnormalities of autonomic function, such as changes in sweating, skin color and texture, and skin temperature are less common but may be prominent features of partial peripheral nerve injury, particularly in the still poorly understood "reflex sympathetic dystrophies."

The compression neuropathies will be discussed in a proximal-to-distal sequence, beginning with radiculopathies (spinal root lesions) which, in the instrumental musician at least, most often occur in the neck, affecting the upper limb. Since the majority of these are associated with cervical disc degeneration and spondylosis, they are more prevalent in older musicians. Symptoms of cervical radiculopathy may be severe and acute in onset or, more commonly, may be insidious or intermittent. Characteristically, the symptoms include pain, usually identifiable as originating in the neck and radiating distally in a specific distribution down the arm, sensory loss or paresthesia in similar distribution, and sometimes motor dysfunction. In the majority of studies in the general population, C-6 and particularly C-7 are the most frequently affected (28). Among the musicians we have evaluated (24), C-8 radiculopathy was surprisingly common although the numbers are small. The involvement of the small muscles of the hand in C8-T1 radiculopathy might bring the instrumental musician to medical attention at an earlier stage than other groups.

This 42-year-old right-handed professional violinist has a history of trauma to the lower back from an athletic injury and underwent lumbar laminectomy 12 years previously after developing footdrop. A myelogram performed at that time was carried up to the cervical region and showed a small defect at C5-6. At that time he was also having some symptoms in the neck and a year later had severe right arm and shoulder pain associated with right hand paresthesia. Examination then showed only slight hyperreflexia in the left leg. An EMG was said to show fibrillations in two C5-6 innervated muscles. A repeat myelogram 1 year later showed minimal left greater than right indentation of the dye column at C5-6. Since that time he has had recurrent problems with the right arm. Two years previously he developed pain in the left arm with weakness of the left ring and little fingers. He also noted a tendency of the little finger to tremble in certain positions. Examination revealed moderate restriction of neck mobility. There was slight weakness of right forearm pronators. There was more substantial weakness involving the intrinsic left hand muscles, both ulnar- and median-innervated. There was very mild impairment of sensation on the right index and middle fingers and on the left little and ring fingers. Right arm reflexes were all slightly less brisk than those on the left. Lower limb reflexes were symmetrical and quite brisk with downgoing toes. An EMG showed mild chronic neurogenic motor unit potential changes in right C-6 and C-7 distribution and more prominent changes in C-8 distribution on the left. The cervical spine x-rays showed extensive degenerative changes at C3-4 through C7-T1. The final diagnosis was bilateral chronic cervical radiculopathy. A conservative program including physical therapy has provided modest symptomatic relief. The patient would not consider surgery.

The diagnosis is made from the clinical picture. X-ray of the cervical spine, neuroimaging procedures such as myelography, CT scan, and MRI, as well as

EMG, may be useful. Conservative treatment with initial immobilization, physical therapeutic techniques including exercise, and analgesics is usually effective. Surgery may be required when pain is unrelenting or progressive neurological dysfunction occurs.

Peripheral nerves can be compressed at the level of the brachial plexus, giving rise to what has been called thoracic outlet syndromes (TOS). The controversies surrounding this diagnosis are well known and the interested reader is referred to a number of publications which have dealt with this diagnosis and the attendant controversies (29–32). For the purposes of this discussion, it is assumed that this entity exists and that it is possible to make a reasonable diagnosis based upon the clinical picture. The true neurogenic TOS, which is characterized by clinically and electrically identifiable sensory and motor dysfunction, will not be further reviewed since it is a rare disorder and has not, to my knowledge, been reported in a musician. We will focus on the symptomatic form (31) (which others may call the "disputed" form) (32) of TOS, in which the symptoms of arm pain, paresthesia, usually along the ulnar forearm and hand, and motor dysfunction are generally unaccompanied by objective sensory, motor, and reflex loss. The symptoms are usually positional and can characteristically be reproduced by maneuvers which further compromise the fibers of the brachial plexus. I have found that the most effective maneuver in instrumentalists, at least, is downward traction on the affected arm, adding some internal rotation at the shoulder as well. A substantial percentage of patients with symptomatic TOS have a characteristic neck and upper trunk appearance which has been called the "droopy shoulder" configuration (33,34). This consists of a long, relatively thin neck and shoulders which slope downward and forward at rest (Fig. 5.2). Obviously, not all persons with this configuration will have symptoms of TOS, but it does seem to predispose to this symptom complex. I have not found the other TOS maneuvers, such as the Adson and the hyperabduction position, with or without hand exercise, to be as helpful in eliciting symptoms, but this experience is not universal (30). Whether it is important to be able to obliterate the radial pulse with these or any other maneuvers is also controversial but in my experience bears little relationship to the production of symptoms, and I do not rely on it at all. Unfortunately, there are as yet no adequate ancillary studies which allow us to confirm the diagnosis of TOS (32). Studies, however, can and often should be done to exclude other diagnoses with which this can easily be confused. X-rays of the neck may reveal cervical ribs or elongated lateral processes and will also confirm the droopy shoulder configuration. EMG and, less commonly, SEP may be helpful in excluding other causes of similar symptoms. Treatment is also controversial; we always begin with a conservative program of exercises to modify posture and strengthen the shoulder elevators. Increasing postural awareness during playing and with other activities may also be of benefit. Some have advocated bracing for the droopy shoulder posture (34). The question of surgery arises in the patient who does not respond to these measures. Once again there is controversy regarding not only the utilization of surgery at all but also the type of procedure to be carried out. We have had excellent success with surgery in carefully selected patients who have

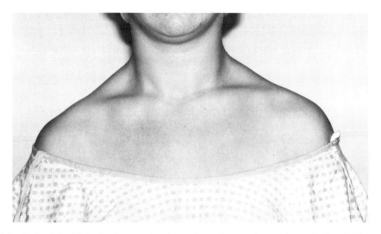

FIG. 5.2. A pianist with typical upper trunk configuration and symptoms in the right arm suggestive of droopy shoulder syndrome.

failed to respond to other measures. In our series (24), of the 27 patients with TOS, 19 responded favorably to conservative treatment and 2 underwent surgery, both successfully. With regard to both diagnosis and treatment, one can only advise thorough evaluation and careful consideration of appropriate diagnostic and therapeutic options.

This 38-year-old dulcimer and autoharp performer has had numbness and tingling in the left hand and pain in the left arm while playing over the last 4 months. Neurological examination was normal. Symptoms were reproduced by downward traction on the left arm and while playing the autoharp particularly. Several months of rigorous physical therapy were unsuccessful and indeed her symptoms worsened. She subsequently underwent left first rib resection with complete resolution of her symptoms and returned to a playing schedule which was even more intense than she had ever attempted previously. She has remained asymptomatic for 5 years.

Of the three major nerves derived from the brachial plexus which supply the upper extremity, the median nerve is the most frequently affected by compression, and the site of entrapment is usually at or distal to the wrist in the carpal tunnel. This is the most common entrapment neuropathy in the general population and other than the thoracic outlet syndrome appears to be the most common in performing artists as well (10,24). There has been disagreement as to whether this specific mononeuropathy is causally related to hand use (35,36), and there is no convincing evidence that repetitive hand or wrist movement contributes to its prevalence in performing artists. The carpal tunnel is formed by the arcade of wrist bones dorsally and laterally, with a firm ligament, the flexor retinaculum, forming the roof ventrally. The median nerve, which passes through the carpal tunnel, is subject to entrapment by the surrounding flexor tendons (particularly in the presence of any inflammation) and by the overlying ligament, especially when it is swollen or thickened. The canal may actually vary in size, and it has been suggested that this may be a predisposing factor to the carpal tunnel syndrome (CTS) (37). Clinically, in performing artists and others, the typical features include pain and paresthesia, usually limited to the thumb, index and middle fingers, and the radial half of the ring finger, although many patients cannot differentiate and describe tingling in all of the fingers. Pain may be not only in the hand but also more proximal. The symptoms characteristically occur at night and often awaken the patient from sleep. Symptoms may also occur with daily activities such as holding a book, newspaper, or telephone, and instrumentalists describe aggravation of symptoms with playing. Objective sensory loss may be mild or absent, especially in early cases, and atrophy or weakness are relatively uncommon except in later stages. Eliciting distal paresthesia by tapping over the median nerve at the wrist (Tinel's sign) and provoking symptoms by passively flexing the wrists for 1 minute (Phalen's maneuver) may be helpful in supporting the diagnosis. Both of these maneuvers may be positive, however, in those who have no other clinical or electrical evidence of median neuropathy, and both may be notably absent in those with even severe symptoms and signs. The diagnosis is confirmed in almost all cases by electrodiagnostic testing. Nonsurgical measures include splinting of the wrists, particularly at night, antiinflammatory medication, diuretics, and sometimes local corticosteroid injection. Modification of activity may be all that is required. When these measures fail, surgical decompression is almost invariably effective. In performing artists particularly, surgery must be followed by carefully supervised rehabilitation. In our experience, unless surgery has been delayed with resulting severe sensorimotor deficits, successful return to performance is the rule. Of the eight patients with CTS whom we have reported (24), three have responded to conservative measures, and five have had excellent surgical results.

A 59-year-old right-handed pianist noted right hand numbness 3 years previously and subsequently developed left hand numbness as well. This would generally occur at night and would occasionally awaken her. Nine months previously she began to have shooting pains in the hands, especially when playing the piano. Pain and numbness became more constant. EMG suggested median neuropathy at the wrists. Examination revealed no muscle atrophy and no convincing weakness. Sensory examination was also normal, including 2-point discrimination. The reflexes were normal. Tinel's sign was positive bilaterally but the Phalen maneuver was negative. She delayed surgical treatment for several years but subsequently underwent bilateral carpal tunnel release and has been asymptomatic since then.

The median nerve may be entrapped more proximally in the forearm. In the pronator syndrome (38,39), pain and some tenderness may be more prominent in the upper forearm and paresthesia, while in the same distribution as in carpal tunnel syndrome, is not so characteristically nocturnal. Weakness may involve not just the thenar muscles but also the long flexor of the thumb particularly. As with CTS, the relationship to hand usage is uncertain but it seems likely that repeated forceful pronation, particularly, may predispose to this disorder (39). Modification of activity, local measures including corticosteroid injection and surgery are treatment options. Entrapment of the anterior interosseous branch of the median nerve causes weakness of the long flexor of the thumb and index finger and sometimes of the middle finger, along with weakness of the pronator quadratus. This is a pure motor branch, and hence no sensory symptoms are to be expected. Anterior interosseous neuropathy is a relatively uncommon disorder, and there is certainly no evidence that it is more likely to occur in instrumentalists, although excessive muscular exercise has been blamed in several reports. Once again, conservative measures are tried initially, following which surgery may be considered for persisting symptoms and signs.

This 39-year-old harpist had an episode of right forearm pain 10 years previously, diagnosed as tendinitis. This responded to rest and a nonsteroidal antiinflammatory drug. Six months previously she developed pain in the right forearm, accompanied by numbness and tingling primarily in the right thumb, index, and middle fingers. This occurred during a series of rehearsals and concerts in which she had to tune several harps repeatedly. This required vigorous and repeated pronation and supination of the right forearm. There was marked tenderness in the right upper forearm over the proximal pronator teres. Pain was elicited by resistive pronation of the right forearm. Neurological examination was normal. An EMG was also normal, including needle electrode examination of several median-innervated muscles. The tentative diagnosis was right pronator syndrome. Conservative treatment and rest ultimately led to complete recovery. She has used a special tuning device since that time.

The ulnar nerve is also subject to compression, usually in the region of the elbow. Confusing terminology in the literature has led to considerable imprecision in diagnosis. Compression of the ulnar nerve may occur as it passes through the condylar groove between the olecranon and the medial epicondyle of the humerus. Here the nerve is easily palpated and is readily traumatized, a phenomenon that we all have experienced in hitting the "funny bone." Just beyond this, the nerve enters the cubital tunnel, formed by muscle and connective tissue structures which can entrap the ulnar nerve at that level as well. Clinical differentiation between involvement at the condylar or ulnar groove and the cubital tunnel may be impossible, and electrodiagnostic studies may not provide clear distinction. Differentiation may be important, however, in determining the appropriate therapy. Previous elbow trauma, a tendency to lean on the elbow, prolonged elbow flexion (which reduces the capacity of both the condylar groove and the cubital tunnel), and repeated flexion and extension of the elbow may predispose to ulnar neuropathy at either site. In a portion of the normal population, the ulnar nerve may slip out of the condylar groove with elbow flexion, moving alongside or anterior to the medial epicondyle. This may be responsible for localized ulnar neuropathy in some cases. It is probably important to note that ulnar neuropathy in violinists and violists is almost invariably in the left arm (24,40), suggesting that sustained flexion may be more important than repeated flexion and extension. The patient with ulnar neuropathy again has the expected pain, usually along the ulnar (little finger) aspect of the forearm and hand, sensory disturbance of the little finger and ulnar half of the ring finger as well as the ulnar third of the hand, and weakness of the ulnar-innervated intrinsic muscles of the hand, less commonly of the forearm. Nerve conduction studies and needle electrode examination are often helpful but less reliably confirm or localize the site of injury than in carpal tunnel syndrome. Once again, treatment is aimed at reducing the trauma to the ulnar nerve by modifying position or activity and avoiding elbow pressure. Choice of surgical treatment may depend upon the exact site of compression. Most commonly, transposition of the nerve is performed for involvement at the condylar groove, with or without medial epicondylectomy. Some have suggested that simple decompression may suffice for cubital tunnel entrapment. Our results would support this approach. Charness et al. (40) have reported excellent results in thirteen patients (four bilateral) with conservative and, when necessary, surgical treatment.

An 18-year-old right-handed violin student was seen for left arm pain which developed while he was practicing 6 hours per day at a music camp. The pain decreased when he stopped playing, but the next month he developed recurrent pain along with tingling in the left little and ring fingers. The symptoms persisted, and he also complained of some weakness in the left fingers. Neurological examination showed only a very subtle sensory deficit in the left ring finger, most readily demonstrated by testing pin sharpness on the ulnar compared to radial half of the finger. An EMG suggested left ulnar neuropathy at the elbow but was not definitive. He underwent transposition of the left ulnar nerve with medial epicondylectomy. However, by this time he had virtually abandoned his career and had entered medical school. During the next several years his left arm gradually improved and he once again took up the violin. He is currently in a major symphony orchestra and has no left arm symptoms.

The ulnar nerve may be compressed more distally in the wrist or hand. Although this is relatively uncommon, it has been reported in flutists (42), and I have seen it in one violinist (24). In these cases sensory loss may not be present, depending on the exact site of the injury, and weakness is the predominant feature. Playing position may be a contributing factor.

Any of the digital nerves may be susceptible to compression. Since there are no motor fibers in the digital nerves, the symptoms are entirely sensory, consisting of segmental numbness in the distribution of the compressed digital branch and pain. These injuries are most likely to occur from external pressure, usually against the instrument. A tight grip is probably the major underlying cause. It may occur in the left index finger of a violinist or violist from pressure against the neck of the instrument and in the same finger in a flutist (43) from pressure against the flute. A cellist patient had numbness of the tip of the right thumb, along the ulnar aspect of the distal phalanx, from pressure on the bow stick. A percussionist who was practicing four mallet techniques on the marimba developed compression involving a digital nerve of the middle finger. These are generally reversible if the technique can be altered. In flutists, technique for holding the instrument may be changed, and a temporary cushion may be devised to protect the site of compression.

This 18-year-old right-handed flute student was seen for evaluation of left hand pain and numbness associated with playing the flute. Three years previously she broke her left index finger and after returning to the flute she developed her current symptoms. She began to have pain at the MCP joint of the left index finger, radiating proximally toward the radial wrist and forearm, and numbness of the left index finger occurring after playing for about 1 hour. Examination revealed mild tenderness on palpation of the index finger MCP joint. Thoracic outlet maneuvers did not reproduce her symptoms. There was a mild but consistent decrease in sensitivity to pinprick over the radial aspect of the left index finger dorsally. Examination while playing the flute revealed pressure of the instrument on the index finger along the radial aspect of the proximal phalanx (Fig. 5.3). Modification of technique and an orthotic device led to virtually complete resolution of her symptoms.

Other examples of mononeuropathy in the upper limb may be found in the literature, including radial mononeuropathies. A particularly vexing and controversial syndrome is associated with alleged entrapment of the posterior interosseous branch in the "radial tunnel" (44). This disorder, also known as "resistant tennis elbow," is characterized by pain with little or no weakness or sensory loss and presents problems similar to those encountered in the TOS as outlined above. Many patients so described have had elbow and forearm pain associated with repetitive forceful arm motion and have tenderness distal to the lateral epicondyle. Pain is aggravated by resistive supination or extension of the middle finger with the elbow extended but there are few, if any, firm neurological signs. Despite careful evaluation of dozens of patients with these symptoms and signs, I have not been able to confirm a single case by electrodiagnostic studies. Other equally uncommon focal neuropathies may

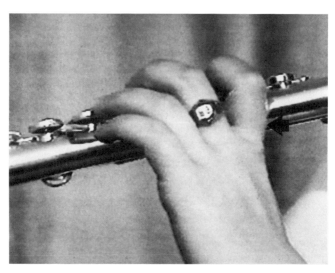

FIG. 5.3. 18-year-old flutist with digital neuropathy involving the radial aspect of the left index finger due to pressure against the instrument.

occasionally be encountered, such as the reported entrapment of the posterior cutaneous nerve of the upper arm in a drummer (45).

Similarly, occasional mononeuropathies in the lower extremity may occur in performers. Two cases of saphenous mononeuropathy have been reported in viola da gamba players, secondary to pressure of the instrument against the inner aspect of the lower leg (46,47). Since this instrument should be cradled and not tightly gripped, this mononeuropathy is again presumably due to excessive tension or poor technique. Peroneal nerve compression has also been described in a guitarist (48).

Cranial mononeuropathies may also be peripheral in origin. The only one which seems causally related to playing is one which involves the segmental sensory branches supplying the lip of wind players. Most of these are localized to the sensory fibers compressed by the mouthpiece of a brass or wind instrument and presumably result from pressure against the dental arch. While numbness is often a presenting complaint, these instrumentalists usually also describe lip dysfunction which may be due to impaired sensory feedback or to some associated impairment of lip muscles. We have found these extremely difficult to analyze, but fortunately they seem to respond to reduction in playing time or change in repertoire; occasional patients have had to take a complete respite from the instrument for several weeks.

An 18-year-old right-handed trombonist began having numbness of the right upper lip while he was playing up to 8 hours per day during his first year at a conservatory. He describes this as a feeling like Novocain which occurs whenever he plays, particularly higher notes and louder volume. He also complains of a feeling of roughness which he detects on the inner surface of the right upper lip with his tongue or externally with his finger. When the problem is most severe he feels as if a small portion of his right upper lip is "flapping" inside the mouthpiece. Examination revealed no clear asymmetry of motor function and there was no definite asymmetry of sensation on the lip, either externally or in the mouth. On playing the instrument he tended to hold it tilted to the right so that asymmetric pressure was exerted. With prolonged playing he developed slight numbness on the right upper lip within the area covered by the mouthpiece (Fig. 5.4). Attempts have been made to alter playing technique and practice habits.

Occupational Cramp: A Focal Dystonia

The final type of neurological disorder in musicians to be discussed is the occupational cramp or focal dystonia. This particularly troublesome disorder is the least understood and the most difficult to treat of all those which afflict performers. Interest in this entity, known by such terms as occupational neurosis, craft palsy, and professional impotence, goes back at least to the nineteenth century. The most common and familiar form is writer's cramp. To my knowledge, the first reference to a musician so affected dates from 1840 (49). The investigators of the nineteenth century, exemplified by Gowers (50) and Poore (51), recognized this as a nervous system disorder, although they could not localize the process definitively to the

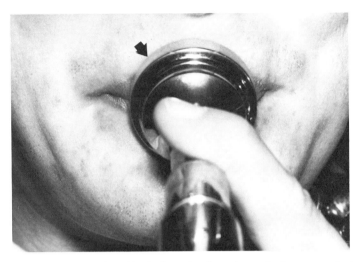

FIG. 5.4. 18-year-old trombonist with playing-related numbness in the segment of the right upper lip underlying the mouthpiece (*arrow*).

central or peripheral nervous system. The contribution of psychic factors was also clearly recognized at that time. Indeed, for the better part of this century, occupational cramp has been considered by the majority of practitioners to be largely psychogenic; this view is still held by many, despite convincing evidence to the contrary. A detailed discussion of this controversy is beyond the scope of this chapter, but the interested reader is referred to the work of Marsden and others (52,53).

The typical musician with occupational cramp first notes difficulty with muscular control, speed, or dexterity in the fingers or hand, or less commonly in the muscles of the lips, tongue, or jaw (26,27,54–56). In our series (27), the patients have characteristically been in the fourth or fifth decade of life and hence have generally been playing for 25 or more years. This is also the only disorder among musicians in which men have outnumbered women by a 2 to 1 margin. In addition to impaired control, patients may complain of stiffness, tightness, cramping, or fatigue. A small number of patients in our series have had significant pain, more often at some point after the onset of impaired control and perhaps secondary to attempts at compensation for the motor control disorder. Some (57,58) have emphasized the frequency of pain and believe that the painful overuse syndromes are basically similar in pathophysiology to the occupational cramp; others disagree (26,59). As the disorder progresses, involuntary movements are often noted. Newmark and Hochberg (26) have emphasized the frequency of certain specific patterns of dystonia in particular instrumental groups, such as the involuntary flexion of little and ring fingers of the right hand in pianists. We have seen a variety of abnormal patterns and involuntary movements (Fig. 5.5–5.6) and indeed have been more struck by the differences among various patients than by their similarities.

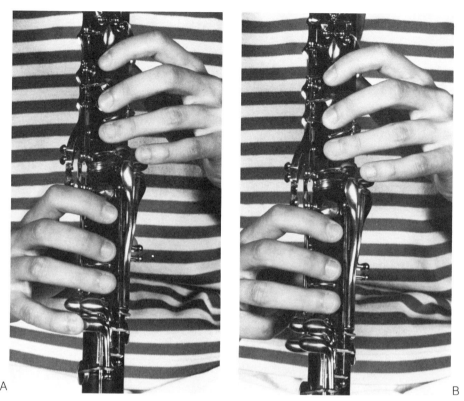

FIG. 5.5. 29-year-old clarinetist with history (1½ years) of difficulty controlling the right little finger while playing. A: Hand position as she begins to play. B: After playing less than 1 minute, the right little finger begins to curl involuntarily, pulling the finger off the key.

Typically, but not invariably, the involuntary movements and cramp occur only with specific tasks. In our series (27) more than 50% were associated only with instrumental playing, and other activities which involve the same muscle groups could be carried out without difficulty. Sometimes this task specificity disappears as the disorder progresses. Another change that occurs with time is that the cramp or involuntary movement begins earlier after initiation of the activity. Whereas the instrumentalist may be able to play for 15 to 20 minutes at first, as the problem evolves the ability to play unimpeded diminishes and ultimately the movement disorder may be noted immediately upon attempting to play the first note. A similar pattern has been noted in writer's cramp.

The diagnosis is made by characteristic history. Because many, if not most, of these are task specific, it is clear that the evaluation must include observation of the instrumentalist in the act of playing. Failure to do so will almost invariably lead to the erroneous conclusion that the problem is imagined or hysterical, since the neurological examination is otherwise normal in the vast majority. At times the impair-

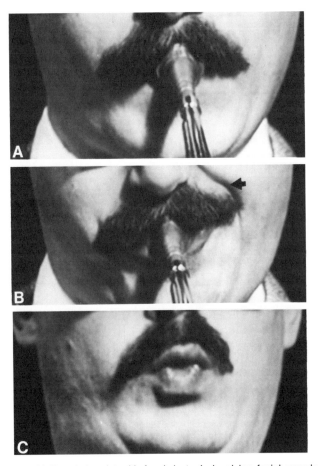

FIG. 5.6. 36-year-old French hornist with focal dystonia involving facial muscles. A: He pre-pares to blow into the mouthpiece. Note symmetry of facial contour. B: As air is emitted, the facial muscles pull to the left, with deepening of the left nasolabial fold (*arrow*). Air leaks through the slightly separated lips on the left. C: He is able to whistle without similar facial muscle spasm. (From Lederman RJ, *Med Probl Perform Art* 1988; 3:48. Courtesy of Hanley and Belfus, Inc.)

ment in motor control can be quite subtle, and one may have to listen and watch repeatedly for minor changes in the ability to carry out certain patterns of activity. One violist noted difficulty only with certain ascending passages; as he played these repeatedly, one could distinguish an occasional missed note which, in a less expert performer, would have been considered a minor technical inadequacy. In this case it clearly represented the loss of ability to carry out a fingering sequence (first, third, second through fourth, etc.) which previously had been easily accomplished.

At the present time there are no reliable tests which allow confirmation of the diagnosis. While an occasional patient with focal dystonia may have a lesion involving the basal ganglia (60), the rule in focal dystonias is that no structural lesion can be identified. Recording of muscle activity in the affected limb may show sustained or poorly modulated discharge with simultaneous activation of agonists and antagonists (cocontraction) (61,62). Recently, a technique for demonstrating a physiologic abnormality of reciprocal innervation in the affected limb has been reported (63). If this finding can be confirmed in a large number of patients with focal dystonia, it may provide a very valuable marker and may also serve further to confirm the "organic" nature of the disorder.

The precise etiology and pathophysiology of occupational cramp remains unknown. Certainly overuse in its broadest sense plays some role. Those who develop these disorders use the affected part for some task involving repetitive or sustained activity, usually associated with the afflicted patient's occupation. This, however, cannot be the only factor, since only a small percentage of those who have similar levels of such activity develop occupational cramp. Gowers noted the frequency with which writers who had a rigid or cramped style of writing would develop the occupational cramp. Some musicians who have developed this disorder appear to have had a great deal of tension or rigidity in their playing techniques, but this is clearly not the only predisposing condition and may not even be an important one.

The question of a relationship between focal dystonia and prior trauma to peripheral tissues has been raised (26,64,65). We have seen a small number of patients with apparent nerve entrapment associated with focal dystonia as well as a few cases following mechanical or soft tissue trauma (27). These include a pianist who developed severe occupational cramp after a fractured wrist and a harpist who developed a hand cramp after a burn injury. This relationship has been likened to that of development of causalgia after peripheral nerve injury but the mechanism remains quite uncertain (64).

Treatment of the occupational cramp in musicians remains as much a problem today as it was at the time of Gowers (50) and Poore (51) 100 years ago. Both of these authors advocated a period of rest from the offending activity. Gowers specifically stated that the earlier this commenced after onset of the cramp, the more likely that rest would be effective, and the shorter the period of rest needed to be. Gowers also pointed out that unless the style of writing (in the case of writer's cramp), could be changed to a freer manner, the disorder would likely recur. Unfortunately, in musicians, this is not even as easy as it could be in the writer. Gowers recommended that writers switch to the opposite hand. Obviously this is not usually an option in the musician, although I have seen one violinist who did successfully switch from playing right-handed to a left-handed technique. Gowers also noted that the opposite hand could become similarly affected in about half of the cases. In this particular violinist, the occupational cramp did in fact subsequently affect the opposite hand. Because of the technical limitations of playing style in most, if not all, instruments, changing to a "freer" manner of playing is not so simple. In fact, we have found that rest from the offending activity has not been particularly useful. A French horn player with occupational cramp involving the lip stopped playing for 12 years and virtually the moment he picked up the horn again, the cramp recurred

(27). Other therapeutic techniques today, including a variety of drugs (66,67) such as anticholinergics, dopamine receptor agonists and antagonists, psychotherapy and behavioral techniques (68,69), and local injections of botulinum toxin (70) have been only marginally more successful than the strychnine, application of voltaic electrical stimulation, and hypodermic morphia or cocaine of Gowers and Poore (50,51). Among our patients, successes have been characterized by being able to continue playing at an adequate level, but none of the musicians has been satisfied with the degree of recovery or can be considered cured. Sometimes, accommodations can be made by changes in repertoire, favoring slower pieces or merely slow tempi, or refingering difficult passages.

PREVENTION OF NEUROLOGICAL PROBLEMS IN PERFORMERS

We have discussed in some detail the treatment of the various neurological disorders affecting performing artists but have neglected the more important approach—prevention. Unfortunately, there are few, if any, data upon which to base a preventative approach, only common sense and conjecture. One would assume that, if most performers and students describe increases in practice time or intensity of practice, changes of instrument or technique, new repertoire, unrelated activity or trauma, or emotional stress as precipitating events for development of their problems, then avoidance of these should reduce the chance of injury. Obviously this is not often going to be possible. We do believe, however, that sensible practice habits, including frequent breaks and reasonable total practice and playing time; good general body conditioning; specific attention to maintenance of good posture, strength, and flexibility of the required muscles; warm-up and cool-down programs before and after practice and playing sessions; and gradual rather than sudden changes in duration and intensity of playing are helpful in reducing the incidence of both musculoskeletal and neurological problems. However, no evidence so far available substantiates this assumption. Indeed, a possibly relevant study in industry, in which a regular exercise program was prescribed to one group of workers, suggests that this did not reduce the frequency of injury, although the participants generally felt better (71). In other industrial settings, ergonomic changes in certain tasks have been found to be effective in reducing the occurrence of work-related injury (72,73).

FUTURE DIRECTIONS IN RESEARCH ON NEUROLOGICAL
PROBLEMS OF PERFORMING ARTISTS

We have reviewed above the bulk of what is known about the specific neurological problems which affect performing artists and which impact most frequently on their ability to carry out their particular art. Much of the concern with the relationship between nervous system function and performing arts has been mentioned only in passing. As discussed in the opening paragraph of this chapter, the precise central and peripheral nervous system functions which enable the performer to create and recreate the master works of music, dance, and drama are incompletely understood. This can provide a rich and fertile ground for investigation. It is no overstatement to assert that understanding the complexities of sensory perception, the interpretative and emotional content, and the neuromuscular processes involved in execution of the arts would be tantamount to understanding much of human behavior in general. It is not proposed that we discuss here the methods by which this lofty goal might be achieved. Rather, we might look at some of the specific problems reviewed and consider briefly some investigative goals which may be achievable in the coming decade.

The areas of investigation may be divided into three sections. The first deals with the epidemiology of neurological problems in performing artists. Among the goals of epidemiology are the assessment of disease frequency (incidence and prevalence) in a specific group or population, determination of risk factors influencing the development of certain disorders, and disease prognosis, including both the natural history and the effects of treatment. Implicit in any study of disease frequency is the need for accuracy in diagnosis and case ascertainment. The larger the population being surveyed, the more likely it is that both of these suffer. Individual practitioners carrying out epidemiologic surveys are more likely to render consistent diagnoses, although consistency does not always ensure diagnostic accuracy. Survey instruments such as questionnaires depend upon patient reporting of information, which may or may not be accurate and yet often these are the only practical methods of obtaining information from large groups. Individual physician-patient contact is more likely to provide diagnostically accurate information, but is increasingly impractical for larger groups. Consistency of information gleaned from both types of studies would be reassuring as far as data reliability is concerned. Risk factor analysis also depends upon accuracy of diagnosis and on the thoroughness with which all potential contributory factors are investigated. Identification of a specific risk factor for a disease requires that data regarding the presence or absence of that risk factor be available. As an example in the performing arts, one might ask whether hand size could be a contributory factor to development of playing-related pain in instrumentalists or, much more specifically, carpal tunnel syndrome in pianists. The answer could not be obtained without having information in the survey regarding hand size; just how specific this information would have to be (e.g., glove size versus measurements of individual digit length, width, girth, and span) is uncertain. The problems of disease prognosis and analysis of the effects of treatment may be even more difficult. The factors of disease severity and duration at the time of diagnosis or initiation of treatment, the skill and enthusiasm with which treatments are provided, the well-recognized placebo effect, and the assessment of success of treatment outcome are all variables that must be taken into account. The tools of the epidemiologist to carry out both risk factor analysis and assessment of natural history include both the retrospective and the prospective study. Each of these requires careful planning and include the use of a "control."

There is currently a need for information on the frequency with which neurological problems occur in performing artists as well as a need for risk factor analysis and determination of natural history. There are many reasons for believing that performing artists provide an excellent population to study epidemiologically. They form an easily identifiable group, tend to be observant, sensitive, and analytical, are highly motivated, and also tend to be very interested in health issues. At the same time, performers may be reluctant to participate in surveys and other research efforts, as has been noted in some such attempts (22,23). A number of explanations have been offered for this reluctance, but it does complicate the efforts to obtain data on large groups of performers. My own view is that this reticence is diminishing but still influences efforts in this regard.

Little information is available regarding the mechanisms by which the major neurological problems outlined above develop in performing artists. A substantial body of knowledge is available, however, regarding the conditions in which compression neuropathies may occur in other groups. It has already been mentioned that there is still controversy as to whether the most common focal compression neuropathy, carpal tunnel syndrome, is or is not related to occupational hand usage. A few relevant studies have looked at different occupations or hobbies involving varying levels of hand use (74,75). Musicians would seem to be an ideal group to study. Wagner (76) has looked at various hand characteristics in "successful" musicians versus those with technical or musculoskeletal problems, but not with a specific concern regarding focal neuropathies. The risk factors for development of compression neuropathies need to be enumerated, including anatomical and physiological data as well as information on the role of position and technique. A variety of approaches can be utilized for this. There is still room for clinical evaluation, including analysis of body size and configuration, strength, conditioning, flexibility, and other anatomical variants. Sophisticated techniques such as magnetic resonance imaging and computed tomographic scanning may provide additional insight into the internal anatomy and may be adaptable for studies in different positions. For instance, the capacity of specific compartments or passages through the limb may be assessable by such methods. Physiologic data from electrodiagnostic studies may also provide valuable information on susceptibility of nerves to compression in different positions. Inconsistency of results in previous studies of thoracic outlet syndrome, carpal tunnel syndrome, and ulnar neuropathy at the elbow may be resolved by further refinements of technique. Ergonomic studies and newer techniques of motion analysis may also be applied to the compression neuropathies and may provide important information on risk factors and mechanisms of development.

It should also be obvious from prior discussion in this chapter that a great deal of information is needed regarding the occupational cramp or focal dystonias. There is currently widespread and renewed interest in motor control and its disorders in humans and through animal investigations. This knowledge certainly can be applied to the focal dystonias but, as has been mentioned above, there is not even universal agreement that the occupational cramps do in fact represent focal (often task-specific) dystonias. Investigation into the anatomic localization of the defect and the physiologic mechanisms would be greatly enhanced by development or identification of an animal model for occupational cramp. Once again, analysis of risk factors, both biological and psychological, is needed.

Prevention and treatment is the third area of urgent need. In many ways this is dependent on the collection of data from the first two areas. By recognizing and understanding the epidemiology and pathophysiology of such disorders, specific treatment and prevention strategies can be designed more readily. However, as in all fields of medicine, we can ill afford to await full understanding of disease mechanisms before developing treatment and prevention protocols. For example, it has fortunately not been necessary to understand the reasons for selective involvement of motor neurons by the poliomyelitis virus to be able largely to prevent this devastating illness. Certainly, advances in both prevention and treatment are greatly enhanced by the acquisition of knowledge of the basic mechanisms of disease production. The most acute need in performing arts medicine, in my view, is the development of an effective approach to occupational cramp. While not the most common affliction of the performer, it is the most consistently unyielding to therapeutic efforts. Neuroanatomical, neurophysiological, neuropharmacological, and neuropsychological techniques should all be brought to bear on this most troublesome problem.

The initial steps toward effective therapy and prevention have been facilitated by the many successful dialogues among health care professionals, teachers, and performers. Mutual educational efforts must continue to attempt to overcome the persisting communication barriers among these groups.

The past 10 to 15 years have witnessed a dramatic increase in interest in the health problems of performing artists (77). While much of the literature remains descriptive, scientific methods of investigation are beginning to be applied to it. If performing arts medicine follows the example of many other areas of scientific inquiry, the next decade could easily provide information of immense interest and importance. Let's hope this is the case.

REFERENCES

1. Blau JN, Henson RA. Neurological disorders in performing musicians. In: Critchley M, Henson RA, eds. *Music and the brain: studies in the neurology of music.* London: William Heinemann, 1977;301–322.
2. Horenstein S. Neuromuscular and related aspects of musical performance. *Cleve Clin Q* 1986;53:53–60.
3. Lockwood A. Medical problems of musicians. *N Engl J Med* 1989;320:221–227.
4. Knishkowy B, Lederman RJ. Instrumental musicians with upper extremity disorders: a follow-up study. *Med Probl Perform Art* 1986;1:85–89.
5. Newmark J, Lederman RJ. Practice doesn't necessarily make perfect: incidence of overuse syndromes in amateur instrumentalists. *Med Probl Perform Art* 1987; 2:142–144.
6. Fry HJH. Occupational maladies of musicians: their cause and prevention. *Internat J Music Educ* 1984;2:59–63.
7. Newmark J, Hochberg FH. "Doctor, it hurts when I play:" painful disorders among instrumental musicians. *Med Probl Perform Art* 1987;2:93–97.

8. Quoted in Crofton I, Fraser D. *A dictionary of musical quotations.* New York: Schirmer Books, 1985;119.
9. Albert ML. *Clinical neurology of aging.* New York: Oxford University Press, 1984.
10. Hochberg FH, Leffert RD, Heller MD, Merriman L. Hand difficulties among musicians. *JAMA* 1983;249:1869–1872.
11. Manchester RA. The incidence of hand problems in music students. *Med Probl Perform Art* 1988;3:15–18.
12. Dawson WJ. Hand and upper extremity problems in musicians: epidemiology and diagnosis. *Med Probl Perform Art* 1988;3:19–22.
13. Critchley M. Musicogenic epilepsy. In: Critchley M, Henson RA, eds. *Music and the Brain: studies in the neurology of music.* London: William Heinemann, 1977;344–353.
14. Alajouanine TH. Aphasia and artistic realization. *Brain* 1948;71:229–241.
15. Dalessio DJ. Maurice Ravel and Alzheimer's disease. *JAMA* 1984;252:3412–3413.
16. Henson RA. Maurice Ravel's illness: A tragedy of lost creativity. *Br Med J* 1988;296:1585–1588.
17. Calabrese LH. AIDS in the performing arts. *Med Probl Perform Art* 1987;2:113–116.
18. Raeburn S. Occupational stress and coping in a sample of professional rock musicians II. *Med Probl Perform Art* 1987;2:77–82.
19. Brandfonbrener AG, MacLean IC, Johnsen JA. Myasthenia gravis in wind players: two case studies. *Med Probl Perform Art* 1988;3:155–157.
20. Benton AL. The amusias. In: Critchley M, Henson RA, eds. *Music and the Brain: Studies in the neurology of music.* London: William Heinemann, 1977;378–397.
21. Brust JCM. Music and language: Musical alexia and agraphia. *Brain* 1980;103:367–392.
22. Caldron PH, Calabrese LH, Clough JD, Lederman RJ, Williams G, Leatherman J. A survey of musculoskeletal problems encountered in high-level musicians. *Med Probl Perform Art* 1986;1:136–139.
23. Fishbein M, Middlestadt SE, Ottati V, Straus S, Ellis A. Medical problems among ICSOM musicians: Overview of a national survey. *Med Probl Perform Art* 1988;3:1–8.
24. Lederman RJ. Peripheral nerve disorders in instrumentalists. *Ann Neurol* 1989,26:640–646.
25. Lederman RJ. Nerve entrapment syndromes in instrumental musicians. *Med Probl Perform Art* 1986;1:45–48.
26. Newmark J, Hochberg FH. Isolated painless manual incoordination in 57 musicians. *J Neurol Neurosurg Psychiatry* 1987;50:291–295.
27. Lederman RJ. Occupational cramp in instrumental musicians. *Med Probl Perform Art* 1988;3:45–51.
28. Yoss RE, Corbin KB, MacCarty CS, Love JG. Significance of symptoms and signs in localization of involved root in cervical disc protrusion. *Neurology* 1957;7:673–683.
29. Lascelles RG, Mohr PD, Neary D, Bloor K. The thoracic outlet syndrome. *Brain* 1977;100:601–602.
30. Roos DB. Thoracic outlet syndromes: symptoms, diagnosis, anatomy and surgical treatment. *Med Probl Perform Art* 1986;1:90–93.
31. Lederman RJ. Thoracic outlet syndromes: review of the controversies and a report of 17 instrumental musicians. *Med Probl Perform Art* 1987;2:87–91.
32. Wilbourn AJ, Porter JM. Thoracic outlet syndromes. *Spine: State of the Art Reviews* 1988;2:597–626.
33. Clein LJ. The droopy shoulder syndrome. *Can Med Assoc J* 1976;114:343–344.
34. Swift TR, Nichols FT. The droopy shoulder syndrome. *Neurology* 1984;34:212–215.
35. Armstrong TJ, Silverstein BA. Upper extremity pain in the workplace—role of usage in causality. In: Hadler NM, ed. *Clinical concepts in regional musculoskeletal illness.* New York: Grune and Stratton, 1987;333–354.
36. Hadler NM. Is carpal tunnel syndrome an injury that qualifies for Workers' Compensation insurance? In: Hadler NM, ed. *Clinical concepts in regional musculoskeletal illness.* New York: Grune and Stratton, 1987;355–360.
37. Bleeker ML, Bohlman M, Moreland R, Tipton A. Carpal tunnel syndrome: role of carpal canal size. *Neurology* 1985;35:1599–1604.
38. Kopell HP, Thompson WAL. Pronator syndrome: a confirmed case and its diagnosis. *N Engl J Med* 1958;259:713–715.
39. Morris HH, Peters BH. Pronator syndrome: clinical and electrophysiological features in seven cases. *J Neurol Neurosurg Psychiatry* 1976;39:461–464.

40. Charness ME, Barbaro NM, Olney RK, Parry GJ. Occupational cubital tunnel syndrome in instrumental musicians. *Neurology* 1987;37(Suppl 1):115.
41. Feindel W, Stratford J. The role of the cubital tunnel in tardy ulnar palsy. *Can J Surg* 1958;1:287–300.
42. Wainapel SF, Cole JL. The not-so-magic flute: two cases of distal ulnar nerve entrapment. *Med Probl Perform Art* 1988;3:63–65.
43. Cynamon KB. Flutist's neuropathy. *N Engl J Med* 1981;305:961.
44. Lister GD, Belsole RB, Kleinert HE. The radial tunnel syndrome. *J Hand Surg* 1979;4:52–59.
45. Makin GVJ, Brown WF. Entrapment of the posterior cutaneous nerve of the arm. *Neurology* 1985;35:1677–1678.
46. Schwartz E, Hodson A. A viol paresthesia. *Lancet* 1980;2:156.
47. Howard PL. Gamba leg. *N Engl J Med* 1982;306:115.
48. Mladinich EK, DeWitt J. A newly recognized occupation palsy. *JAMA* 1974;228:695.
49. Romberg MH. *A manual of the nervous diseases of man.* Translated by EH Sieveking, Vol 1. London: Sydenham Society, 1853;320–324.
50. Gowers WR. *A manual of diseases of the nervous system*, 2nd ed, Vol II, 1893. Reprinted by Hafner Publishing Company, Darien CT: 1970;710–730.
51. Poore GV. Clinical lecture on certain conditions of the hand and arm which interfere with the performances of professional acts, especially piano-playing. *Brit Med J* 1887;1:441–444.
52. Sheehy MP, Marsden CD. Writers' cramp—a focal dystonia. *Brain* 1982;105:461–480.
53. Rosenbaum F, Jankovic J. Focal task-specific tremor and dystonia: categorization of occupational movement disorders. *Neurology* 1988;38:522–527.
54. Critchley M. Occupational palsies in musical performers. In: Critchley M, Henson RA, eds. *Music and the brain: studies in the neurology of music.* London: Heinemann, 1977;365–377.
55. Merriman L, Newmark J, Hochberg FH, Shahani B, Leffert R. A focal movement disorder of the hand in six pianists. *Med Probl Perform Art* 1986;1:17–19.
56. Hays B. "Painless" hand problems of string-pluckers. *Med Probl Perform Art* 1987;2:39–40.
57. Fry HJH. Overuse syndrome in musicians—100 years ago: an historical overview. *Med J Aust* 1986;145:620–625.
58. Fry H, Hallett M. Focal dystonia (occupational cramp) masquerading as nerve entrapment or hysteria. *Plast Reconstr Surg* 1988;82:908–910.
59. Lederman RJ. Overuse syndrome in musicians. *Med J Aust* 1987;146:390.
60. Marsden CD. The focal dystonias. *Clin Neuropharmacol* 1986;9 (Suppl 2):549–560.
61. Marsden CD, Rothwell JC. The physiology of idiopathic dystonia. *Can J Neurol Sci* 1987;14:521–527.
62. Cohen LG, Hallett M. Hand cramps: clinical features and electromyographic patterns in a focal dystonia. *Neurology* 1988;38:1005–1012.
63. Panizza ME, Hallett N, Nilsson J. Reciprocal inhibition in patients with hand cramps. *Neurology* 1989;39:85–89.
64. Schott GD. Induction of involuntary movements by peripheral trauma: an analogy with causalgia. *Lancet* 1986;2:712–715.
65. Scherokman B, Husain F, Cuetter A, Jabbari B, Maniglia E. Peripheral dystonia. *Arch Neurol* 1986;43:830–832.
66. James I, Cook P. Bromocriptine for horn players' palsy. *Lancet* 1983;1:1450.
67. Fahn S, Marsden CD. The treatment of dystonia. In: Marsden CD, Fahn S, eds. *Movement disorders 2.* London: Butterworths, 1987;359–382.
68. Liversedge LA, Sylvester JD. Conditioning techniques in the treatment of writer's cramp. In: Eysenck HD, ed. *Behaviour therapy and the neuroses.* New York: Pergamon Press, 1960;327–333.
69. LeVine WR. Behavioral and biofeedback therapy for a functionally impaired musician: a case report. *Biofeedback Self Regul* 1983;8:101–107.
70. Cohen L, Hallett M, Geller B, Dubinsky R, Meer J, Baker M, Hochberg F. Treatment of focal dystonias of the hand with botulinum toxin injection. *Neurology* 1987;37(Suppl 1):123.
71. Silverstein BA, Armstrong TJ, Longmate A, Woody D. Can in-plant exercise control musculoskeletal symptoms? *J Occup Med* 1988;30:922–927.
72. Tichauer ER. Some aspects of stress on forearm and hand in industry. *J Occup Med* 1966;8:63–71.
73. Ohara H, Aoyama H, Itani T. Health hazard among cash register operators and the effects of improved working conditions. *J Human Ergol* 1976;5:31–40.

74. Birkbeck MQ, Beer TC. Occupation in relation to the carpal tunnel syndrome. *Rheumatol Rehab* 1975;14:218–221.
75. Nathan PA, Meadows KD, Doyle LS. Occupation as a risk factor for impaired sensory conduction of the median nerve at the carpal tunnel level. *J Hand Surg* 1988;13B:167–170.
76. Wagner C. Success and failure in musical performance: biomechanics of the hand. In: Rochmann FL, Wilson FR, eds. *The biology of music making: proceedings of the 1984 Denver conference*. St. Louis: MMG Music, Inc., 1988;154–179.
77. Lederman RJ. Performing arts medicine. *N Engl J Med* 1989;320:246–248.

Textbook of Performing Arts Medicine, edited
by R. T. Sataloff, A. Brandfonbrener, and
R. Lederman. Raven Press, Ltd.,
New York © 1991.

6

Diagnosis and Surgical Treatment of the Hand

*†Richard G. Eaton and †† †William B. Nolan

*Professor of Clinical Surgery, College of Physicians and Surgeons of Columbia
University, Director, †The Hand Center, Roosevelt Hospital,
New York, New York 10019 ††St. Luke's-Roosevelt Hospital Center,
New York, New York 10025

GENERAL PRINCIPLES OF MANAGEMENT

Hands are man's unique and highly personal instruments. As a functioning unit, their perception and control begin in the cerebral cortex. Through a remarkably ingenious mechanical and neural system they are capable of infinite combinations of positions and pressures. The hands may be called upon to roll off an arpeggio, interpret braille, split a diamond, or shatter a brick. Manual performance, however, is profoundly influenced by training, experience, and imagination. Since these functions are stored and dispensed by the brain and nervous system, performance is also significantly influenced by emotion and the psyche. The emotional component of this controlling unit can have either a positive or negative influence on overall human performance.

In addition to normal wear and tear, the hands of artists are frequently called upon to execute movements which must be powerful, subtle, or rapidly repetitive. These demands may far exceed normal manual activity and dexterity. They are thus prone to the afflictions of extended mechanical stress such as tendinitis, synovitis, and arthritis. The burden of emotional stress generated by concern for career limitation may be superimposed on these physical problems.

Diagnostic Considerations

Performance-related hand problems which prompt an artist to seek medical attention usually fall into two broad categories: acute-inflammatory or chronic-degenerative. Inflammatory conditions, acute or subacute, make up the significant majority of these presenting complaints. Overuse conditions are often produced by sudden increases in practice time or intensity. Initially they usually follow recognizable anatomic patterns involving specifically overused and inflamed muscle or tendon units. Fairly rapidly, however, compensatory, self-protective patterns develop. This is done in a subconscious effort to relieve pain and spasm in the afflicted musculotendinous units by transferring the stress to another part of the upper limb.

The cerebral cortex designates a motion and the pathway to execute this motion, through a complex series of neural pathways. When this involves secondary musculotendinous units, new stresses to these areas produce pain in a different anatomic distribution. For instance, if the thumb hurts because of acute basal joint inflammation, the wrist, elbow, and shoulder may be positioned to reduce thumb stress. With prolonged playing, the muscles that stabilize the more proximal joints fatigue and become painful. This compensatory sequence may continue with quite convoluted pain patterns developing until the initial entity is recognized and specific treatment is begun.

The key to effective treatment is precise diagnosis. The diagnosis is based on a comprehensive history as well as physical examination. With a functional knowledge of upper limb anatomy and mechanics, the symptoms may be localized to a specific anatomic site.

History Taking

The patient is always asked about recent or past trauma. Although the symptoms are reported to be of recent onset, they may be the result of an old fracture or soft tissue injury. Radiographs are helpful in assessing the hand for evidence of old trauma or previously undiagnosed degenerative condition.

The patient is also asked about recent changes in practice time or technique. In addition to revealing information about a possible overuse etiology, this is an opportunity to discuss the concept of conditioning with the patient. Just as it is not reasonable to run a marathon without conditioning it is equally unreasonable to suddenly double or triple practice time. All physical activity must be increased gradually to avoid injury. This concept, which is fundamental to sports training, has only recently received the attention of musicians who frequently consider performance a primarily mental effort. It is also important to know and record the patients's practice routines and requirements.

The patient is then asked to quantitate the pain on a scale of one to ten. It is important to establish the level of pain as a baseline for evaluation of primary and secondary (compensatory) sites of pain, as well as effectiveness of treatment. It is also useful in helping the patient establish a reasonable practice or performance schedule during the recovery period. It is important to know on what occasions the pain develops, how long it lasts, and what relieves it.

Physical Examination

The patient must localize the symptoms to one point of maximum tenderness. If the physical examination fails to isolate a particular anatomic area, it is useful to have the musician play the instrument. This will often identify a particular motion which causes discomfort. Stop-action videotape can be used to isolate particular motions which aggravate the symptoms. Often careful analysis and correction of poor or compensatory playing postures is necessary before a permanent cure can be effected.

The physical examination will focus on the specific area of reported symptoms. However, a systematic analysis of the neural, musculotendinous, vascular, skeletal, and ligamentous systems must be done to avoid missing the primary diagnosis. The components of a complete hand examination are well described in many textbooks (1–3). A diagnosis should not be made on the basis of one or two provocative tests without examining all of the other possible systems which could produce similar signs and symptoms. The diagnosis of an upper limb problem is frequently a problem in applied anatomy. With a knowledge of the anatomy and mechanics of each particular system, a specific diagnosis becomes apparent and is confirmed by the physical examination.

The standard components of a complete hand examination include motor and sensory evaluation, tendon and joint excursion, vascular examination, evaluation of pinch and grip strength, and appropriate provocative tests. However, in the case of artists, it is also important to test these systems during repetitive activity. Often an anatomic system fails only when subjected to repeated activity, which is fundamental to artistic performance. This aspect of the examination can be evaluated by having the musician play his or her instrument, and can be quantitated as a length of time or number of repetitions of a specific strength or motion test. There are also diagnostic and exercise devices such as the Baltimore Therapeutic Exercise (BTE) machine, which can test the upper extremity systems and quantitate work performance and fatigue levels.

Treatment Considerations

Early recognition of the primary site of pathology and overuse patterns is vital in order to prevent major distortions in motor patterns. Given that many of the problems experienced by the musician are inflammatory in nature, rest and antiinflammatory medication are important. However, *unless the pain is totally disabling for a musician, complete abstinence from practicing should be discouraged.*

Adequate rest can usually be achieved by a moderate reduction in the duration and intensity of practicing. It must be recognized that performance requires strength, coordination, and conditioning. These attributes diminish rapidly when the musician stops practicing entirely. The musician must then overcome the loss of conditioning as well as the primary problem. It is preferable to establish a length of practice time which does not aggravate the symptoms, even if it is only minutes.

When not practicing, immobilization in splints may be carried out for 2 to 3 weeks. On a one to ten scale for pain (ten equals maximum), playing or practicing up to a four or five level may be allowed before stopping to rest, and will thus assure less strain and allow the patient to maintain a reasonable state of coordination, tissue hardiness, and confidence.

Performance disabilities in artists and musicians have the best prognosis when corrected early, before compensatory patterns, muscle and ligamentous weakness and discouragement set in. Most of the symptomatic ligament strains and tendinitis states will begin to respond within 3 to 4 weeks with a carefully managed rest and antiinflammatory regimen. However, certain specific, painful tendon and nerve entrapment syndromes (i.e., trigger finger, deQuervain's disease, carpal and cubital tunnel syndromes) may not completely reverse, or may recur soon after medical treatment has been discontinued.

When these syndromes have become intractable, there should be serious consideration for surgical correction. Surgical release of the mechanical entrapment syndromes provides an excellent prognosis and should return the performer to rapidly increasing function within 3 to 6 weeks. *Despite the natural reluctance to undergo surgery, repeated courses of unsuccessful conservative treatment serve only to prolong the disability and in time create serious career anxieties.* Fortunately, most entrapment-release surgical procedures are brief, simple, and can be done under local or regional anesthesia on an outpatient basis. In the appropriate instance, with a precise diagnosis, surgery offers a high likelihood of completely resolving the problem with a great reduction in the musician's period of disability.

ACUTE-INFLAMMATORY PROBLEMS

Neural Entrapment

Neural entrapment can occur anywhere from the cervical spine to the fingers. Therefore, appropriate treatment of peripheral neuropathies requires a comprehensive knowledge of upper extremity anatomy. The exact site of injury must be established before suggesting a treatment plan. If the lesion is incorrectly localized, the patient will obtain minimal benefit, regardless of the method of treatment.

The precise level of the neurologic lesion is established with a comprehensive physical examination and electrodiagnostic laboratory testing. Injury to a peripheral nerve results in a unique disturbance of motor or sensory function. Electrodiagnostic testing is extremely valuable in confirming the site of nerve compression, making treatment more precise and effective.

It is important to repeat and record these examinations throughout the course of treatment. Only by reviewing this information can the physician determine the success of treatment or the need to switch to a different modality of therapy. Treatment is frequently divided into nonoperative and operative approaches. Nonoperative treatment includes splints, oral antiinflammatory medications including steroids, and injectable steroids.

When nonoperative treatment does not produce prompt clinical improvement, surgical decompression of the nerve is in the best interest of the patient. Of particular importance is the presence of motor paralysis. When this occurs, operative decompression should not be delayed beyond 3 months. Prolonged compression of a peripheral nerve may result in permanent neural damage with atrophy and fibrosis of the denervated muscle. Most compression neuropathies that do not respond to conservative treatment within 3 months rarely will improve without surgical decompression.

Entrapment neuropathies are known to occur at particular sites between the cervical spine and fingers (4). The examining physician must have a complete knowledge of the signs and symptoms of each entity (Table 6.1) (5). Two sites of compression are commonly seen in performing artists: carpal tunnel and cubital tunnel syndromes.

Carpal Tunnel Syndrome

Carpal tunnel syndrome is the most common nerve entrapment syndrome in the upper extremity. This is a result of certain unique anatomic features. The median nerve enters the hand through the carpal tunnel (Fig. 6.1). The tunnel is composed of a dorsal bony carpal arch and is enclosed on the palmar surface by the transverse carpal ligament. This is a rigid fibro-osseous sheath, enclosing the median nerve along with nine tendons and their nutrient synovium.

The arrangement of these ten structures in the carpal tunnel, with the median nerve lying most superficial, permits compression of the nerve between the flexor tendons and the transverse carpal ligament. In addition, any structure which occupies space in this enclosure can compress the median nerve. This can be synovium, a bony tumor, carpal bone dislocation, an anomalous blood vessel, a ganglion, a lipoma, or fat.

Carpal tunnel syndrome is usually the result of synovial swelling (6). The repetitive motion of the flexors and wrist flexion, commonly part of playing an instrument, may result in hypertrophy of the synovium. An increase in synovial volume inside of this limiting space results in median nerve compression.

The patient will report numbness and tingling in the distribution of the median nerve, on the palmar aspects of the thumb, index, middle, and radial half of the ring fingers. The symptoms are frequently worse at night. In recumbency, there is a redistribution of interstitial body fluid and synovial swelling increases. In addition, during sleep the patient's wrist frequently relaxes into flexion. The median nerve is compressed as it enters the congested carpal tunnel across the prominent proximal edge of the transverse carpal ligament. Symptoms are usually relieved if the patient shakes the hands and moves the fingers or even gets up and walks around.

TABLE 6.1. *Evaluation of entrapment neuropathies*

Compression syndrome	Anatomic location	Signs and symptoms
Nerve Root and Brachial Plexus		
Cervical root	Cervical vertebrae	Distally-radiating pain with neck rotation, sensory and neural deficits appropriate to the cervical root, EMG denervation of proximal muscle groups
Thoracic outlet	First rib, scalenus muscles	Coldness, paresthesia and pain related to subclavian artery and lower trunk of brachial plexus
Radial Nerve		
High radial nerve compression	Spiral groove of humerus, lateral head of triceps	Loss of wrist extension in addition to loss of finger and thumb extension
Posterior interosseous	Arcade of Frohse, radial recurrent artery, radial humeral joint, extensor carpi radialis brevis	Loss of finger and/or thumb extension. No sensory loss
Superficial radial nerve	Elbow and over first dorsal compartment	Sensory disturbance of the thumb without motor loss
Median Nerve		
Pronator teres	Elbow at pronator teres, bicipital aponeurosis	Upper arm pain with resisted pronation
Anterior interosseous	Fibrous edge of superficialas origin	Paralysis of FPL, index FDP, and pronator quadratus
Carpal tunnel	Transverse carpal ligament	Median nerve sensory disturbances, positive Phalen's, intact median nerve extrinsics, thenar atrophy
Ulnar nerve		
Cubital tunnel	Posterior to medial epicondyle	Decreased FCU and FDP V plus sensory changes, ulnar intrinsic weakness/atrophy
Guyon's tunnel	Volar carpal ligament	Sensory and ulnar intrinsic changes

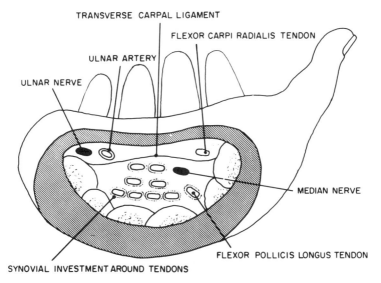

TRANSVERSE CARPAL LIGAMENT

FLEXOR CARPI RADIALIS TENDON

ULNAR ARTERY

ULNAR NERVE

MEDIAN NERVE

FLEXOR POLLICIS LONGUS TENDON

SYNOVIAL INVESTMENT AROUND TENDONS

FIG. 6.1. The carpal tunnel is shown in cross section. The median nerve lies superficial to the flexor tendons (*large filled circle*). Synovial hypertrophy or other space-occupying lesions result in median nerve compression within this closed space.

The symptoms can often be reproduced by placing the wrist in flexion, the Phalen test (Fig. 6.2). Tapping on the palmar surface of the wrist may also result in tingling in a median nerve distribution (Tinel's sign). With prolonged or severe compression, there may be motor loss with atrophy of the thenar muscles and decreased pinch strength as well as sensory impairment.

Electrodiagnostic studies may show a decreased nerve conduction velocity across the wrist and denervation of the thenar intrinsic muscles. However, approximately 25% of patients can have normal studies (7). This study is useful in confirming the clinical diagnosis and in differentiating between carpal tunnel syndrome and more proximal sites of compression. In addition to the space-occupying lesions listed above, systemic conditions have been associated with this entrapment syndrome, including diabetes mellitus, alcoholism, amyloidosis, and pregnancy. Transient symptoms of median nerve compression have also been reported in patients with a history of a distal radius fracture (8,9).

In the absence of muscle atrophy, a trial of conservative therapy is appropriate with splinting and antiinflammatory medication. Splinting consists of placing the wrist in a neutral or slightly extended position. The splint is worn at night for at least 3 weeks.

Antiinflammatory medication can be injected into the carpal tunnel or given orally. Injection of a corticosteroid into the carpal tunnel must be done with great care. The needle can damage the nerve, and skin depigmentation or atrophy may occur due to the steroid. While injection of the carpal tunnel has advocates (10), it

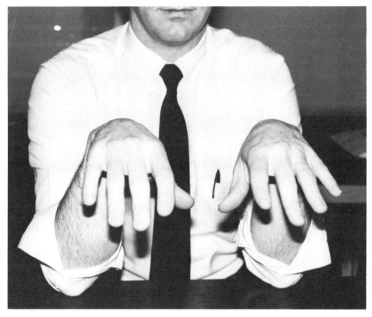

FIG. 6.2. Phalen's maneuver is demonstrated. The patient is instructed to hold the wrists in a flexed position for 60 seconds. The time and description of symptoms are recorded.

has been estimated that in the absence of a reversible systemic etiology such as pregnancy, 65% to 90% of patients will have some recurrence of symptoms (11). The use of nonsteroidal antiinflammatory medication is of limited benefit in the treatment of this problem. In the case of pregnancy, treatment should be conservative as the majority of patients will stop having symptoms when postpartum hormonal changes resolve.

The indication for surgical release of the nerve is failure of conservative measures. If symptoms persist beyond 3 months, or if there is evidence of motor loss, there should be prompt surgical decompression to avoid a permanent disability. Decompression of the carpal tunnel is accomplished by division of the transverse carpal ligament. This can be done with local or regional anesthesia on an outpatient basis. Postoperatively, the wrist is splinted in slight extension for 2 weeks. Full finger motion is encouraged during the period of wrist immobilization. The length of time necessary for recovery of the median nerve depends on the severity of the nerve compression. Frequently, patients report almost immediate relief from the symptoms of night pain and painful tingling. If the nerve has sustained internal injury secondary to severe or prolonged compression, recovery takes months rather than hours and is variable, depending on the regenerative capacity of the individual and the condition of the nerve.

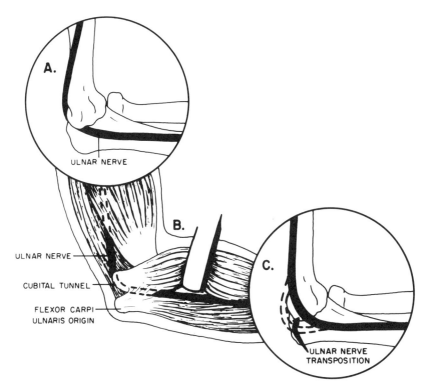

FIG. 6.3. A: The ulnar nerve is seen passing behind the medial epicondyle of the humerus, through the cubital tunnel. B: The relationship of the ulnar nerve to the surrounding muscle and fascial structures is demonstrated. The ulnar nerve may be compressed as it passes through the cubital tunnel or beneath the fascial origin of the flexor carpi ulnaris. C: With an anterior transposition, the ulnar nerve is placed outside of the cubital tunnel, and held in that position by a fascial sling.

Cubital Tunnel Syndrome

The cubital tunnel begins in the ulnar groove behind the medial epicondyle of the humerus (Fig. 6.3[A]). The ulnar nerve is superficial in this location and can be easily palpated with the elbow in flexion. The ulnar nerve passes posteriorly behind the medial epicondyle and through the cubital tunnel, which changes shape and volume during elbow flexion and extension. It then passes between the aponeurotic origins of the wrist and finger flexor muscles, which often become swollen with prolonged activity, such as playing the violin (Fig. 6.3[B]). A neuropathy may result from compression as the nerve passes across the medial intramuscular septum from the anterior to the posterior compartment of the arm, by subluxation of the ulnar nerve across the epicondyle with elbow flexion, or by adhesion fixation of the nerve secondary to elbow joint inflammation (12,13).

The patient complains of pain on the ulnar side of the elbow with tingling in the fourth and fifth fingers. The pain may be provoked by elbow flexion and resisted wrist or individual finger flexion. The pain may radiate proximally or distally into the little finger and ulnar side of the ring fingers. Weakness of the flexor carpi ulnaris (FCU), little finger profundus, and ulnar intrinsic muscles may be present. Intrinsic muscle wasting is a sign of prolonged or severe compression and should be treated by surgical decompression as soon as the diagnosis is established.

Nonoperative treatment consists of padding the elbow and using protective splints to prevent full elbow flexion which tightens the FCU and stretches the nerve as it passes through the cubital tunnel, and stretches the ulnar nerve around the condyle. Oral antiinflammatory medications are occasionally of benefit. Injections in this area risk injury to the ulnar nerve.

If nonoperative measures fail to relieve the symptoms, surgical treatment consists of decompression at the sites of entrapment. Surgical decompression should correct all possible mechanical causes of ulnar neuropathy. Ulnar nerve irritation or compression syndromes are produced by pressure on the nerve on passage across the medical septum above the epicondyle, by compression within the fibro-osseous cubital tunnel, upon entrance into the flexor muscles, or by traction on the nerve fixed by adhesions at any point in its passage posterior to the epicondyle. Complete removal of the nerve from the precarious gauntlet through which it must pass stands the best chance of correcting all pathology. Section of the aponeurotic roof of the canal and medial septum plus neurolysis will correct several of these conditions, but will not relieve the traction problem. It may even create new postsurgical adhesions along the course of the nerve. Published results of such simple decompression procedures do not compare favorably with procedures which include transposition of the nerve out of this bony posterior canal into an anterior position (14).

Considerable controversy exists among surgeons regarding the anterior subcutaneous as opposed to the anterior submuscular transposition. In our experience, a specific technique is used which includes maintaining the nerve anteriorly by creation of a facial septum posterior to the transposed nerve (Figure 6.3[C]) (15). It has the advantage of allowing early elbow motion and does not involve detaching parts of the flexor muscle origins as a means of maintaining the nerve in an anterior position. Placing the transposed nerve beneath this muscle mass may create a new potential site for compression and fixation. Such a technique also requires several weeks of elbow immobilization while the muscle reattachments heal.

Severe and prolonged nerve compression with marked sensory and motor defects frequently indicate major intraneural fibrosis which may not completely respond to any type of decompression surgery. However, relief of pain and significant improvement in sensory and motor deficits can usually be expected by improvement in neuronal circulation following decompression and release of nerve fixation.

Using the subcutaneous transposition with a reconstructed medial septum permits immediate elbow motion. Pain and paresthesia are usually immediately reversed. Recovery of full sensation and motor power depend upon regeneration of nerve fibers from the point of compression and is directly related to the degree of compression and distance to regenerate. Maximum recovery can take as long as 12 months but is usually less than 6 months.

Tendon Entrapment

The extensor and flexor tendons pass through a fibrous pulley system as they enter the digits. These pulleys are necessary to prevent bowstringing of the tendons across flexed finger joints. The pulley systems are necessary to improve the efficiency of the tendons in flexing or extending a joint with the minimal amount of tendon excursion. However, at the site where the flexor tendons enter the pulley system in the distal palm there is considerable friction and with overuse, varying degrees of inflammation may ensue.

As with the carpal tunnel syndrome, these canals are relatively tight, limiting spaces. Under various pathologic conditions, the tendon synovium may hypertrophy and become swollen. This results in a caliber discrepency between the volume of the tendons and the volume of the canal. This impairs excursion of the tendon, causes pain, and may result in snapping or triggering as the digit flexes or extends. This condition tends to occur at predictable sites, where the canal is relatively constricted and the tendons are bulbous (Fig. 6.4).

Repetitive flexion and extension of the digits and thumb are common to playing musical instruments. This probably explains the frequency with which trigger finger and deQuervain's stenosing tenosynovitis occur in this group of professional musicians.

Trigger Thumb and Fingers

Tenosynovitis in the thumb or fingers is a common cause of hand problems in the professional musician. It is more common in women than in men. It is occasionally

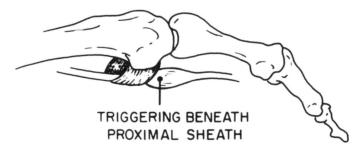

TRIGGERING BENEATH
PROXIMAL SHEATH

FIG. 6.4. A frequent site of tendon entrapment is beneath the A-1 pulley (*filled circle*), where the fibro-osseous tunnel of the finger is relatively constricted and the flexor tendons relatively bulbous.

associated with systemic diseases such as diabetes, rheumatoid arthritis, and gout (16). However, in the musician, repetitive flexion and extension of the digit probably contribute to the frequency with which it occurs.

Triggering or snapping occurs as the patient tries to flex and extend the digit. The constriction of the fibro-osseous tunnel is associated with an increase in the diameter of the flexor tendons at the level of the metacarpol phalangeal (MP) joint (17). Localized inflammation of the tendon sheath at the entrance to the flexor sheath produces transient locking of the tendon. Often the patient localizes the snapping to the proximal interphalangeal joint of the fingers or the interphalangeal joint of the thumb. When this is reported, the physician should always think of triggering as a possible etiology.

If the swelling around the tendon becomes great enough, it is impossible for the tendons to glide past the point of constriction. The digit is then locked in either flexion or extension. This is referred to as a "locked trigger." Triggering occurs most frequently in the middle and ring fingers.

Nonoperative treatment consists of oral steroids or a local injection of steroid into the fibro-osseous tunnel at the level of the MP joint. This may result in relief of the symptoms. It should never be done in the treatment of children or to treat a locked trigger.

Recurrences frequently occur after steroid treatment. Failure to achieve complete relief in 3 to 4 weeks is an indication for surgical release of the tendon sheath, a simple and reliable surgical procedure that permanently relieves the symptoms.

Surgical treatment involves a small incision over the appropriate MP joint and division of the proximal pulley under direct vision (Fig. 6.5). The surgery is done with local anesthesia, and the patient is then asked to flex and extend the digit. A full range of motion confirms that the problem has been corrected. The hand is placed in a soft dressing and the sutures are removed at approximately 10 days. Full active motion is usually achieved within 1 month.

deQuervain's Disease

Stenosing tenosynovitis of the first dorsal compartment of the wrist is another common cause of wrist and hand pain in the performing artist (Fig. 6.6) (18). The patient reports pain associated with thumb motion, localized on the radial side of the wrist. There is frequently swelling over the first dorsal compartment, at the level of the radial styloid process.

Pianists often report severe pain with "thumb under" motions, where the thumb is flexed beneath the fingers to strike a key in sequence after the little finger. In fact, this motion is similar to Finkelstein's sign (Fig. 6.7), the classic provocative test for this problem. Both "cross-overs" and the Finkelstein's sign stretch the adbuctor pollicus longus and extensor pollicis brevis tendons, which causes pain in the first dorsal compartment.

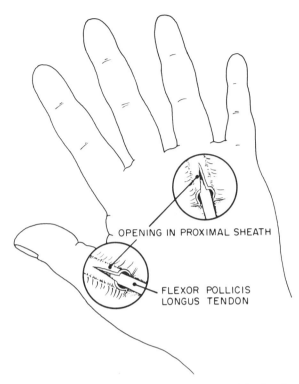

FIG. 6.5. The location of the surgical release of the A-1 pulleys of the thumb and ring finger is shown. The skin incisions are made within a skin crease and centered over the MP joints (*filled circles*).

When these symptoms are reported, it is important to examine the basal (carpo-metacarpal) joint of the thumb, which can produce similar complaints. These problems are differentiated by x-rays and physical examination of the basal joint. It is also important to examine the patient for evidence of tenosynovitis of the second dorsal compartment, intersection syndrome (19).

Nonoperative treatment consists of oral steroids or local steroid injection, or systemic anti-inflammatory medication in combination with a splint that immobilizes the wrist and thumb. This treatment usually results in relief of pain. However, in the absence of a medically correctable condition that is responsible for deQuervain's, such as pregnancy or an endocrinopathy, the symptoms frequently recur with the resumption of activity (20).

Surgical decompression of the first dorsal compartment is done with local or regional anesthesia on an outpatient basis. The wound is allowed to heal for 2 weeks with the wrist held in a plaster shell. The prognosis following surgery is excellent (21).

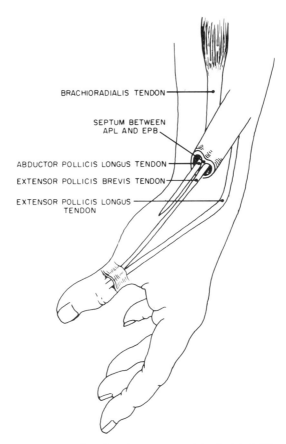

BRACHIORADIALIS TENDON

SEPTUM BETWEEN
APL AND EPB

ABDUCTOR POLLICIS LONGUS TENDON

EXTENSOR POLLICIS BREVIS TENDON

EXTENSOR POLLICIS LONGUS
TENDON

FIG. 6.6. The anatomy of the first dorsal compartment is depicted. The abductor pollicis longus and extensor pollicis brevis tendons are contained in this compartment. An increase in tendon diameter caused by synovitis will restrict movement of the tendons in the tunnel and cause pain.

CHRONIC-DEGENERATIVE PROBLEMS

The second general category of performance-related hand problems includes the chronic-degenerative disorders. Osteoarthritis is the most common problem in this category. It is frequently seen in the general population. The incidence of hand involvement in the general population increases with age. In the age group of 18 to 24 years, less than 3% of people have radiographic evidence of an arthritic hand condition. However, by age 75, 80% of men and 90% of women have arthritic changes (22). In the vast majority of the population, the radiographic changes seldom have clinical significance. However, the performing artist frequently subjects the hands to forces that can exacerbate an arthritic condition and become a source of disability.

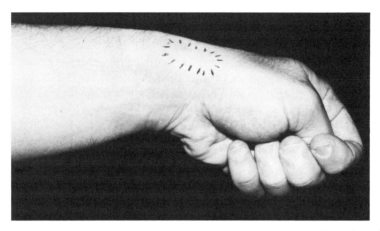

FIG. 6.7. Finkelstein's sign for deQuervain's disease is demonstrated. The thumb is positioned in the palm, and the wrist is moved in an ulnar direction. This stretches the abductor pollicis longus and the extensor pollicis brevis tendons and causes pain over the first dorsal compartment.

Osteoarthritis is the result of ordinary wear of a joint surface, posttraumatic damage to a joint surface, or joint destruction accelerated by ligament laxity. Pain is the primary manifestation of this process. It is poorly localized and results in weakness and decreased motion. In addition to the voluntary loss of motion which results from pain, with joint destruction the mechanical characteristics of the joint and surrounding ligaments change. The joint becomes stiff with a loss of flexion or extension. The degenerative type of osteoarthritis ultimately results in a loss of motion with a visible deformity around the joint. However, it may occasionally become acutely swollen and painful.

Basal Joint Arthritis

The thumb with its unique range of motion and power, heads the list for chronic or degenerative problems in the hands of performing artists. The highly mobile basal joint of the thumb owes its great range to its trapeziometacarpal "saddle" articulation, nature's version of the mechanical universal joint. Such mobility, however, has its price, as this joint develops earlier and significantly more disabling degenerative changes than other joins of the hand (22). In a random radiographic sampling of women past 50 years of age, one in six demonstrated moderate to advanced osteoarthritic changes in the thumb trapeziometacarpal joint.

Such osteoarthritis is seldom symptomatic in musicians whose major hand posturing is in a position of abduction (away from the palm or index finger). The saddle joint is stable and well-seated in this position. However, problems may develop with this joint in movements in which the thumb is in flexion or adduction. This is the position of pinching against the index finger or the "thumb under" maneuver while playing the piano.

In the adducted and flexed position (pinch), two negative events occur. First, the metacarpal shifts out of the center of the saddle where it is most stable. Second, it is in this position that the thumb usually transmits its greatest force. Prolonged pinching causes the metacarpal base to slide up on one horn of the saddle, creating significant compression on this small area of cartilage.

Prolonged and repetitious compression in time may cause loss of cartilage or aggravate existing arthritic changes, leading to the pain and stiffness of osteoarthritis. The patient complains of pain and weakness that is worse with activity and relieved by rest. The pain is diffuse, and is frequently localized to the radial side of the wrist. The point of maximum tenderness can be identified by pressing directly over the trapeziometacarpal thumb joint. Decreased pinch strength and lateral subluxation (attempted dislocation) of the metacarpal on the trapezium are also frequently present. A radiograph with attempted lateral subluxation is called a stress view (Fig. 6.8A–6.8B). These radiographs, which induce lateral subluxation of the metacarpal on the trapezium, are useful in demonstrating the degree of joint capsule laxity.

Radiographs are utilized to determine the degree of degeneration (stage of degeneration) (Fig. 6.9). Radiographic staging of degenerative arthritis is important because it helps to establish the extent of damage which in turn helps determine the type of reconstructive surgery necessary, should symptoms become intractable (Table 6.2) (23).

In stage I the joint is hypermobile and inflamed. Radiographs show less than one-third subluxation of the joint and normal articular contours. With acute inflammation, molded splints and antiinflammatory medications frequently resolve the symptoms. If symptoms persist, reconstruction of the volar ligament restores stability, resolves the pain, and reduces further degeneration (24). In stage II, early cartilage damage is present. Radiographs show more than one-third subluxation, joint space narrowing and calcific fragments along the joint margins less than 2 mm in size. Clinically, stage II is similar to stage I and its treatment is the same.

Stage III has significant joint space narrowing and articular degeneration. Larger debris with fragments greater than 2 mm in size is seen. All involvement noted on the x-ray is confined to the trapeziometacarpal joints. The scaphotrapezial joint has no visible degenerative changes. In this stage, stiffness and deformity have developed. Crepitus may be noted with twisting of the basal joint. Thenar muscular atrophy and decreased key pinch strength may be present. Conservative treatment is similar to stages I and II.

If conservative treatment of stage III fails to relieve the symptoms, relief can be obtained by reconstructive surgery. Arthroplasty, which reconstructs the ligaments and interposes soft tissue between the irregular joint surfaces has been highly successful. Four weeks immobilization in a cast and 2 to 3 months of therapy are required for optimal results.

Stage IV is a diffuse arthrosis with involvement of both the thumb trapezio-

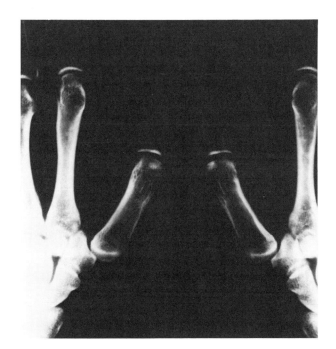

A

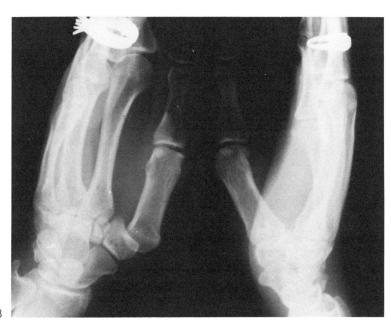

B

FIG. 6.8. A: The stress view is a posteroanterior x-ray of both thumbs, with the patient pushing the radial sides of the tips of the thumbs against each other. This patient demonstrates a lateral shift of the thumb metacarpals off of the trapezium. **B:** The stress view is repeated after the patient has had a ligament reconstruction on the right side. Note how the metacarpal is now seated in an anatomic position on the trapezium, compared to the left side which continues to demonstrate instability.

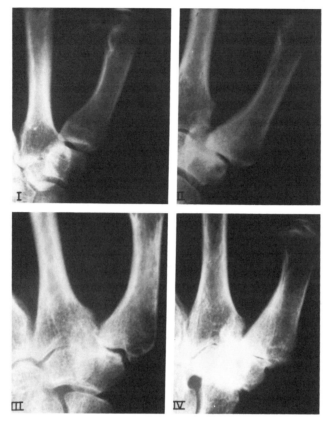

FIG. 6.9. The four stages of articular disease at the trapeziometacarpal joint are shown. Stage I includes less than one-third subluxation of the trapeziometacarpal joint and normal articular contours. Stage II shows evidence of early degenerative changes such as small bony fragments at the joint margins. Stage III reveals marked joint space narrowing, larger debris (greater than 2 mm), and sclerosis along the joint margins. Stage IV is pantrapezial disease.

metacarpal and scaphotrapezial joints. There is severe joint space destruction associated with cystic and sclerotic subchondral bone changes of all the trapezial joint facets. Clinically, these patients have signs and symptoms similar to stage III patients. Treatment for this advanced stage includes trapezial resection, implant arthroplasty, and ligament reconstruction. Our preference is to use a perforated silicone implant (25). The silastic spacer maintains the functional length of the thumb and provides for ligamentous stability of the implant and joint.

Distal Interphalangeal Joint Osteoarthritis

The distal interphalangeal joints (DIP) of the fingers are the most frequent site of osteoarthritis in the human skeleton (Fig. 6.10). The prominent spurs flanking the

TABLE 6.2. *Evaluation and treatment of thumb basal joint osteoarthritis*

Stage*	Clinical findings/x-rays	Treatment
Stage I	Pain and swelling, normal articulations	Splints and antiinflammatories, and/or ligament reconstruction
Stage II	Pain and swelling plus instability $>1/3$ of joint surface and calcifications >2 mm	Same as stage I
Stage III	Pain and deformity. Articular destruction of trapeziometacarpal joints	Interposition arthroplasty
State IV	Same as stage III, thumb held in adducted posture. Degeneration of both trapeziometacarpal and scaphotrapezial joints	Implant replacement of trapezium

*This is radiographic staging for prognostic evaluation. Ultimate staging is based on direct visualization of joint surfaces.

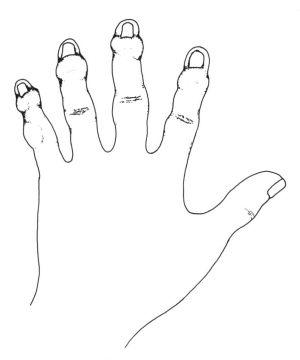

FIG. 6.10. Osteoarthritis at the level of the distal interphalangeal joints is demonstrated. This is the most common site of degenerative arthritis in the body. Enlargement and deformity of these joints is referred to as Heberden's nodes. Arthritic changes at the proximal interphalangeal joint, as seen on the little finger, are called Bouchard's nodes.

base of the fingernail (Heberden's nodes) are conspicuous external manifestations of the osteoarthritic process of cartilage loss and irregularity of the subjacent joint surfaces (26).

These processes predominantly involve women, but fortunately have no predilection for musicians. Heberden's nodes may begin to appear in the fifth decade and are painful in only a moderate number of patients. There is degeneration of the articular cartilage with narrowing of the joint space. The nodes represent hypertrophic bone formation of the condyles of the middle phalanx and adjacent base of the distal phalanx. There may be lateral angulation with erosion of the joint surface. These changes are best seen on posteroanterior and lateral radiographs.

Pain, when present, is usually intermittent, lasting 3 to 4 weeks at a time and quite responsive to antiinflammatory medications, particularly aspirin. Often patients complain more of the appearance than of pain. For those with persistent symptoms, a small dorsal splint may be applied to prevent motion of the joint for a period of 2 to 3 weeks.

Painful distal osteoarthritic joints are relatively uncommon among musicians, with the possible exception of the fifth finger of pianists. Whether the osteoarthritic pain makes playing the piano more difficult or playing the piano brings on the pain is never clear. The angulation of the distal phalanx can also be disabling, especially in the string player who cannot place the finger on the string effectively. Should splinting and antiinflammatory medication not completely relieve the symptoms, very predictable relief of symptoms can be achieved by surgical fusion of the affected joint. The functional loss is minimal, as there is already stiffness of the joint due to pain and arthritic destruction. Fusion also places a deformed joint in a more functional position while completely eliminating the pain.

Ligamentous Laxity of the MP Joint of the Thumb

The thumb of the bow hand of large, upright string instrument players (i.e., cello and bass) is particularly prone to chronic ligament stress. Long hours of continuous longitudinal pressure while "pinching" the bow create varying degrees of stretching of the ligaments of the metacarpophalangeal joint. A very tight gripping technique is particularly stressful for the ligaments.

Biomechanical studies have shown that for each kilogram of force transmitted to the tip of the thumb, 12 times that force crosses the basal joint and 6 times the terminal force crosses the metacarpophalangeal joint. Ligaments provide primary stability for all joints with the adjacent muscles serving as secondary support. With lax or chronically stretched ligaments, however, the thumb MP joint must depend more upon dynamic stabilization through its cone of intrinsic thenar muscles.

Protracted, sustained contraction of both the intrinsic and extrinsic muscles of the hand which stabilize the lax MP joint leads inevitably to muscular fatigue. Early signs of muscle fatigue are cramps and muscle spasm, complaints not uncommon among musicians and writers. A significant number of artists and musicians with hand and arm cramps will, upon careful physical examination, demonstrate significant ligament laxity and joint hypermobility. Short-term splinting and a modification of playing technique will often relieve such symptoms. However, once a ligament has become significantly stretched, it is unlikely to shorten or contract to a more physiologic tension (Fig. 6.11). Surgical management of intractable pain due to ligament laxity involves reconstruction of the ulnar collateral ligament of the MP joint, usually utilizing the palmaris longus tendon as a graft. There is absolutely no residual functional deficit from taking away this "spare" palmaris tendon.

Prolonged and repetitious flexion-adduction (pinching) of the thumb, such as required to grip a bow, stabilize a woodwind instrument, or repeatedly perform the "thumb under" maneuvers when playing piano, may also induce progressive stretching of the palmar ligament at the base of the thumb metacarpal. Chronic incompetence of the capsule of this highly mobile joint leads to pain and accelerated wear of joint surfaces. The body compensates for this ligamentous laxity by recruiting adjacent thumb intrinsic muscles to stabilize this important basal joint. In time,

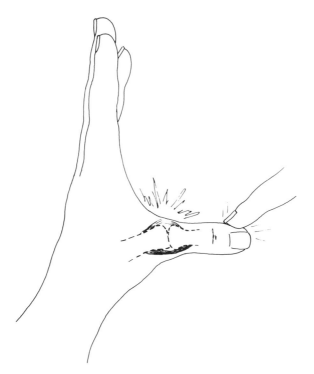

FIG. 6.11. Rupture or laxity of the thumb's ulnar collateral ligament results in an instability of the thumb to radial deviation. The laxity is always compared to the opposite hand's thumb. With an acute injury, radial stress of the proximal phalanx causes pain over the ulnar side of the thumb's MP joint.

these muscles fatigue. This initially results in cramps and may eventually cause severe diffuse pain. Symptomatic hypermobility of the base of the thumb is associated with stage I radiographic changes and is considered "prearthritic", the initial stage of basal joint arthrosis.

Splinting and antiinflammatory medications will relieve minor laxity conditions, but will not cure the major laxity states. It is probable that prolonged laxity predisposes to degenerative changes in this joint.

A predictable correction of the painful hypermobile basal joint of the thumb is through reconstruction of its basal ligament utilizing a strip of adjacent wrist tendon. Use of a strip of this tendon does not produce a functional loss. Postoperative immobilization for 4 weeks is followed by a rapid return to playing. By 3 months after reconstruction, essentially normal function would be expected.

APPROACHING SURGERY

The thought that one has been "sentenced" to surgery is always a shock, particularly when it involves the hands of a musician or artist. Indeed, it is difficult for anyone to be enthusiastic about undergoing surgery. Fortunately, the pathologic conditions discussed in this chapter, if not responsive to conservative management, are quite predictably corrected by surgery, with an excellent long-term prognosis.

The recurring tragedy among musicians is the inordinately long periods of disability so often associated with easily correctable conditions. Months may stretch to years of non- or under-performance, either because of the dread of surgery or lack of information as to the prognosis for this type of surgery.

Except for reconstructive arthroplasties of the basal joint of the thumb, the procedures described in this chapter are simple, minimally painful and highly predictable. The patient should be healed and rehabilitated sufficiently to be utilizing maximum force without pain in a relatively short period of time. It is unfortunate that so many artists endure prolonged disability and career limitations for conditions which are readily amenable to simple surgical procedures.

REFERENCES

1. Kilgore E, Graham W. *The Hand.* Philadelphia, Lea and Febinger, 1977;36–40.
2. American Society for Surgery of the Hand. *The hand examination and diagnosis,* 2nd ed. New York, Churchill Livingstone, 1983;11–47.
3. Chase R. *Atlas of hand surgery.* Philadelphia, W.B. Saunders, 1973;3–22.
4. Eversmann W. Compression and entrapment neuropathies of the upper extremity. *J of Hand Surgery* 1983;8 (part 2):759.
5. Spinner M, Spencer P. Nerve compression lesions of the upper extremity. *Clin Orthop* 1974;104:46.
6. Bruner J. Carpal tunnel syndrome. *Hand* 1972;4:220–223.
7. Buchthal F, Rosenfalck A, Trojaborg W. Electrophysical findings in entrapment of the median nerve at wrist and elbow. *J Neurol Neurosurg Psychiatry* 1974;37:340.
8. Abbott L, Saunders J. Injuries of the median nerve in fractures of the lower end of the radius. *Surg Gynecol Obstet* 1933;57:507.
9. Meadoff N. Median nerve injuries in fractures in the region of the wrist. *Calif Med* 70:252–256.

10. Foster J. Hydrocortisone and the carpal tunnel syndrome. *Lancet* 1960;1:454–456.
11. Eversmann W. *Operative Hand Surgery.* In: Green D, ed. New York, Churchill Livingstone, 1988; 1432.
12. Miller R, Camp P. Postoperative ulnar neuropathy. *JAMA* 1979; 241:1636–1639.
13. Spinner M. *Injuries to the major branches of peripheral nerves of the forearm*, 2nd ed. Philadelphia, W.B. Saunders, 1978;278.
14. Dellon AL. Review of treatment results for ulnar nerve entrapment at the elbow. *J Hand Surgery* 1989;14A:688–700.
15. Eaton R, Crowe J, Parkes JC. Anterior transposition of the ulnar nerve using a non-compressing fiscio-dermal sling. *JBJS* 1980;62-A:820–825.
16. Conklin J, White W. Stenosing tenosynovitis and its possible relation to the carpal tunnel syndrome. *Surg Clin North Am* 1960;40:531–540.
17. Fahey J, Bollinger J. Trigger-finger in adults and children. *J Bone Joint Surg* 1954;36A:1200–1218.
18. Burton R, Littler JW. Tendon entrapment syndrome of the first extensor compartment (De Quervain's disorder). *Curr Probl Surg* 1975;12:32–34.
19. Grundberg A, Reagan D. Pathologic anatomy of the forearm: intersection syndrome. *J Hand Surg* 1985;10A:299–302.
20. Wood T. DeQuervain's disease: a plea for early operation: a report on 40 cases. *Br J Surg* 1954;51: 358–359.
21. Potter P. Stenosing tenovaginitis at the radial styloid (De Quervain's disease). *Ann Surg* 1943;117: 294.
22. Kelsey J.*Upper extremity disorders.* St. Louis: CV Mosby Co., 1980;19–22.
23. Eaton R, Glickel S. Trapeziometacarpal osteoarthritis: staging as a rationale for treatment. *Hand Clinics* 1987;(4)3:455–469.
24. Eaton R, Lane L, Littler JW, Keyser JJ. Ligament reconstruction for the painful thumb carpometacarpal joint: a long term assessment. *J Hand Surg* 1984;9-A:692–699.
25. Eaton R. Replacement of the trapezium for arthritis of the basal articulation. *JBJS* 1979;61(1):76–82.
26. McCarty D. *Arthritis and allied conditions.* Philadelphia, Lea and Febinger, 1979;1164.

Textbook of Performing Arts Medicine, edited by R. T. Sataloff, A. Brandfonbrener, and R. Lederman. Raven Press, Ltd., New York © 1991.

7

Care of the Professional Voice

Robert Thayer Sataloff

Professor of Otolaryngology, Thomas Jefferson University, Philadelphia, Pennsylvania 19103

Professional voice users provide exciting challenges and special responsibilities for physicians and other health care professionals. Professional voice users include not only singers and actors, but also attorneys, politicians, clergy, educators (including some physicians), telephone receptionists, and others. Although they span a broad range of vocal sophistication and voice needs, they share a dependence on vocal endurance and quality for their livelihoods. However, the vocal needs of performing artists are especially great. Professional singers are the Olympic athletes of the voice world, and they will be discussed at length in this chapter, because mastery of the science and art of caring for singers provides the physician with sufficient expertise to treat other professional voice users as well. Although physicians are frequently called upon to care for singers and other voice professionals, most doctors have little or no training in sophisticated analysis and treatment of subtle problems of the voice. Initially, voice complaints may seem vague and subjective, especially to health care professionals unfamiliar with the jargon of singers and actors. However, accurate diagnosis and rational treatment may be achieved through systematic inquiry based on understanding of the anatomy, physiology, psychology and psychoacoustics of voice production. In general, failure to establish a diagnosis for a professional singer with a voice complaint is due to lack of expertise on the part of the physician rather than an imaginary complaint on the part of the singer.

ANATOMY

The anatomy of a singer is not limited to the region between the suprasternal notch and the hyoid bone. Practically all body systems affect the voice. The larynx receives the greatest attention because it is the most sensitive and expressive component of the vocal mechanism, but anatomic interactions throughout the patient's body must be considered in treating the professional voice.

The Larynx

A detailed discussion of laryngeal anatomy is beyond the scope of this chapter. However, it is helpful to think of the larynx as composed of three anatomic units: mucosa, intrinsic muscles, and extrinsic muscles. The vibratory margin of the vocal fold is much more complicated than simply mucosa applied to muscle. This structure consists of five layers (Fig. 7.1) (1). This thin, lubricated, squamous epithelium covering the vocal folds forms the area of contact between the vibrating vocal cords and acts somewhat like a capsule, helping to maintain vocal fold shape. The superficial layer of the lamina propria, also known as Rienke's space, is made up of loose fibrous components and matrix. It contains very few fibroblasts. The intermediate layer of the lamina propria contains more fibroblasts and consists primarily of elastic fibers. The deep layer of the lamina propria is composed primarily of collagenous fibers and is rich in fibroblasts. The vocalis muscle makes up the body of the vocal fold and is one of the intrinsic laryngeal muscles. The region of the intermediate deep layers of the lamina propria is called the vocal ligament, and lies immediately below Reinke's space. Functionally, the various layers have different

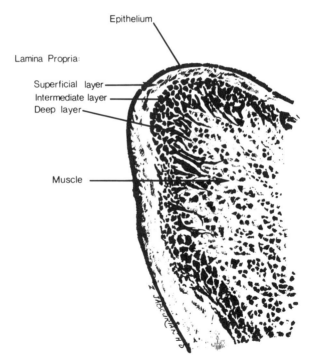

FIG. 7.1. Frontal cross section of a human vocal fold through the middle of the membranous portion (from Hirano M, ref. 1, with permission).

mechanical properties and act somewhat like ball bearings of different sizes in allowing the smooth shearing action necessary for proper vocal fold vibration. Mechanically, they actually act more like three layers consisting of the *cover* (epithelium and Reinke's space), *transition* (intermediate deep layers of the lamina propria), and the *body* (the vocalis muscle). Understanding this anatomy is important because different pathologic entities occur in different layers. Moreover, fibroblasts are responsible for scar formation. Therefore, lesions that occur in the cover (such as nodules, cysts, and most polyps) should permit treatment without disturbance of the intermediate and deep layers, fibroblast proliferation, or scar formation. Intrinsic muscles are responsible for abduction, adduction, and tension of the vocal folds. Extrinsic laryngeal musculature maintains the position of the larynx in the neck. Since raising or lowering the larynx may alter the tension or angle between laryngeal cartilages, the extrinsic muscles are critical in maintaining a stable laryngeal skeleton so that the delicate intrinsic musculature can work effectively. In the trained singer, the extrinsic muscles maintain the larynx in a relatively constant position. Training of the intrinsic musculature results in vibratory symmetry of the vocal folds, producing regular periodicity. This contributes to what the listener perceives as a "trained" voice. The vocal folds may be thought of as the oscillator of the vocal mechanism (2).

The Supraglottic Vocal Tract

The supraglottic larynx, tongue, lips, palate, pharynx, nasal cavity, and possibly the sinuses shape the sound quality produced at the level of the vocal cords by acting as a resonator. Minor alterations in the configuration of these structures may produce substantial changes in voice quality. The hypernasal speech typically associated with a cleft palate or the hyponasal speech characteristic of severe adenoid hypertrophy are obvious. However, mild edema from an upper respiratory tract infection, pharyngeal scarring, or muscle tension changes produce less obvious sound alterations. These are immediately recognizable to a trained vocalist or astute critic, but often elude the laryngologist.

The Tracheobronchial Tree, Lungs, and Thorax

In singing, the lungs supply a constant stream of air that passes between the vocal folds and provides power for voice production. Singers often are thought of as having "big chests." Actually, the primary respiratory difference between trained and untrained singers is not increased total lung capacity, as popularly assumed. Rather, the trained singer learns to use a higher proportion of the air in his lungs, thereby decreasing his residual volume and increasing his respiratory efficiency (3).

The Abdomen

The abdominal musculature is the so-called support of the singing voice, although singers generally refer to their "diaphragm" as their support mechanism. The diaphragm generates inspiratory force. Although the abdomen can perform this function in some situations (4), it is primarily an expiratory-force generator. The abdominal musculature receives considerable attention in vocal training. The purpose of abdominal support is to maintain an efficient, constant power source and inspiratory-expiratory mechanism. There is disagreement among voice teachers as to the best model for teaching support technique. Some experts describe positioning the abdominal musculature under the rib cage, while others advocate distension of the abdomen. Either method may result in vocal problems if used incorrectly; but distending the abdomen (the inverse pressure theory) is especially dangerous because it tends to focus the singer's muscular effort in a downward and outward direction, which is ineffective. Thus, the singer may exert considerable effort, believing he is practicing good support technique, without obtaining the desired effect. Proper abdominal training is essential to good singing, and the physician must consider abdominal function when evaluating vocal disabilities.

The Musculoskeletal System

Musculoskeletal condition and position affect the vocal mechanism and may produce tension or impair abdominal muscle function, resulting in voice dysfunction. Stance deviation, such as from standing to supine, produces obvious changes in respiratory function. However, lesser changes, such as distributing one's weight over the calcaneus rather than forward over the metatarsal heads (a more athletic position), alter the configuration of the abdominal and back musculature enough to influence the voice. Tensing arm and shoulder muscles promotes cervical muscle strain, which can adversely affect the larynx. Careful control of muscle tension is fundamental to good vocal technique. In fact, some methods use musculoskeletal conditioning as the primary focus of voice training.

The Psychoneurological System

The psychological constitution of the singer impacts directly upon the vocal mechanism. Psychological phenomena are reflected through the autonomic nervous system, which controls mucosal secretions and other functions critical to voice production. The nervous system is also important for its mediation of fine muscle control. This fact is worthy of emphasis because minimal voice disturbances may occasionally be the first signs of serious neurologic disease.

HISTORY

Extensive historical background is necessary for thorough evaluation of the singing voice, and the otolaryngologist who sees singers only on occasion cannot reasonably be expected to remember all the pertinent questions. Although some laryngologists feel that a lengthy inquisition is helpful in establishing rapport with professional singers, many of us who see a substantial number of singers per day within a busy practice need a thorough but less time-consuming alternative. A history questionnaire for professional singers can be extremely helpful in documenting all the necessary information, in helping the singers sort out and articulate their problems, and in saving the clinician writing time. During the last few years, the author has developed a questionnaire (5) which has proven helpful (Appendix I). The singer is asked to complete the form in the waiting room before seeing the doctor. No history questionnaire is a substitute for direct, penetrating questioning by the physician; however, the direction of most useful inquiry can be determined from a glance at the questionnaire. Obviating the need for extensive writing permits the physician greater eye contact with his patient and facilitates rapid establishment of the close rapport and confidence that are so important in treating professional singers. The physician is also able to supplement his initial impressions and historical information from the questionnaire with seemingly leisurely conversation during the physical examination. The use of the historical questionnaire has added substantially to the efficiency, consistent thoroughness, and ease of managing these delightful, but often complex patients.

Age

Serious vocal endeavor may start in childhood and endure throughout a lifetime. As the vocal mechanism undergoes normal maturation, the voice changes. The optimum time to begin serious vocal training is controversial. For many years, most people advocated delay of vocal training and serious singing until near puberty in the female and after puberty and voice stabilization in the male. However, in a child with earnest vocal aspirations and potential, it is reasonable to start specialized training early in childhood. Initial instruction should teach the child to vocalize without strain and avoid all forms of voice abuse. It should not permit premature indulgence in operatic bravado. Most experts agree that singing during puberty should be minimized or avoided altogether, particularly by the male. Recent studies indicating the contrary are highly controversial. Voice maturation may occur at any age from the early teenage period to the fourth decade of life. The dangerous tendency for young singers to attempt to sound older than their vocal years frequently causes vocal dysfunction.

All components of voice production are subject to normal aging. Abdominal and general muscular tone frequently decrease, lungs lose elasticity, the thorax loses its distensibility, the mucosa of the vocal tract atrophies, mucous secretions change character, nerve endings are reduced in number, and psychoneurologic functions differ. Moreover, the larynx itself loses muscle tone and bulk and may show depletion of submucosal ground substance in the vocal folds. The laryngeal cartilages ossify and the joints may become arthritic and stiff. The hormonal environment is altered. Vocal range, intensity, and quality all may be modified. Vocal fold atrophy may be the most striking alteration. The clinical effects of aging seem more pronounced in female singers, although vocal fold histologic changes may be more prominent in males. Excellent male singers occasionally extend their careers into their 70s or beyond (6,7). However, some degree of breathiness, decreased range, and other evidence of aging should be expected in elderly voices.

Complaints

Careful questioning as to the onset of vocal problems is needed to separate acute from chronic dysfunction. Often an upper respiratory tract infection will bring a singer to the physician's office, but penetrating inquiry may reveal a chronic vocal problem that is the singer's real concern. It is important to identify acute and chronic problems before beginning therapy so that both patient and physician may have realistic expectations and optimum therapeutic selection. The specific nature of the vocal complaint can provide a great deal of information. Just as dizzy patients rarely walk into the physician's office complaining of "rotary vertigo," singers may be unable to articulate their symptoms without guidance. They may use the term *hoarseness* to describe a variety of conditions that the physician must separate. Hoarseness is a coarse or scratchy sound most often associated with abnormalities of the leading edge of the vocal folds, such as laryngitis or mass lesions. Breathiness is a vocal quality characterized by excessive loss of air during vocalization. In some cases, it is due to improper technique. However, any condition that prevents full approximation of the vocal cords can be responsible. Such causes include vocal cord paralysis, a mass lesion separating the leading edges of the vocal cords, arthritis of the cricoarytenoid joint, arytenoid dislocation, unilateral scarring of the vibratory margin, and senile vocal cord atrophy. Fatigue of the voice is inability to continue to sing for extended periods without change in vocal quality. The voice may fatigue by becoming hoarse, losing range, changing timbre, breaking into different registers or, by other uncontrolled aberrations. A well-trained singer should be able to sing for several hours without developing vocal fatigue. Fatigue is often caused by misuse of abdominal and neck musculature or "over-singing," singing too loudly too long. Vocal fatigue may be a sign of general tiredness or of serious illnesses such as myasthenia gravis. Volume disturbance may manifest as inability to sing loudly or inability to sing softly. Each voice has its own dynamic range. Within the course of training, singers learn to sing more loudly by singing more efficiently. They also learn to sing softly, a more difficult task, through years of laborious practice. Most volume problems are secondary to intrinsic limitations of the voice or technical errors in singing, although hormonal changes, aging and neurologic disease are other causes. Superior laryngeal nerve paralysis will impair the ability to sing loudly. This is a frequently unrecognized consequence of herpes infection (8) (such as "cold sores") and may be precipitated by an upper respiratory tract infection. Most singers require only about ten minutes to half an hour to "warm up the voice." Prolonged warm-up time, especially in the morning, is most often caused by reflux laryngitis. Tickling or choking during singing is associated with laryngitis or voice abuse. Often a symptom of pathology of the vocal fold's leading edge, it should contraindicate singing until vocal cord examination. Pain while singing can indicate vocal cord lesions, laryngeal joint arthritis, infection, or gastric acid irritation of the arytenoids; but it is much more commonly caused by voice abuse with excessive muscular activity in the neck rather than acute pathology on the leading edge of a vocal cord, and it does not require immediate cessation of singing pending medical examination.

Date of Next Important Performance

If a singer seeks treatment at the end of his busy season and has no pressing engagements, management of the voice problem should be relatively conservative and designed to assure long-term protection of the larynx, the most delicate part of the vocal mechanism. However, the physician and patient rarely have this luxury. Most often, the singer needs treatment within a week of an important engagement, and sometimes within less than a day. Younger singers fall ill shortly before performances, not due to hypochondria or coincidence, but rather from the immense physical and emotional stress of the preperformance period. The singer is frequently working harder and singing longer hours than usual. Moreover, he may be under particular pressure to learn new material and to perform well for a new audience. Furthermore, he may be sleeping less than usual because of additional time rehearsing or because of the discomforts of a strange city. Seasoned professionals make their living by performing regularly, sometimes several times a week. Consequently, *any* time they get sick is likely to precede a performance. Caring for voice complaints in these situations requires highly skilled judgment and bold management.

Professional Singing Status and Goals

In order to choose a treatment program, the physician must understand the importance of the singer's voice in long-term career plans, the importance of the upcoming concert, and the consequences of canceling the concert. Injudicious prescription of voice rest can be almost as damaging to a vocal career as can ill-advised performance. Although a singer's voice is his most important commodity, other factors distinguish the few successful artists from the multitude of less successful singers with equally good voices. These include musicianship, reliability, and "professionalism." Canceling a concert at the last minute may seriously damage a performer's reputation. Reliability is especially critical early in a singer's career. Moreover, an expert singer often can modify his performance to decrease the strain on his voice. No singer should be allowed to perform in a manner that will permit serious injury to his vocal cords; but in the frequent borderline cases, the condition of the larynx must be weighed against other factors affecting the singer as an artist.

Amount and Nature of Vocal Training

It is important to establish how long a singer has been singing seriously, especially if his active performance career predates the beginning of his vocal training. Active amateur singers frequently develop undesirable techniques that are difficult to modify. Extensive voice use without training or premature training with inappropriate repertoire may underlie persistent vocal difficulties later in life. The number of years a singer has been training his or her voice may be a fair index of vocal proficiency. A person who has studied voice for a year or two is somewhat more apt to have gross technical difficulties than is someone who has been studying for 20 years. However, if training has been intermittent or discontinued for some time, technical problems are common. In addition, methods vary among voice teachers. Hence, a student who has had many teachers commonly has numerous technical insecurities or deficiencies responsible for vocal dysfunction. This is especially true if the singer has changed to a new teacher within the preceding year. The physician must be careful not to criticize the patient's current voice teacher in such circumstances. It often takes years of expert instruction to correct bad habits.

Everyone speaks more often than he sings, yet most singers report little speech instruction. Even if a singer uses his voice flawlessly while practicing and performing, voice abuse at other times may result in damage that affects singing.

Type of Singing and Environment

The "Lombard effect" is the tendency to increase vocal intensity in response to increased background noise. A well-trained singer learns to compensate for this tendency and to avoid singing at unsafe volumes. Singers of classical music usually have such training and frequently perform with only a piano, where the balance can be controlled well. However, singers performing in large halls, with orchestras, or in operas early in their careers tend to oversing and strain their voices. Similar problems occur during outdoor concerts because of the lack of auditory feedback. This phenomenon is seen even more among "pop" singers. Pop singers are often in a uniquely difficult position; often despite little vocal training, they enjoy great artistic and financial success and endure extremely stressful demands on their time and their voices. They are required to sing in large halls not designed for musical performance, amidst smoke and other environmental irritants, accompanied by extremely loud background music. One frequently neglected key to survival for these singers is the proper use of monitor speakers. These direct the sound of the singer's voice toward the singer on the stage and provide acoustical feedback. In addition to the usual investigation, it is important to determine whether the pop singer utilizes monitor speakers, and whether they are loud enough for the singer to hear. Amateur singers are often no less serious about their music than are professionals, but they generally have less ability to compensate technically for handicaps produced by illness or other physical disability. It is rare that an amateur suffers a great loss from postponing a performance or from permitting a replacement to sing. In most cases, the amateur singer's best interest is served through conservative management directed at long-term maintenance of good vocal health. A great many singers who seek physicians' advice are primarily choral singers. They often are enthusiastic amateurs, untrained, but dedicated to their musical recreation. They should be handled like amateur solo singers, educated specifically about the Lombard effect, and cautioned to avoid the excessive volume so common in a choral environment. One good way for a singer to monitor loudness is to cup the hand to the ear. This adds about 6 dB to the perception of one's own voice and can be a very helpful guide in noisy surroundings (9). Young professional singers are often hired to augment amateur choruses. Feeling that the professional quartet has been hired to "lead" the rest of the choir, they often make the mistake of trying to accomplish that goal by singing *louder* than others in their sections. Such a singer should be advised to lead the section by singing each line as a soloist giving a voice lesson to the two people standing beside him, and as if there were a microphone in front of him recording his performance for his voice teacher. This approach usually will not only preserve his voice, but will also produce a better choral sound.

Rehearsal

Vocal practice is as essential to the singer as exercise is to the athlete. Proper vocal practice incorporates scales and specific exercises designed to maintain and develop the vocal apparatus. Simply singing songs and giving performances without routine studious concentration on vocal technique is not adequate for the performing singer. The physician should know whether the singer practices daily, whether he practices at the same time daily, and how long he practices. Most serious singers practice for at least 1 to 2 hours per day. If a singer routinely practices in the late afternoon or evening but frequently performs in the morning (religious services, school classes, teaching voice, choir rehearsals, etc.), one should inquire into his warm-up procedures preceding such performances. Singing "cold," especially at unaccustomed hours of the morning, may result in the use of minor muscular alterations to compensate for vocal insecurity due to inadequate preparation. Such crutches can result in voice dysfunction. Similar problems may occur from instances of voice use other than formal singing. Schoolteachers, telephone receptionists, sales people, and others who speak extensively often derive great benefit from 5 or 10 minutes of vocalization of scales first thing in the morning. Although singers rarely practice their scales too long, they frequently perform or rehearse excessively. This is especially true immediately before a major concert or audition, when physicians are most likely to see acute problems. When a singer has hoarseness and vocal fatigue and has been practicing a new role for 14 hours a day for the last 3 weeks, no simple prescription is going to solve his problem. However, a treatment regimen can usually be designed to carry the performer safely through his or her musical obligations.

Voice Abuse in Singing

A detailed discussion of vocal technique in singing is beyond the scope of this chapter. However, the most common technical errors involve excessive muscle tension in the tongue, neck and larynx, inadequate abdominal support, and excessive volume. Inadequate preparation can be a devastating source of voice abuse, and may result from limited practice, limited rehearsal of a difficult piece, or limited vocal training for a given role. The latter error is tragically common. In many situations, voice teachers are to blame, especially in competitive academic environments. Both singer and teacher must resist the impulse to show off the voice in works that are either too difficult for the singer's level of training or simply not suited to the singer's voice. Singers are habitually unhappy with the limitations of their voices. At some time or another most baritones wish they were tenors and walk around proving they can sing high Cs in "Vesti la giubba." Singers with other vocal ranges have similar fantasies. Attempts to make the voice something that it is not, or at least that it is not yet, are frequently harmful.

Voice Abuse in Speaking

Dissociation of one's speaking and singing voice is probably the most common cause of voice abuse problems in excellent singers. Too frequently, all the expert training in support, muscular control, and projection is not applied to a singer's speaking voice. Unfortunately, the resultant voice strain impacts on the singing voice as well as the speaking voice. Such damage is especially prone to occur in noisy rooms and in cars, where the background noise is deceptively high. Backstage greetings after a lengthy performance can be particularly devastating. The singer usually is exhaused and distracted. The environment is often dusty and dry, and there generally is a noisy crowd. Similar conditions prevail at postperformance parties, where smoking and alcohol worsen matters. These situations should be avoided by any singer with vocal problems and should be controlled through awareness at other times. Three particularly destructive vocal activities are worthy of note. Cheerleading requires extensive screaming under the worst possible physical and environmental circumstances. It is a highly undesirable activity for anyone considering serious vocal endeavor. This is a common conflict in younger singers because the teen who is the high school choir soloist frequently turns out also to be student council president, yearbook editor, captain of the cheerleaders, etc. Conducting, particularly choral conducting, can also be deleterious. An enthusiastic conductor, especially of an amateur group, frequently ends up singing all four parts intermittently, at volumes louder than the entire choir, for lengthy rehearsals. Conducting is a common avocation among singers, but must be done with expert technique and special precautions to avoid voice injury. Hoarseness or loss of soft voice control after conducting a rehearsal suggests voice abuse while conducting. Teaching singing may also be hazardous to vocal health. It can be done safely; but it requires skill and thought. Most teachers teach seated at the piano. Late in a long, hard day, this posture is not conducive to maintenance of optimal abdominal and back support. Usually, teachers work with students continually positioned to the right or left of the keyboard. This may require the teacher to turn the neck at a particularly sharp angle, especially when teaching at an upright piano. Teachers also often demonstrate vocal materials in their students' vocal ranges, rather than their own, illustrating bad as well as good technique. If a singing teacher is hoarse or has neck discomfort or deterioration of soft singing control at the end of a teaching day (assuming that the teacher warms up before beginning voice lessons), voice abuse should be suspected. Helpful modifications include teaching with a grand piano, sitting slightly sideways on the piano bench, or alternating student position to the right and left of the piano to facilitate better neck alignment. Retaining an accompanist so that the teacher can stand rather than teach from behind a piano, along with many other helpful modifications, is possible.

General Health

Singing is an athletic activity and requires good conditioning and coordinated interaction of numerous physical functions. Maladies of any part of the body may be reflected in the voice. Failure to exercise to maintain good abdominal muscle tone and respiratory endurance is particularly harmful, in that deficiencies in these areas undermine the power source of the singing voice. Singers generally will attempt to compensate for such weaknesses by using inappropriate muscle groups, particularly in the neck, that result in vocal dysfunction. Similar problems may occur in the well-conditioned vocalist in states of fatigue. These are compounded by mucosal changes that accompany excessively long hours of hard work. Such problems may be seen, even in the best singers, shortly before important performances in the height of the concert season.

There is a popular but untrue myth that great opera singers must be obese. However, the vivacious, gregarious personality that often distinguishes the great performer seems to be accompanied frequently by a propensity for excess, especially culinary excess. This excess is as undesirable in the vocalist as it is in most other athletic artists, and it should be avoided from the start of one's vocal career. However, attempts to effect weight reduction in an established singer are a different matter. The vocal mechanism is a finely tuned, complex instrument and is exquisitely sensitive to minor changes. Substantial fluctuations in weight frequently result in deleterious alterations of the voice, although these are usually temporary. Weight reduction programs for established singers must be monitored carefully and designed to reduce weight in small increments over long periods of time. A history of sudden recent weight change may be responsible for almost any vocal complaint. In addition, appropriate and attractive body weight is becoming particularly important in the opera world as this formerly theater-based art form moves to television and film media.

Singers usually will volunteer information about upper respiratory tract infections and "postnasal drip," but the relevance of other maladies may not be obvious. Consequently, the physician must seek out pertinent history. Acute upper respiratory tract infection causes inflammation of the mucosa, alters mucosal secretions, and makes the mucosa more vulnerable to injury. Coughing and throat-clearing are particularly traumatic vocal activities and may worsen or provoke hoarseness associated with a cold. Postnasal drip and allergy may produce the same response. Infectious sinusitis is associated with discharge and diffuse mucosal inflammation, resulting in similar problems, and may actually alter the sound of a singer's voice, especially his own perception of his voice. Futile attempts to compensate for disease of the supraglottic vocal tract, in an effort to return the sound to normal, frequently result in laryngeal strain. The expert singer compensates by monitoring his technique rather than his sound, or singing "by feel" rather than "by ear."

Dental disease, especially temporomandibular joint dysfunction, introduces muscle tension in the head and neck, which is transmitted to the larynx: directly, through the muscular attachments between the mandible and the hyoid bone, and indirectly, as generalized increased muscle tension. These problems often result in decreased range, vocal fatigue and change in the quality or placement of a voice. Such tension often is accompanied by excess tongue muscle activity, especially pulling the tongue posteriorly. This hyperfunctional behavior acts through hyoid attachments to disrupt the balance among the intrinsic and extrinsic laryngeal musculature.

Reflux laryngitis is common among singers because of the high intra-abdominal pressures associated with proper support and because of lifestyle requirements. Singers frequently perform at night. They generally refrain from eating before performances, because a full stomach compromises effective abdominal support. They compensate at postperformance gatherings late at night and then go to bed with full stomachs. Chronic arytenoid and vocal cord irritation by reflux of gastric juice may be associated with dyspepsia; the key features are a bitter taste and halitosis upon awakening in the morning, a dry or "coated" mouth, often a scratchy sore throat or a feeling of a "lump in the throat," hoarseness and the need for prolonged vocal warm-up. The physician must be alert to these symptoms and ask about them routinely; otherwise, the diagnosis will be missed, often because people who have had this problem for many years or for a lifetime do not even realize it is abnormal. Hearing loss is often overlooked as a source of vocal problems. Auditory feedback is fundamental to singing. Interference with this control mechanism may result in altered vocal production, particularly if the singer is unaware of his hearing loss.

Any condition that alters abdominal function, such as muscle spasm, constipation or diarrhea, interferes with support and may result in a voice complaint. These symptoms may accompany infection or anxiety.

The human voice is an exquisitely sensitive messenger of emotion. Highly trained singers learn to control the effects of anxiety and other emotional stresses on their voices under ordinary circumstances. However, in some instances this training may break down, or a performer may be inadequately prepared to control his voice under specific stressful conditions. Preperformance anxiety is the most common example; but insecurity, depression and other emotional disturbances are also generally reflected in the voice. Anxiety reactions are mediated in part through the autonomic nervous system and result in a dry mouth, cold clammy skin, and thick secretions. These reactions are normal, and good vocal training, coupled with assurance that there is no abnormality or disease, generally overcomes them. However, long-term poorly compensated emotional stress and exogenous stress (from agents, producers, teachers, parents, etc.) may cause substantial vocal dysfunction and may result in permanent limitations of the vocal apparatus. These conditions must be diagnosed and treated expertly. Hypochondriasis is uncommon among professional singers, despite popular opinion to the contrary.

Endocrine Dysfunction

Endocrine problems are worthy of special attention. The human voice is extremely sensitive to endocrinologic changes. Many of these are reflected in alterations of fluid content of the lamina propria just beneath the laryngeal mucosa. This causes alteration in the bulk and shape of the vocal folds and results in voice change. Hypothyroidism (10–14) is a well-recognized cause of such voice disorders, although the mechanism is not well understood. Hoarseness, vocal fatigue, muffling of the voice, loss of range, and a feeling of a lump in the throat may be present even with mild hypothyroidism. Even when thyroid function tests are within the low-normal range, this diagnosis should be entertained, especially if thyroid-stimulating hormone levels are in the high-normal range or are elevated. Thyrotoxicosis may result in similar voice disturbances (14). Voice changes associated with sex hormones are encountered commonly in clinical practice and have been investigated more thoroughly than have other hormonal changes. Although there appears to be a correlation between sex hormone levels and depths of male voices (higher testosterone and lower estradiol levels in basses than in tenors) (15), the most important hormonal considerations in males occur during the maturation process. When castrato singers were in vogue, castration at about the age of 7 or 8 years resulted in failure of laryngeal growth during puberty, and voices that stayed in the soprano or alto range boasted a unique quality of sound (16). Failure of a male voice to change at puberty is uncommon today and usually is psychogenic (17). However, hormonal deficiencies such as those seen in cryptorchidism, delayed sexual development, Klinefelter's syndrome, or Frölich's syndrome may be responsible. In these cases, the persistently high voice may be the complaint that brings the patient to medical attention. Voice problems related to sex hormones are seen most commonly in female singers. Although vocal changes associated with the normal menstrual cycle may be difficult to quantify with current experimental techniques, there is no question that they occur (18–21). Most of the ill effects are seen in the immediate premenstrual period and are known as "laryngopathia premenstrualis." This condition is common and is caused by physiologic, anatomic and psychologic alterations secondary to endocrine changes. The vocal dysfunction is characterized by decreased vocal efficiency, loss of the highest notes in the voice, vocal fatigue, slight hoarseness, and some muffling of the voice, and it is often more apparent to the singer than to the listener. Submucosal hemorrhages in the larynx are common (21). In many European opera houses, singers are excused from singing during the premenstrual and early menstrual days ("grace days"). This practice is not followed in the United States. Although ovulation inhibitors have been shown to mitigate some of these symptoms (20), in some women (about 5%) birth control pills may deleteriously alter voice range and character even after only a few months of therapy (22–25). When oral contraceptives are used, the voice should be monitored closely. Under crucial performance circumstances, oral contraceptives may be used to alter the time of menstruation, but this practice is justified only in unusual situations. Estrogens are helpful in postmenopausal singers but should not be generally given alone. Sequential replacement therapy is the most physiologic and should be used under the supervision of a gynecologist. Under no circumstances should androgens be given to female singers, even in small amounts, if there is any reasonable therapeutic alternative. Clinically, these drugs are most commonly used to treat endometriosis. Androgens cause unsteadiness of the voice, rapid changes of timbre, and lowering of fundamental voice frequency (26–31). The changes are irreversible. In rare instances, androgens may be produced by pathologic conditions such as ovarian or adrenal tumors, and voice alterations may be the presenting symptoms. Rarely, they may also be secreted during an otherwise normal pregnancy. Pregnancy frequently results in voice alterations known as "laryngopathia gravidarum." The changes may be similar to premenstrual symptoms or may be perceived as desirable changes. In some cases, alterations produced by pregnancy are permanent (32,33). Although hormonally induced changes in the larynx and respiratory mucosa secondary to menstruation and pregnancy are discussed widely in the literature, the author has found no reference to the important alterations in abdominal support. Muscle cramping associated with menstruation causes pain and compromises abdominal contraction. Abdominal distention during pregnancy also interferes with abdominal muscle function. Any singer whose abdominal support is compromised substantially should be discouraged from singing until the abdominal disability is resolved. Hormonal disturbances in other segments of the diencephalic-pituitary system may also result in vocal dysfunction. In addition to the thyroid and the gonads, the parathyroid, adrenal, pineal, and pituitary glands are included in this system. Other endocrine disturbances may alter voice as well. For example, pancreatic dysfunction may result in xerophonia (dry voice), as in diabetes mellitus. Thymic abnormalities can lead to feminization of the voice (34).

Exposure to Irritants

Any mucosal irritant can disrupt the delicate vocal mechanism. Allergies to dust and mold are aggravated commonly during rehearsals and performances in concert halls, especially older concert halls, because of the numerous curtains, backstage trappings and dressing room facilities that are rarely cleaned thoroughly. Nasal obstruction and erythematous conjunctivae suggest generalized mucosal irritation. The drying effects of cold air and dry heat may also affect mucosal secretions, leading to decreased lubrication and a "scratchy" voice and tickling cough. These symptoms may be minimized by nasal breathing, which allows inspired air to be filtered, warmed and humidified. Nasal breathing rather than mouth breathing whenever possible is proper vocal technique. While back stage between appearances during rehearsals, aspiration of dust and other irritants may also be controlled by wearing a protective mask, such as those used by carpenters, or a surgical mask that does not contain fiberglass. This is especially helpful when set construction is going on in the rehearsal area. A history of recent travel suggests other sources of direct mucosal irritation. The air in airplanes is extremely dry, and airplanes are noisy (35). Singers must be careful to avoid talking loudly and to maintain nasal breathing during air travel. Environmental changes can also be disruptive. Las Vegas is infamous for the mucosal irritation caused by its dry atmosphere and smoke-filled rooms. In fact, the resultant complex of hoarseness, vocal "tickle," and fatigue is referred to as "Las Vegas voice." A history of recent travel should also suggest "jet lag" and generalized fatigue, which may be potent detriments to good vocal function.

Smoke

The deleterious effects of tobacco smoke on mucosa are indisputable. It causes erythema, mild edema, and generalized inflammation throughout the vocal tract. Both smoke itself and the heat of the cigarette appear to be important. Marijuana produces a particularly irritating, unfiltered smoke, which is inhaled directly, causing considerable mucosal response. Smoking should not be permitted by the serious singer. Singers who refuse to stop smoking marijuana should at least be advised to use a water pipe to cool and partially filter the smoke. Some singers are required to perform in smoke-filled environments and may suffer the same effects as the smokers themselves. In some theaters, it is possible to place fans upstage or direct the ventilation system so as to create a gentle draft toward the audience, clearing the smoke away from the stage. "Smoke eaters" installed in some theaters are also helpful.

Drugs

A history of alcohol abuse suggests the probability of poor vocal technique. Intoxication results in incoordination and decreased awareness, which undermine vocal discipline designed to optimize and protect the voice. The effect of small amounts of alcohol is controversial. Although many experts oppose it because of its vasodilatory effect and consequent mucosal alteration, many singers do not seem to be adversely affected by small amounts of alcohol, such as a glass of wine with supper on the day of a performance. However, many singers have mild sensitivities to certain wines or beers. If a singer develops nasal congestion and rhinorrhea after drinking beer, for example, he should be made aware that he probably has a mild allergy to that particular beverage and should avoid it prior to singing.

Singers frequently acquire antihistamines to help control "postnasal drip" or other symptoms. The drying effect of antihistamines may result in decreased vocal cord lubrication, increased throat clearing, and irritability leading to frequent coughing. Antihistamines may be helpful to some singers, but they must be used with caution.

When a singer is already taking antibiotics at the time he seeks the attention of a physician, it is important to find out the dose and the prescribing physician, if any, as well as whether the singer frequently treats himself with inadequate courses of antibiotics. It is not uncommon for singers to develop "sore throats" shortly before performances and to start themselves on inappropriate antibiotic therapy, which they generally discontinue following their performance.

Diuretics are also popular among some singers. They are often prescribed by gynecologists at the request of the singers to help deplete excess water in the premenstrual period. Unsupervised use of these drugs may result in dehydration and consequent mucosal dryness.

Hormone use, especially oral contraceptives, must be mentioned specifically during the physician's inquiry. Women frequently will not routinely mention hormones when asked if they are taking any medication. Vitamins are also frequently not mentioned. Most vitamin therapy seems to have little effect on the voice. However, high-dose vitamin C (5 to 6 g a day), which is used by some people to prevent upper respiratory tract infections, seems to act as a mild diuretic and may lead to dehydration and xerophonia (36).

Cocaine use is increasingly common, especially among pop musicians. It can be extremely irritating to the nasal mucosa, causes marked vasoconstriction, and may alter the sensorium, resulting in decreased voice control and a tendency toward vocal abuse.

Foods

Various foods are said to affect the voice. Traditionally, milk and ice cream are avoided by singers before performances. In many people, they seem to increase the amount and viscosity of mucosal secretions. Allergy and casein have been implicated, but no satisfactory explanation has been established. Restriction of these foods in a singer's diet before he sings may be helpful in some cases. Chocolate may have the same effects, and should be viewed similarly. Singers should be asked about eating nuts. This is important not only because some people feel they produce effects similar to those of milk products and chocolate, but moreover because they are extremely irritating if aspirated. The irritation produced by aspiration of a small organic foreign body may be severe and impossible to correct rapidly enough to permit performance. Highly spiced foods may also be direct mucosal irritants. In addition, they seem to aggravate reflux laryngitis. Coffee and other beverages containing caffeine also aggravate gastric reflux and seem to alter secretions and necessitate frequent throat-clearing in some people. In large quantities they may also cause hyperactivity and tremor. Fad diets, especially rapid weight-reducing diets, are notorious for causing voice problems. Lemon juice and herbal teas are both felt to be beneficial to the voice. Both may act as demulcents, thinning secretions, and may very well be helpful. When inquiring about foods, it is also useful to know whether the singer eats immediately before singing. A full stomach may interfere with abdominal support or may result in reflux of gastric juice during abdominal muscle contraction.

Surgery

A history of laryngeal surgery in a professional singer is a matter of great concern. It is important to establish exactly why the surgery was done, by whom it was done, whether intubation was necessary, and whether ancillary speech training was instituted if the lesion was associated with voice abuse (vocal nodules). If the vocal dysfunction that brought the singer to the physician's office dates from the immediate postoperative period, significant surgical trauma must be suspected.

Otolaryngologists frequently are asked about the effects of tonsillectomy upon the voice. Singers may come to the physician following tonsillectomy and complain of vocal dysfunction. There is no question that removal of tonsils can alter the voice (37,38). Tonsillectomy changes the configuration of the supraglottic vocal tract. In addition, scarring alters pharyngeal muscle function, which is trained meticulously in the professional singer. Singers must be warned that they may have permanent voice changes following tonsillectomy. These can be minimized by dissecting in the proper plane to lessen scarring. It generally takes 3 to 6 months for the singer's voice to stabilize or return to normal following surgery. As with any procedure for which general anesthesia may be needed, the anesthesiologist should be advised preoperatively that the patient is a professional singer. Intubation and extubation should be done with great care and with nonirritating plastic rather than rubber tubes.

Surgery of the neck, such as thyroidectomy, may result in permanent alterations in the vocal mechanism through scarring of the extrinsic laryngeal musculature. The strap muscles are important in maintaining laryngeal position and stability of the laryngeal skeleton and should be retracted rather than divided whenever possible. A history of recurrent or superior laryngeal nerve injury may explain a hoarse, breathy, or weak voice. However, in rare cases a singer can compensate even for recurrent laryngeal nerve paralysis and have a nearly normal voice. Thoracic and abdominal surgery interferes with respiratory and abdominal support. Following these procedures, singing should be prohibited until pain has subsided and healing has occurred sufficiently to allow normal support. Frequently, it is advisable to institute abdominal exercises prior to resuming vocalizing. Singing without proper support is worse for the voice than not singing at all. The author requires that his singers be able to do ten sit-ups before resuming singing following abdominal or thoracic surgery. Other surgical procedures may be significant if they necessitate intubation or if they affect the musculoskeletal system so that the singer has to change his stance or balance. For example, balancing on one foot after leg surgery may decrease the effectiveness of the singer's support mechanisms.

A comprehensive history frequently reveals the etiology of a singer's problem even before a physical examination is performed. However, a specialized physical examination, often including objective assessment of voice function, is essential (39,40).

PHYSICAL EXAMINATION

As with any of our patients, examination of the professional singer must include an assessment of his general physical condition and a thorough ear, nose, and throat evaluation. As with any athletic activity, singing requires stamina and reasonably good physical conditioning. Any physical condition which impairs normal function of the abdominal musculature is suspect as an etiology for dysphonia. Some such conditions are obvious, such as pregnancy. However, a sprained ankle or broken leg that requires the singer to balance himself in an unaccustomed posture may distract him from maintaining good abdominal support and may result in voice dysfunction. Any neurologic disorder that results in tremor, endocrine disturbances such as thyroid dysfunction or menopause, the aging process, and other systemic conditions also may alter the voice. The physician must remember that maladies of almost any body system may result in voice dysfunction, and he must remain alert to conditions outside the head and neck.

Complete Ear, Nose, and Throat Examination

Examination of the ears must include assessment of hearing acuity. Even a relatively slight hearing loss may result in voice strain as the singer tries to balance his vocal intensity with his associate performers. This is especially true of hearing losses acquired after vocal training has been completed. The effect is most pronounced with sensorineural hearing loss. With conductive hearing loss, singers tend to sing more softly than appropriate rather than too loudly, and this is less harmful.

The conjunctivae and sclerae should be observed routinely during an ear, nose, and throat examination for erythema suggesting allergy or irritation, for pallor suggesting anemia and for other abnormalities such as jaundice. These observations may reveal the problem reflected in the vocal tract even before the larynx is visualized.

The nose should be assessed for patency of the nasal airway, character of the nasal mucosa and nature of secretions, if any. If a singer is unable to breathe through his nose because of anatomic obstruction, he is forced to breathe unfiltered, unhumidified air through his mouth. Pale gray allergic mucosa or swollen infected mucosa in the nose suggests abnormal mucosa elsewhere in the respiratory tract.

Examination of the oral cavity should include careful attention to the tonsils and lymphoid tissue in the posterior pharyngeal wall, as well as to the mucosa. Diffuse lymphoid hypertrophy associated with a complaint of "scratchy" voice and irritative cough may indicate chronic infection. The amount and viscosity of mucosal and salivary secretions should be noted also. Xerostomia (dry mouth) is particularly important. Dental examination should focus not only on oral hygiene, but also on the presence of wear facets suggestive of bruxism (teeth grinding). Bruxism is a clue to excessive tension and may be associated with dysfunction of the temporo-mandibular joints, which should also be assessed routinely. Thinning of the enamel in a normal or underweight patient may be a clue to bulimia. However, it may also occur with excessive ingestion of lemons which some singers eat to help thin their secretions.

Examination of the neck for masses, restriction of movement, excess muscle tension and scars from prior neck surgery or trauma should be carried out. Particular attention should be paid to the thyroid gland. Laryngeal vertical mobility is also important. For example, tilting of the larynx due to partial fixation of strap muscles cut during previous surgery may produce voice dysfunction. So may fixation of the trachea to overlying neck skin. Examination of the cranial nerves should be included. Finding diminished fifth nerve sensation, diminished gag reflex, palatal deviation, or other mild cranial nerve deficits may indicate mild cranial polyneuropathy. Postviral infection neuropathies may involve the superior laryngeal nerve and cause weakness, fatigability, and loss of range in the singing voice. More serious neurologic disease may also be associated with such symptoms and signs.

Laryngeal Examination

Examination of the larynx begins when the singer enters the physician's office. The range, ease, volume, and quality of the speaking voice should be noted. Technical voice classification is beyond the scope of most physicians. However, the physician should at least be able to discriminate substantial differences in range and timbre, such as between bass and tenor or between alto and soprano. Although the correlation between speaking and singing voices is not perfect, a speaker with a low comfortable bass voice who reports that he is a tenor may be misclassified and singing inappropriate roles with consequent voice strain. This judgment should be deferred to an expert, but the observation should lead the physician to make the appropriate referral. Excessive volume or obvious strain during speaking clearly indicates that voice abuse is present and may be contributing to the patient's singing complaint.

Any patient with a voice complaint should be examined by indirect laryngoscopy at least. It is not possible to judge voice ranges, quality, or other vocal attributes by inspection of the vocal cords. However, the presence or absence of nodules, mass lesions, contact ulcers, hemorrhage, erythema, paralysis, arytenoid erythema (reflux), and other anatomic abnormalities must be established. Erythema of the laryngeal surface of the epiglottis is often seen in association with frequent coughing or clearing of the throat and is caused by direct trauma from the arytenoids during these maneuvers. The mirror or a laryngeal telescope often provides a better view of the posterior portion of the vocal folds than is obtained with flexible endoscopy. Stroboscopic examination adds substantially to diagnostic abilities. A stroboscopic light source can be directed at the physician's head mirror, permitting good assessment of laryngeal vibration. Such an examination frequently reveals vibratory irregularities that would be missed by routine examination.

Another helpful adjunct is the operating microscope. Magnification allows visualization of small mucosal disruptions and hemorrhages that may be significant but overlooked otherwise. This technique also allows photography of the larynx with a microscope camera. Magnification may also be achieved through magnifying laryngeal mirrors or by wearing loupes. Loupes usually provide a clearer image than do most of the magnifying mirrors available. Laryngeal telescopes are also extremely useful and allow photography, magnification, stroboscopy and excellent visualization.

Fiberoptic laryngoscopy can be performed as an office procedure and allows inspection of the vocal cords in patients whose vocal cords are difficult to visualize indirectly. In addition, it permits observation of the vocal mechanism in a more natural posture than does indirect laryngoscopy. In the hands of an experienced endoscopist, this method may provide a great deal of information about both speaking and singing voices. The combination of a fiberoptic laryngoscope with a laryngeal stroboscope may be especially useful (41). This system permits magnification, photography, and detailed inspection of vocal fold motion. More sophisticated systems that permit fiberoptic strobovideolaryngoscopy are currently available commercially. They are an invaluable asset and are used routinely by this author (Fig. 7.2). The video system also provides a permanent record, permitting reassessment, comparison over time, and easy consultation with other physicians. A refinement not currently available commercially is stereoscopic fiberoptic laryngoscopy, accomplished by placing a laryngoscope through each nostril, fastening the two together in the pharynx and observing the larynx through the eyepieces (42). This method allows excellent visualization of laryngeal motion in three dimensions. However, it is practical primarily in a research setting. Rigid endoscopy with anesthesia may be reserved for the rare patient whose vocal cords cannot be assessed adequately by other means, or for patients who need surgical procedures to remove or biopsy laryngeal lesions. In many cases this may be done with local anesthesia, avoiding the need for intubation and the traumatic coughing and vomiting that may occur even after general anesthesia administered by mask. Coughing following general anesthesia may be minimized by using topical anesthesia in the larynx and trachea. However, topical anesthetics may act as severe mucosal irritants in a small number of patients. They may also predispose the patient to aspiration in the postoperative

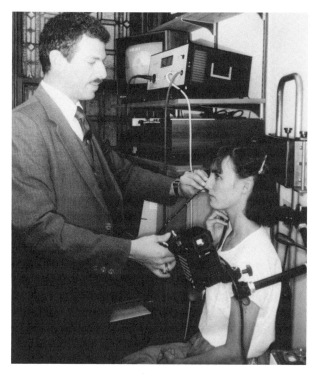

FIG. 7.2. Equipment used for routine office evaluation includes a fiberoptic laryngoscope, video camera with character generator, monitor, stroboscope (Bruel & Kjaer) and video camera. A pulmonary function machine is also partly visible below the video system.

period. If a singer has had difficulty with a topical anesthetic in the office, it should be avoided in the operating room. When used, topical anesthetic should be applied at the end of the procedure. Thus, if inflammation occurs, it will not interfere with microsurgery. Postoperative duration of anesthesia is also optimized. The author has had the least difficulty with a 4% lidocaine preparation (Xylocaine).

OBJECTIVE TESTS

Reliable, valid, objective analysis of the voice is extremely important. Although objective testing is just being developed and has not yet gained wide use in clinical practice, it is as invaluable to the laryngologist as audiometry is to the otologist. Familiarity with some of the measures currently available is extremely helpful.

The Need for Objective Tests

A battery of objective tests that allows reliable, valid, objective assessment of subtle changes in voice function, a "meter of the voice," is needed. This development is necessary not only to treat professional singers, but also to assess the results of laryngeal surgery, treatments for spasmodic dysphonia and other conditions, and to help diagnose the many systemic diseases associated with voice change. Reporting that a patient's voice is "better" without objective measures is as unsatisfactory as reporting that a patient's hearing is "better" without an audiogram. A few objective tests are discussed below. Each of them may be clinically useful in selected circumstances, and they may well be forerunners in a new era of routine, objective voice assessment.

Strobovideolaryngoscopy

Strobovideolaryngoscopy is the single most important technological advance in diagnostic laryngology, with the possible exception of the fiberoptic laryngoscope. Stroboscopic light allows routine, slow-motion evaluation of the mucosal cover layer of the leading edge of the vocal fold. This improved physical examination permits detection of vibratory asymmetries, structural abnormalities, small masses, submucosal scars, and other conditions that are invisible under ordinary light (43). For example, in a patient with a poor voice following laryngeal surgery and a "normal-looking larynx," stroboscopic light reveals adynamic segments that explain the problem even to an untrained observer (such as the patient). The stroboscope is also extremely sensitive in detecting changes caused by fixation from small laryngeal neoplasms in patients who are being followed for leukoplakia, or following laryngeal irradiation. Coupling stroboscopic light with the video camera allows later reevaluation by the laryngologist or by other physicians. A relatively standardized method of subjective assessment of video stroboscopic pictures is in wide clinical use (44,45), allowing comparison of results among various physicians and investigators. Characteristics assessed include fundamental frequency, symmetry of bilateral movements, periodicity, glottal closure, amplitude, mucosal wave, the presence of nonvibrating portions, and other unusual findings (such as a tiny polyp). In addition, objective, frame-by-frame computer analysis is also possible, although not practical (or necessary) on a routine clinical basis, yet.

Other Techniques to Examine Vocal Fold Vibration

Ultra high-speed photography provides similar images but requires expensive, cumbersome equipment and delayed data processing. *Electroglottography* (EGG) uses two electrodes on the skin of the neck above the thyroid laminae. A weak, high-frequency voltage is passed through the larynx from one electrode to the other. Opening and closing of the vocal cords varies the transverse electrical impedance, producing variation of the electrical current in phase with vocal fold vibration. The resultant tracing is called an electroglottogram. It traces the opening and closing of the glottis, and can be correlated with stroboscopic images (46). Electroglottography allows objective determination of the presence or absence of glottal vibrations, easy determination of the fundamental period of vibration, and is reproducible. It reflects the glottal condition more accurately during its closed phase, and quantitative interpretation of the glottal condition is probably not valid (47). EGG shows increasing promise for clinical usefulness (48). *Photoelectroglottography* and *ultrasoundglottography* are less useful clinically, but may be reviewed in Hirano's invaluable book *Clinical Examination of the Voice* (47).

Measures of Phonatory Ability

Objective measures of phonatory ability are among the easiest and most readily available for the laryngologist, helpful in treatment of professional vocalists with specific voice disorders, and extremely useful in assessing the results of surgical therapies. *Maximum phonation time* is measured using a stopwatch. The patient is instructed to sustain the "ah" sound for as long as possible following deep inspiration, vocalizing at a comfortable frequency and intensity. In select cases, the frequency and intensity may be controlled using an inexpensive frequency analyzer and sound level meter. The test is repeated three times, and the greatest value is recorded. Normal values have been determined (47). *Frequency range of phonation* is recorded in semitones and records the vocal range from the lowest note in the modal register (excluding vocal fry) to the highest falsetto note. This is the *physiological frequency range of phonation* and disregards quality. The *musical frequency range of phonation* measures the lowest to highest musically acceptable qualities. Tests for maximum phonation time, frequency range, and many of the other parameters discussed below (including spectrographic analysis) may be preserved on a tape recorder for analysis at a convenient future time and used for pretreatment and posttreatment comparisons. Recordings should be made in a standardized consistent fashion. Frequency limits of *vocal register* may also be measured. The registers are (from low to high): vocal fry, chest, mid, head and falsetto. Overlap of frequency among registers occurs routinely. Testing the *speaking fundamental frequency* often reveals excessively low pitch, an abnormality associated with chronic voice abuse and development of vocal nodules. This parameter may be followed objectively throughout a course of speech therapy. *Intensity range of phonation* (IRP) has proven a less useful measure than frequency range. It varies with fundamental frequency (which should be recorded), and is greatest in the middle-frequency range. It is recorded at sound pressure level (SPL) re: 0.0002 microbar. For normal adults who are not professional vocalists, measuring at a single fundamental frequency, IRP averages 54.8dB for males and 51dB for females (49). Alterations of intensity are common in voice disorders, although IRP is not the most sensitive test to detect them. Information from the above tests may be combined in the *fundamental frequency-intensity profile* (47). *Glottal efficiency* (the ratio of the acoustic power at the level of the glottis to subglottal power) provides useful information but is not clinically practical because it is difficult to measure acoustic power at the level of the glottis. *Subglottic power* is the product of *subglottal pressure* and *airflow rate*. These can be determined clinically. Various alternative measures of glottic efficiency have been proposed, including the *ratio of radiated acoustic power to subglottal power* (50), *airflow intensity profile* (51), and *ratio of the root mean square value of the AC component to the mean volume velocity (DC component)* (52). Although glottal efficiency is of great interest, none of these tests is particularly helpful under routine clinical circumstances.

Aerodynamic Measures

The abdomen and thorax form the "power source" of the voice, propelling a controlled stream of air between the vocal folds. Singers refer to this anatomic complex as the "diaphragm" or "support." Effective, well-trained abdominal-thoracic muscle control and efficient respiratory function are essential to healthy vocalization. Traditional *pulmonary function testing* provides the most readily accessible measures of respiratory function. The most common parameters measured include: (1.) *tidal volume*, the volume of air that enters the lungs during inspiration and leaves during expiration in normal breathing, (2.) *functional residual capacity*, the volume of air remaining in the lungs at the end of expiration during normal breathing; it may be divided into *expiratory reserve volume* (maximal additional volume that can be exhaled) and *residual volume* (the volume of air remaining in the lungs at the end of maximal exhalation), (3.) *inspiratory capacity*, the maximal volume of air that can be inhaled starting at the functional residual capacity, (4.) *total lung capacity*, the volume of air in the lungs following maximal inspiration, (5.) *vital capacity*, the maximal volume of air that can be exhaled from the lungs following maximal inspiration, (6.) *forced vital capacity*, the rate of airflow with rapid, forceful expiration from total lung capacity to residual volume, (7.) FEV_1, the forced expiratory volume in one second, (8.) FEV_3, the forced expiratory volume in 3 seconds, and (9.) *maximal mid-expiratory flow rate* or *forced mid-expiratory flow*, the mean rate of air flow over the middle half of the forced vital capacity (between 25% and 75% of the forced vital capacity).

In most established singers, routine pulmonary function testing is not helpful. However, in singers and professional speakers with pathology caused by voice abuse, abnormal pulmonary function tests may confirm deficiencies in aerobic conditioning or may reveal previously unrecognized asthma. Testing before and after bronchodilator therapy helps establish this diagnosis. In selected instances, when asthma is suspected clinically, methacholine challenge is justified. Even a mild or moderate obstructive pulmonary disease may have a substantial deleterious effect on the voice; significant asthma may be present, even in the absence of wheezing. Sometimes chronic cough or voice abuse may be the only presenting symptom.

The *spirometer*, readily available for pulmonary function testing, can be used for measuring airflow during phonation. However, it does not allow simultaneous display of acoustic signals, and its frequency response is poor. A *pneumotachograph* consists of a laminar air resistor, a differential pressure transducer, and an amplifying and recording system. It allows measurement of air flow and simultaneous recording of other signals when coupled with a polygraph. A *hot-wire anemometer* allows determination of air flow velocity by measuring the electrical drop across the hot wire. Modern hot-wire anemometers (containing electrical feedback circuitry that maintains the temperature of the hot wire) provide a flat frequency response up to 1KHz and are useful clinically (52).

The four parameters traditionally measured in analyzing the aerodynamic performance of a voice include: *subglottal pressure* (P_{sub}), *supraglottal pressure* (P_{sup}), *glottal impedance*, and *volume velocity of airflow at the glottis*. These parameters and their rapid variations can be measured under laboratory circumstances. However, clinically, their mean value is usually determined. They are related as follows:

$$P_{sub} - P_{sup} = MFR \times GR$$

where MFR is the mean (root mean square) flow rate, and GR is the mean (root mean square) glottal resistance.

When vocalizing an open vowel, the supraglottic pressure equals the atmospheric pressure, reducing the equation to:

$$P_{sub} = MFR \times GR$$

The *mean flow rate* is a useful clinical measure. Using the vowel "ah" sound, it is calculated by dividing the total volume of air used during phonation by the duration of phonation. The subject phonates at a natural pitch and loudness, either over a determined period of time or for a maximum sustained period of phonation. *Air volume* is determined by the use of a mask fitted tightly over the face or by phonating into a mouthpiece while wearing a noseclamp. Measurements may be made using a spirometer, pneumotachograph, or hot-wire anemometer. The normal values for mean flow rate under habitual phonation, which changes in intensity or register, and under various pathologic circumstances have been determined (47). Normal values are available for both adults and children. Mean flow rate is a clinically useful parameter to follow during treatment for vocal nodules, recurrent laryngeal nerve paralysis, spasmodic dysphonia, and other conditions.

Glottal resistance cannot be measured directly, but it may be calculated from the mean flow rate and mean subglottal pressure. Normal glottal resistance is 20 to 100 dyne sec/cm^5 at low and medium pitches and 150 dyne sec/cm^5 at high pitches (50). *Subglottal pressure* is less useful clinically because it requires an invasive procedure for accurate measurement. It may be determined by tracheal puncture, transglottal catheter, or measurement through a tracheostoma using a transducer. Subglottal pressure may be approximated using an esophageal balloon. *Intratracheal pressure*, which is roughly equal to subglottal pressure, is transmitted to the balloon through the trachea. However, measured changes in the esophageal balloon are affected by intraesophageal pressure, which is dependent upon lung volume. Therefore, estimates of subglottal pressure using this technique are valid only under specific, controlled circumstances. The normal values for subglottal pressure under various healthy and pathologic voice conditions have also been determined by numerous investigators (47).

The *phonation quotient* is the vital capacity divided by the maximum phonation time. It has been shown to correlate closely with maximum flow rate (53) and is a more convenient measure. Normative data determined by various authors have been published (47). The phonation quotient provides an objective measure of the effects of treatment and is particularly useful in cases of recurrent laryngeal nerve paralysis and mass lesions of the vocal folds, including nodules.

Acoustic Analysis

Acoustic analysis of voice signals is both promising and disappointing. The skilled laryngologist, speech pathologist, musician or other trained listener frequently infers a great deal of valid information from the sound of a voice. However, clinically useful technology for analyzing and quantifying subtle acoustic differences has not been developed. In many ways, the *tape recorder* is still the laryngologist's most valuable tool for acoustic analysis. Recording a patient's voice under controlled, repeatable circumstances prior to, during, and at the conclusion of treatment allows both physician and patient to make qualitative, subjective acoustic analysis. Objective analysis with instruments may also be made from recorded voice samples. The parameters usually assessed include fundamental frequency (or period), intensity, perturbation, amount and distribution of spectral harmonics, and amount of noise (turbulent air). Very high quality audio recording for computer analysis can be done on videotape using a stereo video recorder, with or without a digital pulse code modulator. *Sound spectrography* is readily available and displays the frequency and harmonic spectrum of a short sample of voice. It also visually records noise. Long-time-averaged-spectrography (LTAS) analyzes spectral distribution of speech samples over time (54), providing some additional information. Although spectrographs demonstrate abnormalities and changes during therapy for vocal nodules or vocal fold paralysis, they are more effective in documenting gross changes that are obvious to the average listener than they are in validating more controversial and subtle alterations in vocal quality, as might be seen in various stages of professional voice training, for example.

In analyzing acoustic signals, the microphone may be placed at the mouth, or it may be positioned in or over the trachea. However, position should be standardized in each office or laboratory (55). Various techniques are being developed to improve the usefulness of acoustic analysis, including inverse filtering and various multidimensional approaches to analysis. Because of the enormous amount of information carried in the acoustic signal, further refinements in objective acoustic analysis should prove particularly valuable for the clinician.

Laryngeal Electromyography

Electromyography requires an electrode system, an amplifier, an oscilloscope, a loudspeaker, and a recording system. Either a needle electrode or a hooked-wire electrode may be used (47). Because of the invasive nature of the procedure, electromyography is rarely utilized in caring for the customary problems of professional voice users. However, it may be extremely valuable in confirming cases of vocal fold paralysis, in differentiating paralysis from arytenoid dislocation, in differentiating recurrent laryngeal nerve paralysis from complete vocal fold paralysis, and in documenting functional voice disorders and malingering.

Psychoacoustic Evaluation

Because the human ear and brain are the most sensitive and complex analyzers of sound currently available, many researchers have tried to standardize and quantify psychoacoustic evaluation. Unfortunately, even definitions of basic terms such as hoarseness and breathiness are still controversial. Standardization of psychoacoustic evaluation protocols and interpretation does not exist. Consequently, although subjective psychoacoustic analysis of voice is of great value to the individual skilled clinician, it remains generally unsatisfactory for comparing research among laboratories or for reporting clinical results.

EVALUATION OF THE SINGING VOICE

The physician's evaluation of the larynx is aided greatly by examination of the singing voice. This is accomplished best by having the singer stand and sing scales, either in the examining room or in the soundproof audiology booth. The physician must be careful not to exceed the limits of his expertise; but if voice abuse or technical error is suspected, or if a difficult judgment must be reached on whether to allow a sick singer to perform, a brief observation of the patient's singing may provide invaluable information. The singer's stance should be balanced, and his weight should be slightly forward. The knees should be bent slightly and the shoulders, torso, and neck should be relaxed. The singer should inhale through his nose. This allows filtration, warming, and humidification of inspired air. In general, the chest should be expanded, but most of the active breathing is abdominal. The chest should not rise substantially, and the supraclavicular musculature should not be involved obviously in inspiration. Shoulders and neck muscles should not be tensed, even with deep inspiration. Abdominal musculature should be contracted before the initiation of the tone. This may be evaluated visually or by palpation (Fig. 7.3). Muscles of the neck and face should be relaxed. Economy is a basic principle of all art forms. Wasted energy, motion, and muscle tension are incorrect and usually deleterious. The singer should be instructed to sing a scale (a five-note scale is usually sufficient) on the "ah" sound, beginning on any comfortable note. Technical errors are usually most obvious as contraction of muscles in the neck and chin, retraction of the lower lip, retraction of the tongue, or tightening of the muscles of mastication. The singer's mouth should be open widely but comfortably. When singing "ah," the singer's tongue should rest in a neutral position with the tip of the tongue lying against the back of the singer's teeth. If the tongue pulls back or

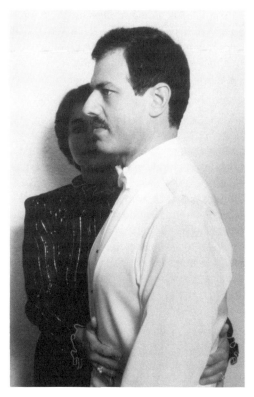

FIG. 7.3. Bimanual palpation of the support mechanism. The singer should expand posteriorly and anteriorly with inspiration. Muscles should tighten *prior* to onset of the sung tone.

demonstrates obvious muscular activity as the singer performs his scales, improper voice use can be confirmed on the basis of positive evidence (Fig. 7.4). The position of the larynx should not vary substantially with pitch changes. Rising of the larynx with ascending pitch is also evidence of technical dysfunction. This examination also gives the physician an opportunity to observe any dramatic differences between the qualities and ranges of the speaking voice and the singing voice. A physical examination summary has proven helpful in organization and documentation (40).

Remembering the admonition to avoid exceeding his expertise, the physician who examines many singers can often glean invaluable information from a brief attempt to modify an obvious technical error. For example, a decision on whether to allow a singer with mild or moderate laryngitis to perform is often difficult. On the one hand, an expert singer has technical skills that allow him to sing around adverse circumstances safely. On the other hand, if a singer does not sing with correct technique and does not have the discipline to modify volume, technique, and repertoire as necessary, his risk of vocal injury may be increased substantially by even mild inflammation of the vocal cords. In borderline circumstances, observation of the singer's technique may help the physician greatly in making a judgment. If the singer's technique appears flawless, we may feel somewhat more secure in allowing him to proceed with performance commitments. More commonly, even good singers demonstrate technical errors when they have laryngitis. In a vain effort to compensate for dysfunction at the vocal cord level, a singer will often modify his technique in the supraglottic or subglottic vocal tract. In the good singer, this usually means going from good technique to bad technique. The most common error involves pulling back the tongue and tightening strap muscles in the neck. Although this increased muscular activity gives the illusion to the singer that he is doing something to make his voice more secure, this technical maladjustment undermines the effectiveness of his support and increases vocal strain. The physician may ask the singer to hold the top note of his five-note scale; while the note is being held, he may simply tell the singer "relax your tongue" and at the same time point toward the singer's abdominal musculature. Most good singers will immediately correct to good technique. If they do, and if upcoming performances are particularly important, we may be able to allow performance with a reminder that meticulous technique is essential. The singer should be advised to "sing by feel rather than by ear," and to consult his voice teacher. He should also be told to conserve his voice except when it is absolutely necessary for him to use it. If a singer is unable to correct promptly from bad technique to good technique, especially if the singer uses excessive muscle tension in the neck and ineffective abdominal support, it is generally safer not to allow performance in the presence of even mild vocal cord pathology. With increased experience and training, the laryngologist may make other observations that assist him in arriving at appropriate treatment recommendations for his singer patients. If treatment is to be instituted, at least a tape recording of the voice is advisable in most cases and essential before any surgical intervention. The author routinely uses strobovideolaryngoscopy for diagnosis and documentation in virtually all cases, as well as many of the objective measures discussed above. Such testing is extremely helpful clinically and medicolegally. Spectrography may be useful in some severe vocal disorders. However, in its present state of development, routine spectrography is of limited help in documenting the subtle differences in voice quality usually involved in caring for professional singers.

OTHER APPROPRIATE EXAMINATION

A general physical examination should be performed whenever there is question as to the patient's systemic health. Debilitating conditions such as mononucleosis may be noticed first by the singer as vocal fatigue. A neurologic assessment may be particularly revealing. The physician must be careful not to overlook dysarthrias and dysphonias characteristic of movement disorders and of serious neurologic disease. Dysarthria is a defect in rhythm, enunciation, and articulation, usually resulting from neuromuscular impairment or weakness such as they occur after a stroke. It may be seen with oral deformities or illness as well. Dysphonia is an abnormality

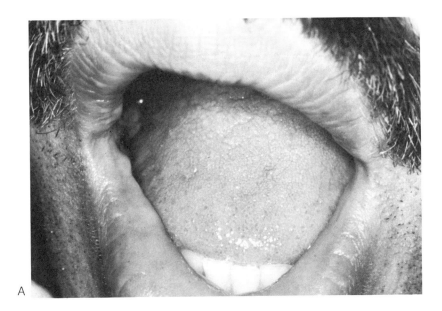

A

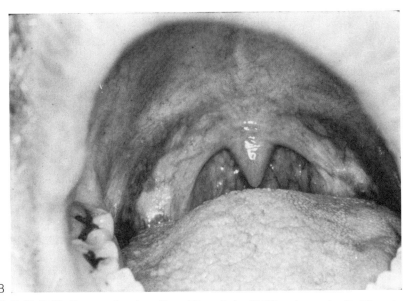

B

FIG. 7.4A–7.4D. Proper relaxed position of the anterior (7.4A) and posterior (7.4B) portions of the tongue. Common improper use with the tongue pulled back from the teeth (7.4C) and raised posteriorly (7.4D).

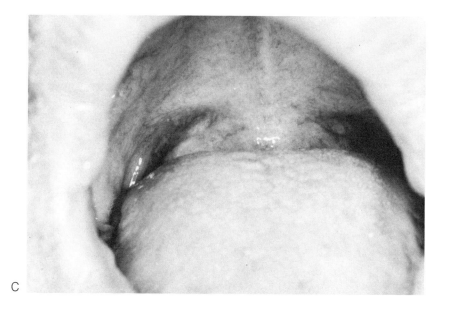

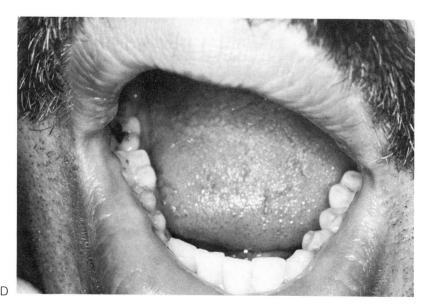

FIG. 7.4. *Continued.*

of vocalization usually originating from problems at the laryngeal level. Physicians should be familiar with the six types of dysarthria, their symptoms and their significance (56,57). Flaccid dysarthria occurs in lower motor neuron or primary muscle disorders such as myasthenia gravis and tumors or strokes involving the brainstem nuclei. Spastic dysarthria is found in upper motor neuron disorders (pseudobulbar palsy) such as multiple strokes and cerebral palsy. Atactic dysarthria is seen with cerebellar disease, alcohol intoxication, and multiple sclerosis. Hypokinetic dysarthria accompanies Parkinson's disease. Hyperkinetic dysarthria may be spasmodic, as in the Gilles de la Tourette syndrome, or dystonic, as in chorea and cerebral palsy. Mixed dysarthria is seen in amyotrophic lateral sclerosis. The classification above actually combines dysphonic and dysarthric characteristics, but it is very useful clinically. The value of a comprehensive neurolaryngological evaluation cannot be overstated (58).

Even "minor" problems may produce disturbing or disabling effects in a professional performer who requires nearly perfect physical function.

COMMON DIAGNOSES AND TREATMENTS

In 2,286 cases of all forms of voice disorders reported by Brodnitz (17), 80% of the disorders were attributed to voice abuse or to psychogenic factors resulting in vocal dysfunction. Organic voice disorders were reported in 20% of the patients. Of women with organic problems, about 15% had identifiable endocrine causes. A somewhat higher incidence of organic disorders, particularly reflux laryngitis and acute infectious laryngitis, may be found more commonly.

Reflux Laryngitis

This form of laryngitis is caused by regurgitation of gastric acid into the hypopharynx. The symptoms discussed above and the bright red, often slightly edematous appearance of the arytenoid mucosa help establish the diagnosis. A barium esophagogram may provide additional information but is not needed routinely. In selected cases, 24-hour pH monitoring provides the best analysis and documentation of reflux. The mainstays of treatment are elevation of the head of the singer's bed (not just sleeping on pillows), antacids and avoidance of eating for 3 or 4 hours before going to sleep. Avoidance of alcohol and coffee are beneficial. Cimetidine, ranitidine or famotidine also may be helpful, if there are no contraindications to their use. In this relatively young patient population, it should be remembered that male infertility is one of the complications (although uncommon) of cimetidine.

Anxiety

Good singers are frequently sensitive and communicative people. When the principal cause of vocal dysfunction is anxiety, the physician can often accomplish much with a few minutes of assurance that there is no organic difficulty and by stating the diagnosis of anxiety reaction. The singer should be counseled that anxiety is normal and that recognition of it as the principal problem frequently allows the performer to overcome it. Tranquilizers and sedatives are rarely necessary and are undesirable because they may interfere with fine motor control. Recently, beta-adrenergic blocking agents such as propranolol hydrochloride (Inderal, Ayerst) have achieved some popularity for treatment of preperformance anxiety. Beta-blockers are not recommended for regular use by this author. They have significant effects on the cardiovascular system and many potential complications, including hypotension, thrombocytopenic purpura, mental depression, agranulocytosis, laryngospasm with respiratory distress, bronchospasm, and others. In addition, their efficacy is controversial. Although they may have a favorable effect in relieving performance anxiety, beta-blockers may produce a noticeable adverse effect on singing performance (59). As blood level of drug established by a given dose of beta-blocker varies widely among individuals, initial use of these agents in preperformance situations may be particularly troublesome. In addition, beta-blockers impede increases in heart rate which are needed as physiologic responses to the psychological and physical demands of performance. Although these drugs have a place under occasional, extraordinary circumstances, their routine use is not only potentially hazardous, but also violates an important therapeutic principle. Performers have chosen a career that exposes them to the public. If such a person is so incapacitated by anxiety that he is unable to perform the routine functions of his chosen profession without chemical help, this should be considered symptomatic of a significant underlying psychological problem. It is not routine or healthy for a performer to be dependent on drugs in order to perform, whether the drug is a benzodiazepine, a barbituarate, a beta-blocker, or alcohol. If such a dependence exists, psychological evaluation should be considered by an experienced arts/medicine psychologist or psychiatrist. Obscuring the symptoms by fostering the dependence is insufficient. However, if the singer is on tour and will only be under a particular laryngologist's care for a week or two, the physician should not try to make major changes in the singer's customary regimen. Rather, he should communicate with the performer's primary laryngologist or family physician and should coordinate appropriate long-term care through him or her.

Muscle Problems

The physician must not exceed the limits of his expertise or responsibility. However, if the physician is trained in singing and notices a minor technical error such as isolated excess muscle tension in the tongue, this may be pointed out. Nevertheless, the singer should be referred back to his voice teacher or to a competent phoniatrist for management of these problems. Abdominal muscle problems should be noted and should also be referred back to the vocal teacher. Of course, any medical cause must be corrected. Dental and temporomandibular joint problems usually can be managed easily by a skilled dentist.

Voice Abuse

When voice abuse is due to extracurricular activities such as conducting, screaming at athletic events, or shouting at children, the physician should advise the patient about measures to protect the speaking voice and consequently the singing voice. However, if it is a matter of strain in the singing or speaking voice under ordinary circumstances, treatment should be deferred to a voice teacher or speech pathologist. In many instances, training the speaking voice will benefit the singer greatly, and physicians should not hesitate to recommend such training.

Vocal Nodules, Cysts, and Polyps

Nodules are caused by voice abuse and are a dreaded malady of singers. Occasionally, laryngoscopy reveals asymptomatic vocal nodules that do not appear to interfere with voice production. In such cases, the nodules should not be treated. Some famous and successful singers have had untreated vocal nodules. However, in most cases nodules result in hoarseness, breathiness, loss of range and vocal fatigue. They may be due to abuse of the speaking voice rather than the singing voice. Voice therapy always should be tried as the initial therapeutic modality and will cure the vast majority of patients even if the nodules look firm and have been present for many months or years. Even in those who eventually need surgical excision of their nodules, preoperative voice therapy is essential to prevent recurrence of the nodules. Caution must be exercised in diagnosing small nodules in patients who have been singing actively. Many singers develop bilateral, symmetrical, soft swellings at the junction of the anterior and middle thirds of their vocal cords following heavy voice use. There is no evidence to suggest that singers with such "physiologic swelling" are predisposed towards development of vocal nodules. At present, the condition is generally considered to be within normal limits. The physiologic swelling usually disappears with 24 to 48 hours of rest from heavy voice use. Care must be taken not to frighten the singer or embarrass the physician by misdiagnosing physiologic swellings as vocal nodules. Nodules carry a great stigma among singers, and the psychological impact of the diagnosis should not be underestimated. When nodules are present, the patient should be informed with the same gentle caution used in telling a patient that he or she has a life-threatening illness.

Submucosal cysts of the vocal folds are probably also traumatic lesions that result in blockage of a mucous gland duct. They often cause contact swelling on the contralateral side and are usually misdiagnosed as nodules initially. Occasionally, they can be differentiated from nodules by strobovideolaryngoscopy when the mass is obviously fluid-filled. More often, they are suspected when the nodule (contact swelling) on the other vocal fold resolves with voice therapy, but the mass on one vocal fold does not resolve. Cysts may also be found on one side (occasionally both sides) when surgery is performed for apparent nodules that have not resolved with voice therapy. The surgery should be performed superficially and with minimal trauma, as discussed below.

Many other structural lesions may appear on the vocal folds, of course; not all respond to nonsurgical therapy. Polyps are usually unilateral, and they often have a prominent feeding blood vessel coursing along the superior surface of the vocal fold and entering the base of the polyp. The pathogenesis of polyps cannot be proven in many cases, but the lesion is thought to be traumatic. At least some polyps start as vocal fold hemorrhages. In some cases, even sizable polyps resolve with relative voice rest and a few weeks of low dose steroid therapy such as triamcinolone 4 mg twice a day. However, most of them require surgical removal. If polyps are not treated, they may produce contact injury on the contralateral vocal fold. Voice therapy should be used to assure good relative voice rest and to avoid abusive behaviors before and after surgery. When surgery is performed, care must be taken not to damage the leading edge of the vocal fold, especially if a laser is used, as discussed below.

Upper Respiratory Tract Infection Without Laryngitis

Although mucosal irritation usually is diffuse, singers sometimes have marked nasal obstruction with little or no sore throat and a "normal" voice. If the laryngeal examination shows no abnormality, a singer with a "head cold" should be permitted to sing. However, he should be advised not to try to duplicate his usual sound, but rather to accept the insurmountable alteration caused by the change in his supraglottic vocal tract. The decision as to whether it is advisable professionally for him to appear under those circumstances rests with the singer and his musical associates. He should be cautioned against throat-clearing as this is traumatic and may produce laryngitis. If a cough is present, nonnarcotic medications should be used to suppress it.

Tonsillitis

Recurrent tonsillitis in professional singers seems particularly problematic. On the one hand, no one is anxious to perform tonsillectomy upon an established singer. On the other hand, a singer cannot affort to be sick for a week five or six times a year. Such incapacitation is too damaging to the singer's income and reputation. In general, the same conservative approach toward tonsil disease used in other patients should be applied to professional singers, and tonsillectomy should not be withheld if it is really indicated. It is particularly important to remove only the tonsil without damaging the surrounding tissues in order to minimize restriction of palatal and pharyngeal motion by scar. A singer must be warned that tonsillectomy may alter the sound of his voice, as discussed above. In addition to recurrent, acute tonsillitis, halitosis caused by uncontrollable tonsillar debris may be an appropriate indication for tonsillectomy, on rare occasion. When gastric reflux, dental disease, metabolic abnormalities and other causes of halitosis have been ruled out and chronic tonsillitis has been established as the etiology, treatment should be offered. Although we do not ordinarily consider halitosis a serious malady, it may be a major impediment to success for people who have to work closely with other people such as singers, actors, dentists, barbers, some physicians, and others. If the problem cannot be cured with medication or with hygiene using a soft toothbrush or water spray to cleanse the tonsil, tonsillectomy is reasonable.

Laryngitis With Serious Vocal Cord Injury

Hemorrhage in the vocal folds and mucosal disruption are contraindications to singing. When these are observed, the therapeutic course includes strict voice rest in addition to correction of any underlying disease. Vocal fold hemorrhage in skilled singers is seen most commonly in premenstrual women using aspirin products. Severe hemorrhage or mucosal scarring may result in permanent alterations in vocal fold vibratory function. In rare instances, surgical intervention may be necessary. The potential gravity of these conditions must be stressed, for singers are generally reluctant to cancel an appearance. As von Leden observed, it is a pleasure to work with "people who are determined that the show must go on when everyone else is determined to goof off" (60). However, patient compliance is essential when serious damage has occurred. At the present time, acute treatment of vocal fold hemorrhage is controversial. Most laryngologists allow the hematoma to resolve spontaneously. Because this sometimes results in an organized hematoma and scar formation requiring surgery, some physicians advocate incision along the superior edge of the vocal fold and drainage of the hematoma in selected cases. Further study is needed to determine optimum therapy.

Laryngitis Without Serious Damage

Mild to moderate edema and erythema of the vocal cords may result from infection or from noninfectious causes. In the absence of mucosal disruption or hemorrhage, they are not absolute contraindications to voice use. Noninfectious laryngitis commonly occurs in association with excessive voice use in preperformance rehearsals. It may also be caused by other forms of voice abuse and by mucosal irritation due to allergy, smoke inhalation, and other causes. Mucus stranding between the anterior and middle thirds of the vocal cords is often indicative of voice abuse. Laryngitis sicca is associated with dehydration, dry atmosphere, mouth breathing and antihistamine therapy. Deficiency of lubrication causes irritation and coughing and results in mild inflammation. If there is no pressing professional need for performance, inflammatory conditions of the larynx are best treated with relative voice rest in addition to other modalities. However, in some instances singing may be permitted. The singer should be instructed to avoid all forms of irritation and to rest his voice at all times except during his warm-up and performance. Corticosteroids and other medications discussed may be helpful. If mucosal secretions are copious, low-dose antihistamine therapy may be beneficial, but it must be pre-scribed with caution and should generally be avoided. Copious, thin secretions are better for a singer than scant, thick secretions or excessive dryness. The singer with laryngitis must be kept well hydrated to maintain the desired character of his mucosal lubrication. Psychological support is crucial. It is often helpful for the physician to intercede on the singer's behalf and to convey "doctor's orders" di-rectly to agents or theater management. Such mitigation of exogenous stress can be highly therapeutic. Infectious laryngitis may be caused by bacteria or viruses. Sub-glottic involvement is frequently indicative of a more severe infection which may be difficult to control in a short period of time. Indiscriminate use of antibiotics must be avoided. However, when the physician is in doubt as to the cause and when a major performance is imminent, vigorous antibiotic treatment is warranted. In this circumstance, the damage caused by allowing progression of a curable condition is greater than the damage that might result from a course of therapy for an unproven microorganism while cultures are pending. When a major concert is not imminent, indications for therapy are the same as for the nonsinger. Voice rest (absolute or relative) is an important therapeutic consideration in any case of laryngitis. When there are no pressing professional commitments, a short course of absolute voice rest may be considered, as it is the safest and most conservative therapeutic inter-vention. This means absolute silence and communication with a writing pad. The singer must be instructed not even to whisper, as this may be an even more trau-matic vocal activity than speaking softly. Whistling through the lips also requires vocalization and should not be permitted. Absolute voice rest is necessary only for serious vocal cord injury such as hemorrhage or mucosal disruption. Even then, it is virtually never indicated for more than 7 to 10 days. Three days is often a sufficient period. There are some excellent laryngologists who do not believe voice rest should be used at all. However, absolute voice rest for a few days may be helpful in patients with laryngitis, especially those gregarious, verbal singers who find it diffi-cult to moderate their voice use to comply with relative voice rest instructions. In many instances, considerations of economics and reputation militate against a rec-ommendation for voice rest. In advising performers to minimize vocal use, Punt counseled, "Don't say a single word for which you are not being paid" (61). This admonition frequently guides the ailing singer away from preperformance conversa-tions and backstage greetings and allows a successful series of performances. Singers also should be instructed to speak softly, as infrequently as possible, often at a slightly higher pitch than usual, to avoid excessive telephone use, and to speak with abdominal support as they would use in singing. This is relative voice rest, and it is helpful in most cases. An urgent session with a speech and language pathologist is extremely helpful in providing guidelines to prevent voice abuse. Nevertheless, the singer must be aware that there is some risk associated with performing with laryngitis, even when singing is possible. Inflammation of the vocal folds is associ-ated with increased capillary fragility and increased risk of vocal fold injury or hemorrhage. Many factors must be considered in determining whether a given con-cert is important enough to justify the potential consequences. Steam inhalations deliver moisture and heat to the vocal cords and tracheobronchial tree and are often useful. Nasal irrigations are used by some people but have little proven value. Gargling also has no proven efficacy, but it is probably harmful only if it involves loud, abusive vocalization as part of the gargling process. Ultrasonic treatments, local massage, psychotherapy, and biofeedback directed at relieving anxiety and decreasing muscle tension may be helpful adjuncts to a broader therapeutic program. However, psychotherapy and biofeedback, in particular, must be expertly supervised, if used at all. Voice lessons given by an expert teacher are invaluable. When there is any question of technical dysfunction, the singer should be referred to his teacher. Even when there is an obvious organic abnormality, referral to a voice teacher is appropriate, especially for younger singers. There are numerous "tricks of the trade" that permit a singer to safely overcome some of the disabilities of mild illness. If a singer plans to proceed with a performance during an illness, he should not cancel his voice lesson as part of his relative voice rest regimen. Rather, a short lesson to assure optimum technique is extremely useful.

Drugs for Vocal Dysfunction

When antibiotics are used, high doses to rapidly achieve therapeutic blood levels are recommended, and a full course of 7 to 10 days should be administered. Erythromycins and tetracyclines may be particularly useful in managing respiratory tract infections (62). Although ampicillin is used commonly, amoxicillin may achieve higher tissue levels more rapidly (63) and may be advantageous, particularly when therapy is instituted shortly before a performance. It is often helpful to start treatment with an intramuscular injection. Antihistamines may be used to treat allergies. However, because they tend to cause dryness and are frequently combined with sympathomimetic or parasympatholytic agents which further reduce and thicken mucosal secretions, they may reduce lubrication to the point of producing a dry cough. This dryness may be more harmful than the allergic condition itself. Mild antihistamines in small doses should be tried between performances, but they should generally not be used immediately before performances if the singer has had no previous experience with them. Their adverse effects may be counteracted to some extent with mucolytic agents. Iodinated glycerol (Organidin, Wallace) is an older mucolytic expectorant that helps liquify viscous mucous and increase the output of thin respiratory tract secretions. Phenylpropanolamine hydrochloride/guaifenesin (Entex) is a useful expectorant and vasoconstrictor that increases and thins mucosal secretions. Guaifenesin (Robitussin) also thins and increases secretions. Humibid (Adams) is currently the most convenient and effective guaifenesin preparation available. These drugs are relatively harmless and may be very helpful in singers who complain of thick secretions, frequent throat-clearing or "postnasal drip." Awareness of postnasal drip is often caused by secretions being too thick rather than too plentiful.

Corticosteroids are potent antiinflammatory agents and may be helpful in managing acute inflammatory laryngitis. Although many laryngologists recommend using steroids in low doses (methylprednisolone 10 mg), the author has found higher doses for short periods of time more effective. Depending on the indication, dosage may be prednisolone 60 mg or dexamethasone 6 mg intramuscularly once, a similar starting dose orally tapered over 3 to 6 days. Regimens such as a Decadron (dexamethasone) dose pack or Medrol (methylprednisolone) Dosepak may also be used. Adrenocorticotropic hormone (ACTH) may also be used to increase endogenous cortisone output, decreasing inflammation and mobilizing water from an edematous larynx (64), although the author has found traditional steroid therapy entirely satisfactory. Care must be taken not to prescribe steroids excessively. They should be used only when there is a pressing professional commitment that is being hampered by vocal fold inflammation. If there is any question that the inflammation may be of infectious origin, antibiotic coverage is recommended.

In the premenstrual period, decreased estrogen and progesterone levels are associated with altered pituitary activity. An increase in circulating antidiuretic hormone results in fluid retention in Reinke's space as well as in other tissues. The fluid retained in the vocal fold during inflammation and hormonal fluid shifts is bound, not free, water (9). Diuretics do not remobilize this fluid effectively, and dehydrate the singer, resulting in decreased lubrication and thickened secretions, but persistently edematous vocal cords. If used, their effects should be monitored closely. Aspirin and other analgesics frequently have been prescribed for relief of minor throat and laryngeal irritations. However, the platelet dysfunction caused by aspirin predisposes to hemorrhage, especially in vocal cords traumatized by excessive voice use in the face of vocal dysfunction. Mucosal hemorrhage can be devastating to a professional voice, and aspirin products should be avoided altogether in singers. Acetaminophen is the best substitute, as even most common nonsteroidal antiinflammatory drugs such as ibuprofen may interfere with the clotting mechanism. Nonsteroidal antiinflammatory drugs cause fewer bleeding problems, and acetaminophen usually does not cause abnormal bleeding. Caruso used a spray of ether and iodoform on his vocal cords when he had to sing with laryngitis. Nevertheless, the use of analgesics is extremely dangerous and should be avoided. Pain is an important protective physiologic function. Masking it risks incurring significant vocal damage which may be unrecognized until after the analgesic or anesthetic wears off. If a singer requires analgesics or topical anesthetics to alleviate laryngeal discomfort, the laryngitis is severe enough to warrant canceling a performance. If the analgesic is for headache or some other discomfort not intimately associated with voice production, symptomatic treatment should be discouraged until singing commitments have been completed. Diphenhydramine hydrochloride (Benadryl), 0.5% in distilled water, delivered to the larynx as a mist, may be helpful for its vasoconstrictive properties, but it is also dangerous because of its analgesic effect and is not recommended by this author. However, Punt advocated this mixture and several modifications of it (61). Other topical vasoconstrictors that do not contain analgesics may be beneficial in selected cases. Oxymetazoline hydrochloride (Afrin) is particularly helpful. Propylene glycol, 5% in a physiologically balanced salt solution may be delivered by large particle mist and can provide helpful lubrication, particularly in cases of laryngitis sicca following air travel or associated with dry climates. Such treatment is harmless and may also provide a beneficial placebo effect. Water or saline delivered via a vaporizer or steam generator is frequently effective and sufficient. This therapy should be augmented by oral hydration which is the mainstay of treatment for dehydration. A singer can monitor his state of hydration by observing his urine color. Dr. Van Lawrence advises his singers to "pee pale."

Most inhalers are not recommended for use in professional voice users. Many people develop contact inflammation from insensitivity to the propellants used in many inhalers. Steroid inhalers used for prolonged periods may result in candida laryngitis. Prolonged steroid use, such as is common in asthmatics, also appears capable of causing wasting of the vocalis muscle.

Respiratory Dysfunction

Respiratory problems are especially problematic to singers and other voice professionals (65). They also cause similar problems for wind instrumentalists. Support is essential to healthy voice production. The effects of severe respiratory infection are obvious, and will not be enumerated. Restrictive lung disease such as that associated with obesity may impair support by decreasing lung volume and respiratory efficiency. Even mild obstructive lung disease can impair support enough to result in increased neck and tongue muscle tension, and abusive voice use capable of producing vocal nodules. This scenario occurs with unrecognized asthma. This may be difficult to diagnose unless suspected, because many such cases of asthma are exercise-induced. Performance is a form of exercise. Consequently, the singer will have normal pulmonary function clinically, and may even have reasonably normal pulmonary function tests at rest in the office. He will also usually support well and sing with good technique during the first portion of a performance. However, as performance exercise continues, pulmonary function decreases, effectively impairing support, and resulting in abusive technique. When suspected, this entity can be confirmed through a methacholine challenge test. Treatment of the underlying pulmonary disease to restore the ability to affect correct support is essential to resolving the vocal problem. Treating asthma is rendered more difficult in professional voice users because of the need in some patients to avoid not only inhalers, but also drugs that produce even a mild tremor which may be audible during soft singing. The cooperation of a skilled pulmonologist specializing in asthma and sensitive to the problems of performing artists is invaluable.

Speech and Language Pathology

An excellent speech and language pathologist is an invaluable asset in caring for professional voice users. However, laryngologists should recognize that, like physicians, speech pathologists have varied backgrounds and experience in treatment of voice disorders. In fact, most speech pathology programs teach relatively little about caring for professional speakers and nothing about professional singers. Moreover, there are few speech pathologists in the United States with vast experience in this specialized area, and there are no fellowships in this specialty for speech pathologists. Speech pathologists often subspecialize. A person who expertly treats patients who have had strokes, stutter, have undergone laryngectomy, or have swallowing disorders will not necessarily know how to optimally manage professional voice users. The laryngologist must learn the strengths and weaknesses of the speech pathologist with whom he works. After identifying a speech pathologist who is interested in treating professional voice users, the laryngologist and speech pathologist should work together closely in developing the necessary expertise. Assistance may be found through laryngologists who treat large numbers of singers, or through educational programs such as the Annual Voice Foundation's Symposium on Care of the Professional Voice. In general, therapy should be directed toward relaxation techniques, breath control, and abdominal support. One approach that has proven particularly useful in singers is described by Georgiana Peacher in *How To Improve Your Speaking Voice* (66). This book provides a good basic orientation for the laryngologist and speech pathologist.

Speech pathology may be helpful even when a singer has no obvious problem in his speaking voice but has significant technical problems singing. Once a person has been singing for several years, it is often very difficult for a singing teacher to convince him to correct certain technical errors. Singers are much less protective of their speaking voices. Therefore, a speech pathologist may be able to rapidly teach proper support, relaxation, and voice placement in speaking. Once mastered, these techniques can be carried over fairly easily into singing through cooperation between the speech pathologist and voice teacher. This "back door" approach has proven extremely useful in the author's experience. For the actor, it is often helpful to coordinate speech pathology sessions with acting lessons, and especially with the training of the speaking voice provided by the actor's voice teacher or coach. Information provided by the speech pathologist, acting teacher, and singing teacher *should* be symbiotic and should not conflict. If there are major discrepancies, bad training from one of the team members should be suspected, and changes should be made.

Singing Teachers

In selected cases, singing lessons may also be extremely helpful in nonsingers with voice problems. The techniques used to develop abdominal-thoracic strength, breath control, laryngeal and neck muscle strength and relaxation are very similar to those used in speech therapy. Singing lessons often expedite therapy and appear to improve the result in some patients.

Laryngologists who frequently care for singers are asked often to recommend a voice teacher. This may put the laryngologist in an uncomfortable position, particularly if the singer is already studying with someone in the community. Most physicians do not have sufficient expertise to criticize a voice teacher; we must be extremely cautious about recommending that a singer change teachers. However, there is no certifying agency that standardizes or assures the quality of a singing teacher. Although we may be slightly more confident of a teacher associated with a major conservatory or music school or of one who is a member of the National Association of Teachers of Singing, neither of these credentials assures excellence, and many expert teachers hold neither position. However, with experience, a laryngologist ordinarily develops valid impressions. The physician should record the name of the voice teacher of each of his patients. He should observe whether the same kinds of voice abuse problems occur with disproportionate frequency in the pupils of any given teacher. He should also observe whose pupils usually have few technical problems and are only seen for acute disease such as upper respiratory infection. Technical problems can cause organic pathology such as nodules. So, any teacher who has a high incidence of nodules among his or her students should be viewed with careful concern. The physician should be particularly wary of teachers who are reluctant to allow their students to consult a doctor. The best voice teachers usually have a very low threshold for referral to a laryngologist if they hear anything disturbing in a student's voice. It is proper for the laryngologist to write a letter to the voice teacher (with the patient's permission), describing his findings and recommendations as he would to a physician, speech pathologist, or any other referring professional. A laryngologist seriously interested in caring for singers should take the trouble to talk with and meet local singing teachers. Taking a lesson or two with each teacher provides enormous insight as well. Taking voice lessons regularly is even more helpful. In practice, the laryngologist will usually identify a few teachers in whom he has particular confidence, especially for patients with voice disorders. He should not hesitate to refer singers to these colleagues, especially those singers who are not already in training.

Pop singers may be particularly resistant to the suggestion of voice lessons. Yet they are in great need of training. It should be pointed out that a good voice teacher can teach a pop singer how to protect and expand his voice without changing its quality or making it sound "trained" or "operatic." The author finds it helpful to point out that singing, like other athletic activities, requires exercise, warm-up, and coaching for anyone planning to enter the "big league" and stay there. Just as no major league baseball pitcher would go without a pitching coach and warm-up time in the bullpen, no singer should try to build a career without a singing teacher and appropriate strength and agility exercises. This approach has proven palatable and effective. Physicians should also be aware of the difference between a voice teacher and a voice coach. A voice teacher trains a singer in singing technique and is essential. A voice coach is responsible for teaching songs, language, diction, style, operatic roles, etc., but is not responsible for exercises and basic technical development of the voice.

SURGERY

A detailed discussion of laryngeal surgery is beyond the scope of this chapter. However, a few points are worthy of special emphasis. Surgery for vocal nodules should be avoided whenever possible and should almost never be performed without an adequate trial of expert voice therapy, including patient compliance with therapeutic suggestions. A minimum of 6 to 12 weeks of observation should be allowed while the patient is using therapeutically modified voice techniques under the supervision of a speech pathologist and possibly a singing teacher. Proper voice use rather than voice rest (silence) is correct therapy. The surgeon should not perform surgery prematurely for vocal nodules, under pressure from the patient for a "quick cure" and early return to performance. Permanent destruction of voice quality is a very real complication. Even following expert surgery, this may be caused by submucosal scarring resulting in an adynamic segment along the vibratory margin of the vocal fold. This situation results in a hoarse voice with vocal cords that appear normal upon indirect examination, although under stroboscopic light the adynamic segment is obvious. There is no reliable cure for this complication. Even large, apparently fibrotic nodules of long standing should be given a chance to resolve without surgery. In some cases the nodules remain but become asymptomatic, with normal voice quality. Stroboscopy in these patients usually reveals that the nodules are on the superior surface rather than the leading edge of the vocal folds during proper, relaxed phonation (although they may be on the contact surface and symptomatic when hyperfunctional voice technique is used and the larynx is forced down).

When surgery is indicated for vocal cord lesions, it should be limited as strictly as possible to the area of pathology. There is virtually no place for "vocal cord stripping" in professional voice users with benign disease. Whenever possible, an incision should be made on the superior edge of the vocal fold, and the lesion should be removed submucosally and superficially to avoid scarring. This is accomplished by staying superficial to the intermediate layer of the lamina propria (Fig. 7.5). Preservation of the mucosa along the leading edge of the vocal cord seems to promote more rapid and better healing. When this is not possible, lesions such as vocal nodules should be removed to a level even with the vibratory margin rather than deeply into the submucosa. This minimizes scarring and optimizes return to good vocal function. Naturally, if there is a question of serious neoplasm, proper treatment takes precedence over voice conservation. Surgery should be done under microscopic control. The use of lasers is controversial at present. There is considerable anecdotal evidence suggesting that healing time is longer and the incidence of adynamic segment formation higher with the laser than with traditional instruments. Furthermore, two recent studies (67,68) raise serious concerns about dysphonia following laser surgery. It has been suggested that such complications may result from using too low a wattage, causing dissipation of heat deeply into the vocal fold, and high power density for short duration has been recommended. Nevertheless, many laryngologists caring for professional voice users are avoiding laser surgery in most cases, pending further study. When the laser is used, a biopsy for evaluation by pathologists should be taken prior to destroying the lesion with a laser. If a lesion is to be removed from the leading edge, the laser beam should be centered in the lesion, rather than on vibratory margin, so that the beam does not create a divot in

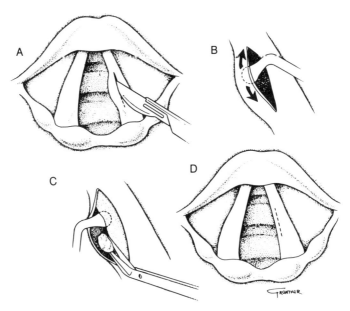

FIG. 7.5. A: Superficial incision is made in superior surface of true vocal fold. B: Blunt dissection is used to elevate mucosa from lesion. Trauma to submucosal tissues is minimized, since they contain fibroblasts that produce scar. C: Only pathologic tissue is excised under direct vision. Mucosa and normal submucosal tissues are preserved. D: Mucosa is reapproximated. Leading edge has not been violated.

the vocal fold (Fig. 7.6). The CO_2 laser (at 1 watt, defocused) is particularly valuable for cauterizing isolated blood vessels responsible for recurrent hemorrhage. Such vessels are often found at the base of a hemorrhagic polyp (Fig. 7.7). At the suggestion of Jean Abitbol, M. D., Paris, France, the author has recently been placing a small piece of ice on the vocal fold immediately prior to and following laser use, to dissipate heat and help prevent edema. There are no studies on the efficacy of this maneuver, and we need more clinical experience before drawing final conclusions; but our preliminary impression is that the ice is helpful. Preliminary findings of an unpublished study performed at Henry Ford Hospital support this impression (69). Voice rest following vocal fold surgery is also controversial. Although some laryngologists do not recognize its necessity at all, most physicians recommend voice rest for approximately 1 week, or until the mucosal surface has healed. Even following surgery, silence for more than a week or 10 days is nearly never necessary and represents a real hardship for many patients.

Too often, the laryngologist is confronted with a desperate singer whose voice has been "ruined" following vocal cord surgery, recurrent or superior laryngeal nerve paralysis, trauma, or some other tragedy. Occasionally, the cause is as simple as a dislocated arytenoid that can be reduced (70). However, if the problem is an adynamic segment, decreased bulk of one vocal cord following "stripping," bowing

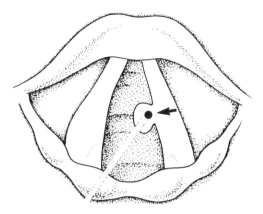

FIG. 7.6. The laser beam is centered in the lesion (*arrow*) so that its most peripheral effects do not disrupt the leading edge of the vocal fold.

caused by superior laryngeal nerve paralysis, or some other serious complication in a mobile vocal cord, great conservatism should be exercised. None of the available surgical procedures for these conditions is consistently effective. If surgery is considered at all, it should be presented to the patient realistically and pessimistically. The patient must understand that the chances of returning the voice to professional quality are very slim, and that there is a chance of making it worse. Zyderm Collagen (Xomed) injection is currently under investigation and shows promise of usefulness in some of these difficult cases (71). However, a great deal more re-

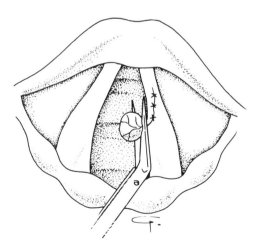

FIG. 7.7. The feeding vessel of a hemorrhagic polyp may be treated with 1 watt defocused laser bursts (each indicated by *X*) of short duration to cauterize the vessel and prevent recurrent hemorrhage.

search will be needed, not only to determine the efficacy, but especially the safety of this material before it can be recommended (72). Occasionally, singers inquire about surgery for pitch alteration. Such procedures (73) have proven successful in specially selected patients (such as those undergoing sex change surgery), but they do not consistently provide good enough voice quality to be performed on a professional voice user.

DISCRETION

The excitement and glamour associated with caring for a famous performer naturally tempt the physician to talk about his distinguished patient. However, this tendency must be tempered. It is not always in a singer's best professional interest to have it known that he has consulted a laryngologist, particularly for treatment of a significant vocal problem. Famous singers and actors are ethically and legally entitled to the same confidentiality we assure for our other patients.

VOICE MAINTENANCE

Prevention of vocal dysfunction should be the goal of all professionals involved in the care of singers. Good vocal health habits should be encouraged in childhood. Screaming, particularly outdoors at athletic events, should be discouraged. Promising young singers who join choirs should be educated to compensate for the Lombard effect. The youngster interested in singing should receive enough training to avoid voice abuse and should receive enthusiastic support for singing works suitable for his age and voice. Singing advanced pieces and "playing" Metropolitan Opera star should be actively discouraged. Training should be continued during or after puberty, and the voice should be allowed to develop naturally without pressure to perform operatic roles prematurely. Excellent regular training and practice are essential, and avoidance of irritants, particularly smoke, should be stressed early. Educating the singer with regard to hormonal and anatomic alterations that may influence the voice allows him to recognize and analyze voice dysfunction, compensating for it intelligently when it occurs. Cooperation among the laryngologist, speech and language pathologist, acting teacher, and singing teacher provides an optimal environment for cultivation and protection of the vocal artist.

ACKNOWLEDGMENTS

The author is indebted to W. B. Saunders for permission to use material from Sataloff, R. T. "Professional Singers: The Science and Art of Clinical Care." *American Journal of Otolaryngology*, 1981,2(3):251–266; to the *Journal of Otolaryngology* for permission to use material from Sataloff, R. T. "Physical Examination of the Professional Singer," *Journal of Otolaryngology*, 1983, 12(5):277–281; to

C. V. Mosby for permission to use material from Sataloff, R. T. "The Professional Voice," in Cummings, C. W., Fredrickson, J. M., Harker, L. A., Krause, C. J., Schuller, D. A. *Otolaryngology-Head and Neck Surgery*, and to Raven Press for permission to use material from Sataloff, R. T., "The Professional Voice," Parts I, II, and III, from the *Journal of Voice*, Volume 1, Numbers 1, 2, and 3. He is also indebted to Joseph Sataloff, M. D., Ronald Bogdasarian, M. D., George Gates, M. D., Barbara-Ruth Roberts, R. N., and Mary Hawkshaw, R. N., for their editorial assistance; to Helen Caputo for preparation of the manuscript; and to Wilbur James Gould, M. D. and Van L. Lawrence, M. D. for their continued advice and support.

APPENDIX I

PATIENT HISTORY: SINGERS

NAME _____ AGE ____ SEX ____ RACE ____
HEIGHT _____ WEIGHT _____ DATE ____
VOICE CATEGORY: ____ soprano ____ mezzo soprano ____ alto
                ____ tenor ____ baritone ____ bass

(If you are not currently having a voice problem, please skip to Question #3)

PLEASE CHECK OR CIRCLE CORRECT ANSWERS

1. How long have you had your present voice problem?
   Who noticed it?
   [self, family, voice teacher, critics, everyone, other ____]
   Do you know what caused it? Yes ____   No ____
   If yes, what?
   Did it come on slowly or suddenly? Slowly ____ Suddenly ____
   Is it getting: Worse ____, Better ____, or Same ____?

2. Which symptoms do you have? (Please check all that apply)
   ____ Hoarseness (coarse or scratchy sound)
   ____ Fatigue (voice tires or changes quality after singing for a short period of time)
   ____ Volume disturbance (trouble singing) softly ____
                                            loudly ____
   ____ Loss of range (high ____ low ____)
   ____ Change in classification (example: voice lowered from soprano to mezzo)
   ____ Prolonged warm-up time (over $1/2$ hrs to warm up voice)
   ____ Breathiness
   ____ Tickling or choking sensation while singing

_____ Other (Please specify) _____

_____

_____

3. Do you have an important performance soon? Yes _____   No _____
   Date(s): _____

4. What is the current status of your singing career?
   Professional _____   Amateur _____

5. What are your long-term career goals in singing?
   [ ] Premiere operatic career
   [ ] Premiere pop music career
   [ ] Active avocation
   [ ] Classical
   [ ] Pop
   [ ] Other [_____]
   [ ] Amateur performance (choral or solo)
   [ ] Amateur singing for own pleasure

6. Have you had voice training? Yes _____   No _____   At what age did you begin?

7. Have there been periods of months or years without lessons in that time?
   Yes _____   No _____

8. How long have you studied with your present teacher?

   Teacher's name:
   Teacher's address:

   Teacher's telephone number:

9. Please list previous teachers and years during which you studied with them:

10. Have you ever had training for your speaking voice?
                            Yes _____   No _____
    Acting voice lessons?   Yes _____   No _____
    How many years?
    Speech therapy   Yes _____   No _____
    How many months?

11. Do you have a job in addition to singing?
           Yes _____   No _____

If yes, does it involve extensive voice use?
    Yes _____   No _____
If yes, what is it? [actor, announcer (television/radio/sports arena), athletic instructor, attorney, clergy, politician, physician, sales person, stock broker, teacher, telephone operator or receptionist, waiter, waitress, secretary, other _____]

12. In your performance work, in addition to singing, are you frequently required to speak?   Yes _____   No _____
    dance?   Yes _____   No _____

13. How many years did you sing actively before beginning voice lessons initially?

14. What types of music do you sing? (Check all that apply)
    _____ Classical   _____ Show
    _____ Night Club   _____ Rock
    _____ Other: (Please specify)_____

15. Do you regularly sing in a sitting position (such as from behind a piano or drum set)?   Yes _____   No _____

16. Do you sing outdoors or in large halls, or with orchestras?
(Circle which one)   Yes _____   No _____

17. If you perform with electrical instruments or outdoors, do you use monitor speakers?   Yes _____   No _____
If yes, can you hear them?   Yes _____   No _____

18. Do you play a musical instrument(s)?   Yes _____   No _____
If yes, please check all that apply:
    _____ Keyboard (Piano, Organ, Harpsichord, Other _____)
    _____ Violin, Viola
    _____ Cello
    _____ Bass
    _____ Plucket Strings (Guitar, Harp, Other _____)
    _____ Brass
    _____ Wind with single reed
    _____ Wind with double reed
    _____ Flute, Piccolo
    _____ Percussion
    _____ Bagpipe
    _____ Accordion
    _____ Other (Please specify): _____

19. How often do you practice?
    Scales: [daily, few times weekly, once a week, rarely, never]

    If you practice scales, do you do them all at once or do you divide them up over the course of a day?
    [all at once, two or three sittings]

    On days when you do scales, how long do you practice them?
    [15, 30, 45, 60, 75, 90, 105, 120, more] minutes

    Songs: [daily, few times weekly, once a week, rarely, never]

    How many hours per day?
    [1/2, 1, 1 1/2, 2, 2 1/2, 3, more]

20. How much are you singing at present (total including practice time) (average hours per day)?
    Rehearsal:
    Performance:

21. Please check all that apply to you:
    ____ Voice worse in the morning
    ____ Voice worse later in the day, after it has been used
    ____ Sing performances or rehearsals in the morning
    ____ Speak extensively (e.g., teacher, clergy, attorney, telephone, work, etc.)
    ____ Cheerleader
    ____ Speak extensively backstage or at post-performance parties
    ____ Choral conductor
    ____ Frequently clear your throat
    ____ Frequent sore throat
    ____ Jaw joint problems
    ____ Bitter or acid taste, or bad breath first thing in the morning
    ____ Frequent "heartburn" or hiatal hernia
    ____ Frequent yelling or loud talking
    ____ Frequent whispering
    ____ Chronic fatigue (insomnia)
    ____ Work around extreme dryness
    ____ Frequent exercise (weight lifting, aerobics, etc.)
    ____ Frequently thirsty, dehydrated
    ____ Hoarseness first thing in the morning
    ____ Chest cough
    ____ Eat late at night
    ____ Ever used antacids
    ____ Under particular stress at present (personal or professional)
    ____ Frequent bad breath
    ____ Live, work or perform around smoke or fumes

_____ Traveled recently: When: _____

                                  Where: _____

Eat any of the following before singing?
    _____ Chocolate   _____ Coffee
    _____ Alcohol   _____ Milk or ice cream
    _____ Nuts   _____ Spiced foods

Other (Please specify):
    _____ Any specific vocal technical difficulties?
    [trouble singing soft, trouble singing loud, poor pitch control, support problems, problems at register transitions, other]
    Describe other:

    _____ Any problems with your singing voice recently prior to the onset of the problem that brought you here?
    [hoarseness, breathiness, fatigue, loss of range, voice breaks, pain singing, others] Describe others:

    _____ Any voice problems in the past that required a visit to a physician?
    If yes, please describe problem(s) and treatment(s):
    [laryngitis, nodules, polyps, hemorrhage, cancer, other]
    Describe other:

22. Your family doctor's name, address and telephone number:

23. Your laryngologist's name, address and telephone number:

24. Recent cold?   Yes _____   No _____

25. Current cold?   Yes _____   No _____

26. Have you been exposed to any of the following chemicals frequently (or recently) at home or at work? (Check all that apply)
    _____ Carbon monoxide   _____ Arsenic
    _____ Mercury   _____ Aniline dyes
    _____ Insecticides   _____ Industrial solvents
    _____ Lead   (benzene, etc.)
    _____ Stage smoke

27. Have you been evaluated by an allergist?   Yes _____   No _____
If yes, what allergies do you have:
[none, dust, mold, trees, cats, dog, foods, other: _____]
(Medication allergies are covered elsewhere in this history form.)
If yes, give name and address of allergist:

28. How many packs of cigarettes do you smoke per day?
Smoking history
_____ Never

_____ Quit. When?
_____ Smoked about _____ packs per day for _____ years.
_____ Smoke _____ packs per day. Have smoked for _____ years.

29. Do you work in a smokey environment?   Yes _____   No _____

30. How much alcohol do you drink? [none, rarely, a few times per week, daily] If daily, or few times per week, on the average, how much do you consume? [1,2,3,4,5,6,7,8,9,10, more] glasses per [day, week] of [beer, wine, liquor]
    Did you used to drink more heavily?   Yes _____   No _____

31. How many cups of coffee, tea, cola or other caffeine-containing drinks do you drink per day?

32. List other recreational drugs you use [marijuana, cocaine, amphetamines, barbiturates, heroin, other _____]:

33. Have you noticed any of the following? (Check all that apply)
    _____ Hypersensitivity to heat or cold
    _____ Excessive sweating
    _____ Change in weight: gained/lost _____ lbs. in _____
                              weeks/ _____ months
    _____ Change in skin or hair
    _____ Palpitation (fluttering) of the heart
    _____ Emotional lability (swings of mood)
    _____ Double vision
    _____ Numbness of the face or extremities
    _____ Tingling around the mouth or face
    _____ Blurred vision or blindness
    _____ Weakness or paralysis of the face
    _____ Clumsiness in arms or legs
    _____ Confusion or loss of consciousness
    _____ Difficulty with speech
    _____ Difficulty with swallowing
    _____ Seizure (epileptic fit)
    _____ Pain in the neck or shoulders
    _____ Shaking or tremors
    _____ Memory change
    _____ Personality change

For females:

Are you pregnant?	Yes _____	No _____
Are your menstrual periods regular?	Yes _____	No _____
Have you undergone hysterectomy?	Yes _____	No _____
Were your ovaries removed?	Yes _____	No _____

At what age did you reach puberty?

Have you gone through menopause?   Yes _____   No _____
If yes, when?

34. Have you ever consulted a psychologist or psychiatrist?
    Yes _____   No _____
    Are you currently under treatment?   Yes _____   No _____

35. Have you injured your head or neck (whiplash, etc.)?
    Yes _____   No _____

36. Describe any serious accidents related to this visit.
    None _____

37. Are you involved in legal action involving problems with your voice?
    Yes _____   No _____

38. List names of spouse and children:

39. Brief summary of ENT problems, some of which may not be related to your present complaint.

PLEASE CHECK ALL THAT APPLY

_____ Hearing loss   _____ Ear pain
_____ Ear noises   _____ Facial pain
_____ Dizziness   _____ Stiff neck
_____ Facial paralysis   _____ Lump in neck
_____ Nasal obstruction   _____ Lump in face or head
_____ Nasal deformity   _____ Trouble swallowing
_____ Mouth sores   _____ Excess eye skin
_____ Jaw joint problem   _____ Excess facial skin
_____ Eye problem
_____ Other: (Please specify)

40. Do you have or have you ever had:
    _____ Diabetes   _____ Seizures
    _____ Hypoglycemia   _____ Psych. therapy
    _____ Thyroid problems   _____ Frequent bad headaches
    _____ Syphilis   _____ Ulcers
    _____ Gonorrhea   _____ Kidney disease
    _____ Herpes   _____ Urinary problems
    _____ Cold sores (fever blisters)   _____ Arthritis or skeletal problems
    _____ High blood pressure   _____ Cleft palate
    _____ Severe blood pressure   _____ Asthma
    _____ Intravenous antibiotics or diuretics   _____ Lung or breathing problems
    _____ Heart attack   _____ Unexplained weight loss

____ Angina   ____ Cancer of (_____)
____ Irregular heartbeat   ____ Other tumor (_____)
____ Other heart problems   ____ Blood transfusions
____ Rheumatic fever   ____ Hepatitis
____ Tuberculosis   ____ AIDS
____ Glaucoma   ____ Meningitis
____ Multiple sclerosis
____ Other illnesses, please specify:

41. Do any blood relatives have:
    ____ Diabetes   ____ Cancer
    ____ Hypoglycemia   ____ Heart disease
    ____ Other major medical problems such as those above.
         Please specify:

42 Describe serious accidents *unless* directly related to your doctor's visit here.
    ____ None
    ____ Occurred with head injury, loss of consciousness or whiplash
    ____ Occurred without head injury, loss of consciousness or whiplash
         Describe:

43. List all current medications and doses (include birth control pills and
    vitamins).

44. Medication allergies
    ____ None   ____ Novocaine
    ____ Penicillin   ____ Iodine
    ____ Sulfa   ____ Codeine
    ____ Tetracycline   ____ Adhesive tape
    ____ Erythromycin   ____ Aspirin
    ____ Keflex/Ceclor/Ceftin   ____ X-ray dyes
    ____ Other. Please specify:

45. List operations
    ____ Tonsillectomy (age ____)   ____ Adenoidectomy (age ____)
    ____ Appendectomy (age ____)   ____ Heart surgery (age ____)
    ____ Other. Please specify:

46. List toxic drugs or chemicals to which you have been exposed:
    ____ Lead   ____ Streptomycin, Neomycin, Kanamycin
    ____ Mercury   ____ Other. Please specify:

47. Have you had x-ray *treatments* to your head or neck (including treatments for acne or ear problems as a child, treatments for cancer, etc.)?
    Yes _____   No _____

48. Describe serious health problems of your spouse or children.
    _____ None

APPENDIX II

LARYNGEAL EXAMINATION

SPEAKING VOICE:

Range: _____ Soprano   _____ Alto   _____ Tenor   _____ Baritone   _____ Bass

Pitch Variability: _____ Normal   _____ Decreased   _____ Increased

Excess Tension: _____ Normal   _____ Minimal   _____ Moderate   _____ Severe
                                  _____ Tongue
                                  _____ Neck
                                  _____ Face

Support: _____ Good   _____ Deficient

Volume: _____ Appropriate   _____ Soft   _____ Loud

Volume Variability: _____ Appropriate   _____ Diminished   _____ Excessive

Quality: _____ Normal   _____ Hoarse   _____ Breathy
           _____ Fatiguable   _____ Diplophonic

Rhythm: _____ Normal   _____ Slow   _____ Fast   _____ Spasmodic
          _____ Stuttering   _____ Dysarthric

Habits: _____ Throat clearing   _____ Coughing

Other:

SINGING VOICE:

Stance: _____ Balanced, proper   _____ Balanced, weight back
          _____ Unbalanced   _____ Knees locked

Breathing: _____ Nasal, unobstructed
             _____ Nasal, partially obstructed
             _____ Oral
             _____ Chest (excessive)
             _____ Abdominal (proper)

Excess Tension: ____ Face ____ Lip ____ Jaw ____ Neck
____ Shoulders ____ Tongue

Tongue Tension: ____ Corrects easily ____ Does not correct easily

Support: ____ Present ____ Practically absent
____ Effective ____ Ineffective
____ Initiated after the tone

Laryngeal Position: ____ Stable ____ Alters ____ High ____ Low

Mouth Opening: ____ Appropriate ____ Decreased ____ Excessive

Vibrato: ____ Regular ____ Irregular ____ Rapid ____ Tremolo

Range: ____ Soprano ____ Alto ____ Tenor ____ Baritone ____ Bass

Register Changes: ____ Controlled ____ Uncontrolled

Quality: ____ Premiere ____ Professional ____ Amateur
____ Pathologic ____ Hoarse
____ Breathy ____ Fatiguable ____ Diplophonic

Technical Errors Present: ____ In all registers ____ Low
____ Middle ____ High

Pitch: ____ Accurate ____ Inaccurate

REFERENCES

1. Hirano M. Structure and vibratory pattern of the vocal folds. In: Sawashima N, Cooper FS, eds. *Dynamic aspects of speech production.* Tokyo: University of Tokyo Press, 1977;13–27.
2. Sundberg J. The acoustics of the singing voice. *Sci Am* 1977;236(3):82–91.
3. Gould WJ, Okamura H. Static lung volumes in singers. *Ann Otol Rhinol Laryngol* 1973;82:89–95.
4. Hixon TJ, Hoffman C. Chest wall shape during singing. In: Lawrence V, ed. *Transcripts of the seventh annual symposium, care of the professional voice,* vol. 1. New York: The Voice Foundation, 1978;9–10.
5. Sataloff RT. Efficient history taking in professional singers. *Laryngoscope* 1984;94:1111–1114.
6. von Leden H. Speech and hearing problems in the geriatric patient. *J Am Geriat Soc* 1977;25:422–426.
7. Ackerman R, Pfan W. Gerotologische untersuchungen zur storunepanfalligkeit der sprechstimme bei berufssprechern. *Folia Phoniat* 1974;25:95–99.
8. Adour K. Personal communication.
9. Schiff M. Comment presented at the seventh symposium on care of the professional voice, the Juilliard School, New York, June 15–16, 1978 (unpublished).
10. Ritter FN. The effect of hypothyroidism on the larynx of the rat. *Ann Otol Rhinol Laryngol* 1964;67:404–416.
11. Ritter FN. Endocrinology. In: Paparella M, Shumrick D, eds. *Otolaryngology,* volume 1. Philadelphia: WB. Saunders, 1973;727–734.
12. Michelsson K, Sirvio P. Cry analysis in congenital hypothyroidism. *Folia Phoniat* 1976;28:40–47.
13. Gupta OP, et al. Nasal pharyngeal and laryngeal manifestations of hypothyroidism. *Ear, Nose and Throat* 1977;56(9):10–21.
14. Malinsky M, et al. Etude clinique et electrophysiologique des alterations de la voix au cours des thyrotoxioses. *Ann Endocrinol* (Paris) 1977;38:171–172.

15. Meuser W, Nieschlag E. Sexualhormone und Stimmlage des Mannes. *Deutsch Med Wochenschr* 1977;102:261–264.
16. Brodnitz F. The age of the castrato voice. *J Speech Hearing Disorders* 1975;40:291–295.
17. Brodnitz F. Hormones and the human voice. *Bull N Y Acad Med* 1971;47:183–191.
18. von Gelder L. Psychosomatic aspects of endocrine disorders of the voice. *J Communication Disorders* 1974;7:257–262.
19. Schiff M. The influence of estrogens on connective tissue. In: Asboe-Hansen G, ed. *Hormones and connective tissue*. Munksgaard Press, Copenhagen 1967;282–341.
20. Wendler J. Zyklusabhangige leistungsschwankungen der stimme und ihre beeinflussung durch ovulationshemmer. *Folia Phoniat* 1972;24:259–277.
21. Lacina V. Der einfluss der menstruation auf die stimme der sangerinnen. *Folia Phoniat* 1968;20:13–24.
22. Dordain M. Etude statistique de l'influence des contraceptifs hormonaux sur la voix. *Folia Phoniat* 1972;24:86–96.
23. Pahn V, Goretzlehner G. Stimmstorungen durch hormonale kontrazeptiva. *Zentralb Gynakol* 1978; 100:341–346.
24. Schiff M. "The pill" in otolaryngology. *Trans Am Acad Ophthalmol Otolaryngol* Jan-Feb 1968;72:76–84.
25. Brodnitz F. Medical care preventive therapy. Panel. In: Lawrence V, ed. *Transcripts of the seventh annual symposium, care of the professional voice*, vol. 3. New York: The Voice Foundation, 1978; 86.
26. Damste PH. Virilization of the voice due to anabolic steroids. *Folia Phoniat* 1964;16:10–18.
27. Damste PH. Voice changes in adult women caused by virilizing agents. *J Speech Hearing Disorders* 1967;32:126–132.
28. Saez S, Francoise S. Recepteurs d'androgenes: mise en evidence dans la fraction cytosolique de muqueuse normale et d'epitheliomas phryngolarynges humains. *C R Acad Sci* (Paris) 1975;280:935–938.
29. Vuorenkoski V, et al. Fundamental voice frequency during normal and abnormal growth, and after androgen treatment. *Arch Dis Child* 1978;53:201–209.
30. Arndt HJ. Stimmstorungen nach behandlung mit androgenen und anabolen hormonen. *Munch Med Wochenschr* 1974;116:1715–1720.
31. Bourdial J. Les troubles de la voix provoques par la therapeutique hormonale androgene. *Ann Otolaryngol* (Paris) 1970;87:725–734.
32. Flach M, Schwickardi H, Simen R. Welchen einfluss haben menstruation and schwangerschaft auf die augsgebildete gesangsstimme? *Folia Phoniat* 1968;21:199–210.
33. Deuster CV. Irreversible stimmstorung in der schwangerscheft. *HNO* 1977;25:430–432.
34. Imre V. Hormonell bedingte stimmstorungen. *Folia Phoniat* 1968;20:394–404.
35. Feder RJ. The professional voice and airline flight. *Ontolaryngology—Head and Neck Surgery* 1984;92(3):251–254.
36. Lawrence V. Medical care for professional voice. Panel. In: Lawrence V, ed.: *Annual symposium, care of the professional voice*, vol. 3. New York: The Voice Foundation, 1978;17–18.
37. Gould WM, Alberti PW, Brodnitz F, Hirano M. Medical care preventive therapy. Panel. In: Lawrence V, ed. *Transcripts of the seventh annual symposium, care of the professional voice*, vol. 3. New York: The Voice Foundation, 1978;74–76.
38. Wallner LJ, Hill BJ, Waldrop W. Voice changes following adenotonsillectomy. *Laryngoscope* 1968;78:1410–1418.
39. Sataloff RT. The professional singer: science and art of clinical care. *Amer J of Oto* 1981;2(3):251–266.
40. Sataloff RT. The professional voice: part II, physical examination. *Journal of Voice* 1987;1(2):191–201.
41. Gould WJ, Kojima H, Lambiase A. A technique for stroboscopic examination of the vocal folds using fiberoptics. *Arch. Otolaryngol* 1979; 105:285.
42. Fujimura O. Stereo-fiberoptic Laryngeal Observation. *J Acoustical Soc Am* 1979;65:70–72.
43. Sataloff RT, Spiegel JR, Carroll LM, et al. Strobovideolaryngoscopy in professional voice users: results and clinical value. *Journal of Voice* 1988;1(4):359–364.
44. Hirano M. Phonosurgery. basic and clinical investigations. *Otologia* (Fukuoka) 1975;21:239–442.
45. Bless D, Hirano M, Feder RJ. Video stroboscopic evaluation of the larynx. *Ear, Nose and Throat Journal* July 1987;66(7):289–296.
46. Leclure FLE, Brocaar ME, Verscheeure J. Electroglottography and its relation to glottal activity. *Folia Phoniat* 1975;27:215–224.

47. Hirano M. *Clinical examination of the voice*. New York: Springer-Verlag, 1981;1–98.
48. Scherer RC, Gould WJ, Titze IR, Meyers AD, Sataloff RT. Preliminary evaluation of selected acoustic and glottographic measures for clinical phonatory function analysis. *Journal of Voice* 1988;2(3):230–244.
49. Coleman RJ, Mabis JH, Hinson JK. Fundamental frequency-sound pressure level profiles of adult male and female voices. *J Speech and Hearing Research* 1977;20:197–204.
50. Isshiki N. Regulatory mechanism of voice intensity variation. *J Speech and Hearing Research* 1964;7:17–29.
51. Saito S. Phonosurgery, basic study on the mechanism of phonation and endolaryngeal microsurgery. *Otologic* (Fukuoka) 1977;23:171–384.
52. Isshiki N. Functional surgery of the larynx. *Official report of the 78th annual convention of the Oto-Rhino-Laryngological Society of Japan, Fuokuoka*, Kyoto University, 1977.
53. Hirano M, Koike Y, von Leden H. Maximum phonation time and air usage during phonation. *Folia Phoniat* 1968;20:185–201.
54. Frokjaer-Jensen B, Prytz S. Registration of voice quality. *Bruel and Kjaer Technical Review* 1976; 3:3–17.
55. Price DB, Sataloff RT. A simple technique for consistent microphone placement in voice recording. *Journal of Voice* 1988;2(3):206–207.
56. Darley F, et al. Differential diagnosis of patterns of dysarthria. *J Speech Hearing Res* 1969;12:246–249.
57. Darley F, et al. Clusters of deviant speech dimensions in the dysarthrias. *J Speech Hearing Res* 1969;12:462–496.
58. Rosenfield DB. Neurolaryngology. *Ear, Nose and Throat Journal* 1987;66(8):323–326.
59. Gates GA, Saegert J, Wilson N, Johnson L, Shepherd A, and Hearnd EM. Effects of beta-blockade on singing performances. *Ann Otol Rhinol Laryngol* 1985;94:570–574.
60. von Leden H. Presentation at the seventh symposium on care of the professional voice, the Juilliard School, New York, June 16, 1978 (unpublished).
61. Punt NA. Applied laryngology—singers and actors. *Proc R Soc Med* 1968;61:1152–1156.
62. Panckey G. Sinusitis, bronchitis, and mycoplasmal pneumonia. In: a symposium on the tetracyclines: a major appraisal. *Bull NY Acad Med* 1978;54:156–164.
63. Neu HC, ed. International symposium on amoxicillin: clinical perspectives. *J Infect Dis* June 1974; 129 suppl:S123–S201.
64. Schiff M. Medical management of acute laryngitis. In: Lawrence V, ed. *Transcripts of the sixth symposium, care of the professional voice*. New York: The Voice Foundation, 1977;99–102.
65. Spiegel JR, Sataloff RT, Cohn JR, Hawkshaw M. Respiratory function in singers: medical assessment, diagnoses, and treatments. *Journal of Voice* 1988;2(1):40–50.
66. Peacher G. *How to improve your speaking voice*. New York: Frederick Fell, 1966;1–135.
67. Abitbol J. Limitations of the laser in microsurgery of the larynx. In: Lawrence VL, ed. *Transactions of the twelfth symposium: care of the professional voice*. New York: The Voice Foundation, 1984; 297–301.
68. Tapia RG, Pardo J, Marigil M, Pacio A. Effects of the laser upon Reinke's space and the neural system of the vocalis muscle. In: Lawrence VL, ed., *Transactions of the twelfth symposium: care of the professional voice*. New York: The Voice Foundation, 1984;289–291.
69. Sheppard L. Personal communication. March 1989.
70. Sataloff RT, Feldman M, Darby KS, et al. Arytenoid dislocation. *Journal of Voice* 1988;1(4):368–377.
71. Ford CN, Bless DM. Collagen injected in the scarred vocal fold. *Journal of Voice* 1988;1(1):116–118.
72. Spiegel JR, Sataloff RT, Gould WJ. The treatment of vocal fold paralysis with injectable collagen: clinical concerns. *Journal of Voice* 1988;1(1):119–121.
73. Isshiki N, Taira T, Tanabe M. Surgical alteration of the vocal pitch. *J Otolaryngology* 1983;12:335–340.

Textbook of Performing Arts Medicine, edited
by R. T. Sataloff, A. Brandfonbrener, and
R. Lederman. Raven Press, Ltd.,
New York © 1991.

8

Ophthalmology and the Performing Arts*

Michael F. Marmor

*Professor and Chairman of the Department of Ophthalmology, Stanford University
Medical Center, Stanford, California 94305*

For most musicians, vision is a vital part of the art. Performance may require physical dexterity and ensemble a trained ear, but vision is the medium through which the wishes of the composer are transferred from page to performer. Even soloists who eschew music on the stage may be closet readers in the privacy of their homes. Vision is less critical for dancers and actors, insofar as sharp acuity is not required for many types of performance. Nevertheless, impaired vision can place limitations on a performer, especially in critical situations such as a dimly lit stage.

This chapter will review some aspects of visual physiology and ocular disease that are of particular relevance to the performer (especially the musician). For the most part, this discussion will concern the effects of aging and intrinsic ophthalmic disease, since the performing arts do not place the eye particularly at risk, but a few occupational hazards will be noted.

OPTICS OF THE EYE

The major visual problems of performers relate to optics of the eye. As shown in Fig. 8.1, the eye consists of a lens system (composed of cornea and lens) and a receptive layer for the image (the retina). Ideally, when the lens in an eye is fully relaxed, the eye should be in perfect focus for faraway objects, a condition called *emmetropia* (Fig. 8.2). However, many people have eyes that are too long or too short for their lens system. *Myopia*, or nearsightedness, results when the eye is too long, so that images of faraway objects come in focus in front of the retina even when the lens is maximally relaxed. Thus, distant objects appear fuzzy while close objects can be seen clearly because the diverging rays can be focused properly on the retina. *Hyperopia*, or farsightedness, results when the eye is too short, so that

---

*Some of the text, and all of the figures in this chapter appeared originally in an article entitled "Vision and the Musician," *Med Probl Perform Art*, 1:117–121, 1986.

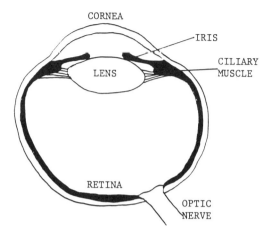

FIG. 8.1. Diagram of the human eye.

the images fall behind the retina when the lens is relaxed. This means that the hyperope must focus just to see things far away and must put more than normal energy into focusing to read or do other close work.

Reading requires that our eyes change focusing power in order to overcome the divergence of rays from letters that are relatively close to us (Fig. 8.3). This is achieved by contracting the ciliary muscle which allows the lens in the eye to bulge into a more spherical shape (with higher refractive power). In youth, the lens is very

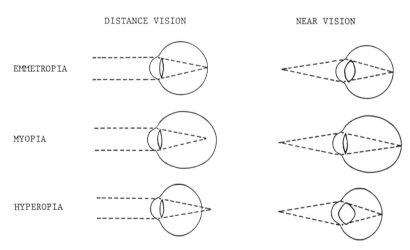

FIG. 8.2. Optical states of the eye. Note the differences in eyeball size and shape. For distance vision, the focusing system is presumed to be fully relaxed; for near vision, the lens has changed shape to the degree necessary for each optical state (from Marmor MF, ref. 2, with permission).

NEAR VISION

YOUTH

OVER AGE 55
(PRESBYOPIA)

CORRECTED
PRESBYOPIA

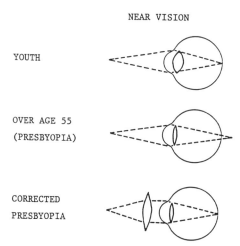

FIG. 8.3. Near vision and presbyopia. The presbyopic lens can no longer adjust enough to focus on near objects unless a reading glass is used (from Marmor MF, ref. 2, with permission).

elastic and becomes very powerful when the ciliary muscle contracts; thus, without changing glasses, an emmetropic child can see clearly far away and also inspect an insect 3 inches from the nose. However, with age, the lens loses elasticity, becomes more yellow, increases in density, and is no longer able to gain much power when the ciliary muscle contracts. Thus, when a person over 50 years old (who sees clearly at distance) tries to read, the lens cannot change enough to compensate. This lack of focusing range is called *presbyopia*, and afflicts everyone by the ages of 45 or 50 years, regardless of whether their basic eye shape is myopic, emmetropic or hyperopic.

Presbyopia is corrected by wearing convex spectacle lenses that bend the rays diverging from a close object, and thereby compensate for the diminished focusing power of an aging human lens. Everyone over age 50 who sees clearly at distance (naturally or with glasses) will need added lens power to read. Some myopes gain this power by simply removing their glasses, but most people must either carry a pair of reading glasses or wear bifocals. Reading glasses or bifocals are ordinarily designed for objects 14 inches away, which is the distance at which most people read.

PRESBYOPIA

The impact of presbyopia on the musician is obvious: glasses that work for distance are no longer effective for reading music. However, the routine solution—wearing reading glasses—may not work well, because music on a stand is generally positioned farther away than a book in a lap. A musician may also need a wider field of view because of the head movement associated with playing. The best solution for the older musician is to have a special pair of glasses made that are set to the exact playing distance and have a larger-than-normal playing segment (if bifocals are used). If the musician has no need to see clearly at distance or to walk around during the music, single vision glasses may be even better than bifocals.

It is important to realize that the near vision segments in a bifocal can be made to fit individual needs (Fig. 8.4). A musician in an orchestra who must periodically look up at the conductor might have bifocals made with a very large bottom section for reading the music and only a small distance segment at the top of the lens. Players who do not wish to wear spectacles could have contact lenses made at the proper power for reading music, but these would not be bifocal, and the performer would have to get on or off the stage in a blur. Bifocal contact lenses exist but do not seat themselves very reliably on most eyes and might be a hazard during a performance.

The key to success in finding the proper music-reading correction is to personalize the glasses (or contact lenses) to each individual's style of play. A musician should carefully measure the distance from eye to music stand before consulting an eye doctor—or better yet, bring the stand right into the doctor's office.

Presbyopia is not a major problem for dancers whose visual cues will never be very close to the eye. Actors will suffer from the need to wear reading glasses, but the disability is no more or less than that which faces anyone in our society over age 50. One implication is that actors must be careful to act the visual age of their characters. An elderly character should either put on glasses to perform a close task or (if myopic) show difficulty with recognition at a distance. A presbyopic actor playing a youthful part must not reveal the need for bifocals.

MYOPIA AND RADIAL KERATOTOMY

Myopia, or nearsightedness, is not a disease of great consequence since it is easily corrected with spectacles or contact lenses. There has been considerable recent publicity about surgical correction of myopia with an operation called radial keratotomy. Since performing artists—especially dancers and actors—represent a group of individuals who may be sensitive about wearing spectacles (or unable to do

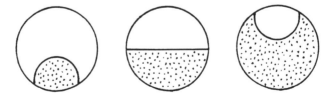

FIG. 8.4. Bifocal lens types with the reading segments shaded. *Left*, conventional bottom segment. *Middle*, executive type bifocal. *Right*, specialized bifocal with a small distance segment on top (from Marmor MF, ref. 2, with permission).

so while working), it is important that they understand the pros and cons of radial keratotomy. It can certainly correct nearsightedness in many individuals, but it is not a panacea and there are definite risks to be recognized. I would advise all performers, even those who do not feel comfortable with contact lenses, to do some careful research before they have a radial keratotomy.

The principle of radial keratotomy is simple. The surgeon makes a radiating set of deep cuts in the cornea, usually extending 90% or more through the wall of the eye. These cuts physically weaken the surface so that the normal fluid pressure inside the eye bulges the cornea slightly and changes its shape. People with moderate degrees of nearsightedness (2 to 5 diopters) stand roughly a 90% chance of achieving 20/40 or better vision without glasses, but many people do not actually achieve 20/20 after radial keratotomy. The operation becomes less predictable with higher degrees of nearsightedness. Even if successful, the radial cuts leave the eye permanently weakened, and the fine scars in the cornea often cause glare which could be particularly unfortunate for a performer working under stage lights. Because intraocular pressure fluctuates during the day, there is a tendency for vision to change slightly from morning to night. Finally, the operation corrects only the cornea and has no effect on the lens. Thus, presbyopia will still supervene around age 45, and the person whose vision has been corrected to spectacle-free distance vision by radial keratotomy is still going to have to wear reading glasses or contact lenses to read music in his or her golden years.

Given these cautions, one can see that radial keratotomy is not a perfect procedure at present levels of technology. While the current success rate of 90% sounds excellent, it means that 10% of patients are not satisfied with the result (and a few will end up considerably worse than they began). This may not be an acceptable risk/benefit ratio for eyes that can get 20/20 vision simply by wearing spectacles or contact lenses. Modern soft lenses are quite easy to tolerate and care for (even disposable ones are available), and the lenses can be changed whenever working conditions or age necessitate a different strength of glasses. I strongly suggest that performers who wish to avoid spectacles should give contact lenses a serious trial before considering the irreversible and potentially problematic solution of radial keratotomy. It is also fair to say that some individuals who cannot tolerate contact lenses (e.g., because of dry eyes) may find radial keratotomy to be an acceptable risk relative to the professional benefits, especially as the procedure improves in safety and predictability. I urge only that the choice be made with full awareness of the risks and alternatives.

GLARE

Glare from obtrusive lighting is a problem for all performers. It may be particularly bothersome to older individuals because the ocular media (especially the lens) become slightly cloudy with age and tend to scatter light. The most obvious solution to glare is to change the lighting, and it is hoped that many theater managers are sufficiently enlightened as to listen to the plight of their charges. However, sometimes this cannot be done because the performance is outdoors (where the ultimate lighting director is often not responsive), or because constraints within the theater prevent further adjustment. One factor that is sometimes ignored is the color of lighting. In general, bluish or white light create more glare than yellowish or warm light because blue wavelengths are scattered more effectively by the lens and ocular media. Thus, warm lighting will be more comfortable for most performers.

There are several ways to shield oneself from glare, although many will not be applicable to performing situations, especially in dance and theater, where visible appliances cannot be worn. The use of a cap or a visor is very effective when the lighting source is overhead. Less obtrusive but similar protection may be obtained by having small shields attached along the top and sides of a spectacle frame. Another approach is the use of dark-tinted or colored spectacles (Fig. 8.5), or the use of tinted hard contact lenses. Most sunglasses are too dark for indoor use, but glasses or lenses with a light yellowish tint filter out the blue end of the spectrum and can reduce the subjective sensation of glare. A variety of ready-made yellowish "high contrast" glasses are available in ski or sports stores, and plastic prescription lenses can be tinted to order by most optical shops. Even ultraviolet-absorbing plastics that appear grossly clear can reduce the sensation of glare in sunlight. Each performer must experiment to find the tint most suited to his or her working conditions. This experimentation might be done with the aid of a local optician willing to demonstrate various colors by tinting lenses, bleaching them if necessary, and tinting them again. Unfortunately, soft lenses generally cannot be tinted, but new varieties may become available.

DARKNESS AND ADAPTATION

There are certain times when the visual problem is simply inadequate lighting. This may occur in an orchestra pit which is dimly lit to avoid bothering the audience

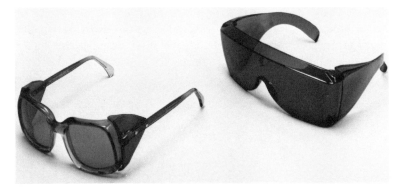

FIG. 8.5. Two types of tinted spectacles with side shields. *Left*, Corning photosensitive lenses (yellowish to reddish). *Right*, Solarshields (amber). Other excellent brands are also available (from Marmor MF, ref. 2, with permission).

or the dancers, on a stage because of theatrical effects, or anywhere during scene changes when the stage goes dark. The fundamental need for theatrical darkness cannot be resolved, but there are some ways that performers and theater managers can minimize the problem.

The retina contains two types of cells that primarily receive light—cones and rods. Cones operate only in moderately bright light to provide color discrimination and sharp reading vision; rods operate only in very dim light and are much less sensitive to red light than to other colors. Thus, reddish light is not only less likely than blue or white light to produce glare, but levels of red light that appear dim to our daylight vision system are virtually invisible to our night vision system. Thus, orange or reddish light can provide satisfactory illumination for visual tasks (such as reading music) while producing relatively little subjective sensation of brightness in the theater at large (where the audience is moderately dark-adapted).

The problems of dark adaptation and night vision differ among the performing arts. Orchestra and solo instrumentalists have no difficulties in this regard (their problems will be from glare or too much light), but pit musicians may suffer from marginal lighting. An experiment that might be considered is a trial of reddish lights in the pit to allow brighter illumination of the music while having relatively less effect on the audience. Dancers and actors work mostly in the light, but encounter dim light in certain staging situations and when the stage lights go off for a scene change. In theater, the effectiveness of a sudden darkness depends in part on the fact that it takes time for visual cells to adjust to the dark. Thus, the audience is temporarily blind in a darkened theater, and by the time their eyes adjust, the performers have left the stage. Unfortunately, the performers are equally affected by the transition, and some dim or reddish offstage lighting (shielded by black curtains that do not reflect) may be needed to help them find the way.

Lighting transitions will be especially difficult for individuals with impaired adaptation ability. This is not as rare as might be imagined, especially among older individuals. The elderly eye is routinely less sensitive to dim lighting than the youthful eye, and the problems of adjustment are compounded by optical concerns such as cataract. Severe night blindness is uncommon, but can occur in disorders such as retinitis pigmentosa and advanced glaucoma (although the loss of side and central vision in these disorders will be much more of a disability). Since there is no specific cure or prosthesis for impaired dark adaptation, the best solutions are awareness of the pathophysiology, compensation with a longer time for adjustment and better lighting.

CATARACTS

Cataracts are a relatively common abnormality in the elderly, and some degree of lens yellowing is present in virtually every eye over 70 years old. Significant cataracts may occur at younger ages from a congenital predisposition, from certain diseases such as diabetes or chronic uveitis (inflammation inside the eye), or from the effects of chronic steroid usage (systemically or as eyedrops). The term cataract is a general one, and simply means opacification of the lens without specifying degree. Thus, a mild degree of cataract may be present without major visual symptoms or disability. The significance of cataract to a performer (and indeed to any individual) depends on the degree to which it interferes with his or her ability to function, rather than on the doctor's assessment of "severity."

Cataracts can be bothersome in general, for two reasons. First, even a mildly cloudy lens will scatter light and reduce sensitivity to subtle contrasts. Thus, even though visual acuity may still be satisfactory, the affected performer may have increased difficulty with glare and adaptation. Second, as the cataract becomes more dense, visual acuity gradually diminishes. To some degree these symptoms can be countered by the techniques discussed above or by adjusting the power of glasses, but eventually a point may be reached where the performer's art is compromised. Then it is time to consider surgery.

Cataract surgery is an excellent operation with a success rate of about 95%. This is high enough to make surgery very worthwhile when a patient feels disabled by poor vision, but rare complications do occur, and the operation should not be performed until and unless the performer feels significantly compromised by the cataracts. There are several techniques for removing cataracts, and each has its advocates; skill and sensitivity of the surgeon are more important factors than the particular technique used. Most patients nowadays will have a lens implant (intraocular lens) put in after the cataract is removed to eliminate the need for thick spectacle lenses or contact lenses. Exceptions would be the very young or a few individuals with associated eye disease. The intraocular implants are very stable nowadays, and are usually placed behind the iris (posterior chamber intraocular lens).

Modern cataract surgery is done on an outpatient basis, and there are few limitations on postoperative activity. Vigorous exercise and manuevers that raise venous pressure in the head are proscribed for a time, but most performers (who are not so active) will be able to work within a few days. Even dancers and vigorously-blowing wind musicians can return to full activity within several weeks, and there is no evidence that intraocular lenses pose a long-term hazard (unless an eye is directly traumatized). Thus, cataract surgery should not be taken lightly but neither should it be feared by the older performer who stands to gain by improved vision.

THE VISUALLY IMPAIRED PERFORMER

Visual impairment is obviously not unique to musicians, as opposed to other performers, but the musician faces the special difficulty of performing a visual task under conditions where conventional optical aids may not work. The basic principle of most visual aids for reading is to magnify objects at the price of bringing them closer to the eyes. For mild degrees of visual impairment, for example, the simple prescription of extra strong reading glasses will suffice to make reading possible, but books may have to be held 7 inches from the face instead of 14 inches. This approach will work for music as well (if one sits twice as close to the stand, the print is optically twice as large) but there are practical limitations posed by the technique of playing certain instruments. A string bass player may not be able to get within 6 inches of the stand without falling off the stool; a violinist playing too close would have an unreasonable risk of knocking the music over; a brass player might find horn and music facing in different directions.

If circumstances allow it, the use of a strong reading correction and close placement of the music is the easiest and best solution to poor vision, but when that is not practical, other options may be considered. For example, the music can be enlarged xerographically. However, there are limitations to this approach: nobody wants to play with a page measuring 4 feet by 6 feet perched on an artist's easel, and if enlarged music is cut apart to the size of ordinary pages, the page turns become frequent and often unacceptable musically. Professor Leland C. Smith at Stanford University currently has a project underway to develop a computer program that will automatically print large-type music with reasonable page turns (Fig. 8.6).

If one cannot get close to the music, why not use a telescope? One can purchase small telescopic lenses that mount on the upper portion of spectacles, so that the hands remain free for performing. However, the high magnification produced by a telescope makes focusing very critical and any degree of head movement disruptive (think how difficult it is to stabilize high-power binoculars). It would be difficut for most musicians to use a telescopic aid (particularly one with a small field of view) and follow a line of music satisfactorily, let alone find the start of the next line. A telescope might help a visually impaired musician to peer up occasionally at the conductor, but I suspect that the problems of motion will render this unsatisfactory. Furthermore, following a conductor is not nearly as difficult a visual task as reading music, since our eyes may recognize broad hand movements even when they cannot resolve the tip of a baton.

Visual impairment has less specific implications for dancers and actors. Both may be able to perform much of their repertoire despite having poor acuity, as long as their roles do not demand recognition of small objects. When the loss of acuity is severe, the limitations will be obvious and of a sort not unique to performers.

One aspect of visual loss that may have special implications in the stage arts is loss of side vision. Blind spots and tunnel vision may occur from vascular occlusions in the eye or brain, from tumors, from glaucoma, and from dystrophies such as retinitis pigmentosa. The presence of large areas of peripheral blindness or of true tunnel vision can be very disabling (and hazardous) because the individual will fail to see objects on the ground or to the side while looking straight ahead. Thus, a dancer might fail to see a marking on the stage and could get injured in a fall or collision. An actor would have trouble moving about a crowded stage. There are no satisfactory optical aids for this type of visual problem, but many of the underlying diseases are treatable, so prompt and thorough ophthalmologic evaluation is important.

Finally, the issue of ocular cosmesis should be noted. Sagging lids, scarred or deviating eyes, or removed eyes with poor appearance or mobility may all pose a

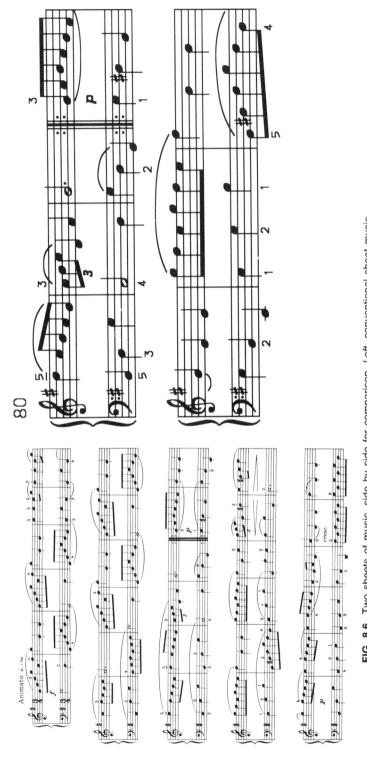

FIG. 8.6. Two sheets of music, side by side for comparison. *Left*, conventional sheet music (minuet courtesy of J.S. Bach). *Right*, computer-enlarged music (courtesy of L.C. Smith) (from Marmor MF, ref. 2, with permission).

real disability to a performer who lives in the public view. It is beyond our scope to discuss the myriad of cosmetic defects that may occur, but it is important to recognize that most of these problems can be effectively managed by ophthalmic plastic and reconstructive surgery.

OCCUPATIONAL HAZARDS TO THE EYE

Neuromuscular disorders and stress-related psychologic disorders are common among performing artists, but there are relatively few risks of ophthalmologic injury or disease. One obvious concern, but one fortunately rather rare in practice is direct trauma from an errant violin bow, baton, or broken violin string in the orchestra, an elbow or finger on the dance floor, or some sharp object on the stage. Most musicians have learned to seat themselves defensively so that the danger is minimal, and professional actors and dancers choreograph their movements with care.

A less obvious problem, but one of which physicians who care for performers should be aware, is the hazard to susceptible individuals from elevated ocular venous pressure while blowing hard on a wind instrument or hanging the head downward (e.g., during a modern dance configuration). For healthy people, blowing hard, straining, or standing on one's head causes no ill effects in the eye; however, if the intraocular blood vessels are unusually fragile, there is a theoretical risk of bleeding. This risk is present when abnormal and fragile new blood vessels grow under or into the retina ("neovascularization"). Neovascularization can occur in diabetic retinopathy (Fig. 8.7), as a sequel to venous occlusive disease in the eye,

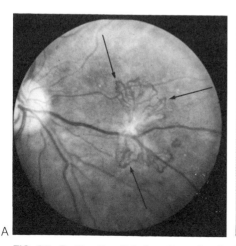
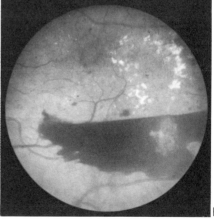

A   B

FIG. 8.7. Proliferative diabetic retinopathy. A: An area of abnormal new vessel growth (neovascularization) (*arrows*). B: Intraocular hemorrhage from diabetic neovascularization (from Marmor MF, ref. 2, with permission).

and in some forms of age-related macular degeneration. In all of these disorders, the neovascularization has a high risk of bleeding on its own and, irrespective of wind playing or dancing, should be treated promptly with laser photocoagulation. After treatment, the chances of bleeding will be low in most cases, and wind playing or dancing need not be proscribed except for those with persistent active disease.

What is the risk for wind players or dancers who do not have new vessels, but who have mild diabetes or early macular degeneration? There is a low but finite chance of bleeding in the eye, since neovascularization must start sometime, and since the onset is often insidious and asymptomatic. However, I do *not* believe the danger to the eye is either predictable or imminent, and it is reasonable to keep performing as long as the performer understands the disease process; these individuals should check their vision regularly and have periodic ophthalmologic examinations so that any growth of new vessels will be recognized as soon as possible.

Respiratory and venous back-pressures can stress the blood vessels and produce pressure in the orbit that bulges the eye forward, but they do not exert any direct force on the retina independent of the eye wall. Thus, wind playing or inverted posture do not predispose to retinal detachment, even in individuals who are at unusual medical risk (such as high myopes or people who have had previous cataract surgery). However, elevated venous pressure in or on the eye could well be a hazard in the immediate postoperative period after cataract surgery until the surgical wound has fully healed (about 6 weeks). Similar concerns exist with respect to the rapid head movements and jarring that occur during vigorous dance activity (or stage battles). These activities carry no significant risk to a normal eye, but could precipitate hemorrhage in a susceptible diseased eye or cause wound rupture in a fresh postoperative eye.

Vigorous head movement or head trauma is also a potential cause of retinal detachment in a small group of unusually susceptible eyes (highly myopic eyes, certain eyes that have had cataract surgery, and fellow eyes when the other has suffered a detachment). It is important to understand that detachment occurs most often from *internal* traction by the vitreous gel rather than external trauma—thus the risk in dance or stunt work comes directly from the sudden movements of the head (e.g., from jumping or twirling) which swirl or swish the vitreous inside the eye. The risk of detachment can be (and should be) assessed by ophthalmologists who specialize in retinal surgery and can sometimes be diminished by prophylactic laser photocoagulation. Fortunately, true high-risk characteristics for detachment are rare and are found predominantly in older age groups (in which the vigor of dance or stunt activity is apt to be less).

SUMMARY

Although vision is critical for most performers, especially musicians, performing poses few risks to eyesight. The greatest problems for day-to-day performance relate to presbyopia in the older musician and difficulties with glare and lighting for all performers. Presbyopia is easily relieved with appropriate correction, but this may have to be tailored to the particular playing style and music stand distance of each player. Glare and lighting are harder to control, but experimentation with colored lenses may be worthwhile. If cataracts interfere significantly with a performer's ability to function, surgery with intraocular lens implantation is very effective. The visually impaired musician may have to sit close to the music or try some visual aids to see. In individuals with active retinovascular disease such as proliferative diabetic retinopathy, there may be some risk of intraocular hemorrhage from straining on a wind instrument, vigorous head movement, or inverted posture. Retinal detachment is not a concern except for very high-risk eyes.

REFERENCES

1. Marmor MF. Visual changes with age. In: Caird FI, Williamson J, eds. *The eye and its disorders in the elderly*, Hertfordshire: John Wright & Sons, Ltd, 1986;28–36.
2. Marmor MF. Vision and the musician. *Med Probl Perform Art*. 1986;1:117–121.

Textbook of Performing Arts Medicine, edited by R. T. Sataloff, A. Brandfonbrener, and R. Lederman. Raven Press, Ltd., New York © 1991.

9

Hearing Loss in Musicians

Robert Thayer Sataloff and Joseph Sataloff

Professors of Otolaryngology, Thomas Jefferson University, Philadelphia, Pennsylvania 19103

Good hearing is of extreme importance to all of us, but it is especially critical to the performing artist. Musicians depend on critical hearing not only for daily discourse, but moreover for the required activities of their vocation. Furthermore, many musicians require good hearing at frequencies above those needed for conversational speech; even a small amount of pitch distortion caused by cochlear dysfunction may make it impossible for the singer or string player to tune and match pitches accurately. Consequently, in selective cases, even a mild hearing impairment that would not be troublesome to the practitioner of another profession may be a serious problem to the performing artist. Therefore, it is essential for physicians and performers to recognize the importance of maintaining healthy hearing, to recognize early correctable causes of hearing loss, and to prevent hearing loss from causes such as noise exposure.

CAUSES OF HEARING LOSS

The classification of causes of hearing loss, audiometric technique, and definitions of terms such as dB and dBA have been described in detail in standard textbooks of otolaryngology and in previous works by the authors (1,2), and they will be reviewed only briefly in this chapter. Hearing loss may be hereditary or nonhereditary, and either form may be congenital (present at birth) or acquired. There is a common misconception that hereditary hearing loss implies presence of the problem at birth or during childhood. In fact, most hereditary hearing loss occurs later in life. Otosclerosis, a common, inherited cause of correctable hearing loss, often presents when people are in their 20s or 30s. Similarly, the presence of deafness at birth does not necessarily imply hereditary or genetic factors. A child whose mother had German measles during the first trimester of fetal life or was exposed to radiation early in pregnancy may be born with a hearing loss. Hearing loss may occur because of problems in any portion of the ear, the nerve between the ear and the brain, or the brain. Understanding hearing loss requires a basic knowledge of the structure of the human ear.

ANATOMY AND PHYSIOLOGY OF THE EAR

The ear is divided into three major anatomical divisions: (1.) the outer ear, (2.) the middle ear, and (3.) the inner ear.

The outer ear has two parts: (1.) the trumpet-shaped apparatus on the side of the head: the *auricle* or *pinna*, and (2.) the tube leading from the auricle into the temporal bone: the *external auditory canal*. The opening is called the *meatus*.

The tympanic membrane, or "eardrum," stretches across the inner end of the external ear canal, separating the outer ear from the middle ear. The middle ear is a small cavity in the temporal bone in which three auditory ossicles, malleus (hammer), incus (anvil), and stapes (stirrup) form a bony bridge from the external ear to the inner ear (Fig. 9.1). The bony bridge is held in place by muscles and ligaments. The middle-ear chamber is filled with air and opens into the throat through the eustachian tube. The eustachian tube helps to equalize pressure on both sides of the eardrum.

The inner ear is a fluid-filled chamber divided into two parts: (1.) the *vestibular*

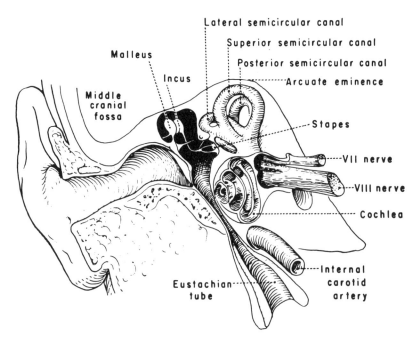

FIG. 9.1. Diagrammatic cross section of the ear. The semicircular canals are connected with maintaining balance.

labyrinth, which functions as part of the body's balance mechanism, and (2.) the *cochlea*, which contains thousands of minute, sensory, hairlike cells (Fig. 9.2). The *organ of Corti* functions as the switchboard for the auditory system. The eighth cranial or acoustic nerve leads from the inner ear to the brain, serving as the pathway for the impulses the brain will interpret as sound.

Sound creates vibrations in the air somewhat similar to the "waves" created when a stone is thrown into a pond. The outer-ear "trumpet" collects these sound waves and funnels them down the external ear canal to the eardrum. The sound waves cause the eardrum to vibrate. The vibrations are transmitted through the middle ear over the bony bridge formed by the malleus, incus, and stapes. These vibrations in turn cause the membranes over the openings to the inner ear to vibrate, causing the fluid in the inner ear to be set in motion. The motion of the fluid in the inner ear excites the nerve cells in the organ of Corti, producing electrochemical impulses that are transmitted to the brain along the acoustic nerve. As the impulses reach the brain, we experience the sensation of hearing.

ESTABLISHING THE SITE OF DAMAGE IN THE AUDITORY SYSTEM

The cause of a hearing loss, like that of any other medical condition, is determined by carefully obtaining a history, making a physical examination, and performing certain laboratory tests. In otology, hearing and balance tests parallel the function of clinical laboratory tests in general medicine. When a hearing loss is classified, the point at which the auditory pathway has broken down is localized, and it is determined whether the patient's hearing loss is conductive, sensorineural, central, functional, or a mixture of these.

Otologic Evaluation

Details of the otologic history, physical examination, and test protocols are available in many otolaryngology texts. Medical evaluation of a patient with a suspected hearing problem includes a comprehensive history; complete physical examination of the ears, nose, throat, head, and neck; assessment of the cranial nerves, including testing the sensation in the external auditory canal (Hitzelberger's sign), audiogram (hearing test); and other tests, as indicated. Recommended additional studies may include blood tests, computed tomography, magnetic resonance imaging, specialized hearing tests such as brain stem evoked response audiometry, tympanometry and central auditory testing, balance testing, and a variety of blood tests for the many systemic causes of hearing loss. All patients with hearing complaints deserve a thorough examination and comprehensive evaluation to determine the specific cause of the problem and to rule out serious or treatable conditions that may be responsible for the hearing impairment. Contrary to popular misconception, not all cases of sensorineural hearing loss are incurable. So "nerve deafness" should be assessed with the same systematic vigor and enthusiasm as conductive hearing loss.

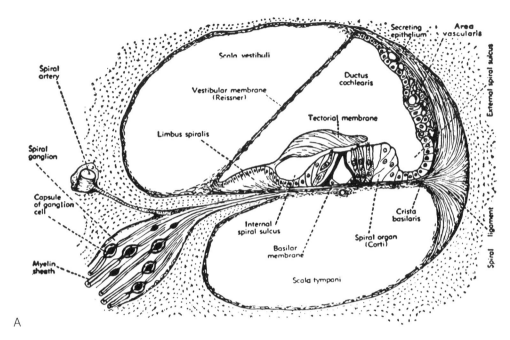

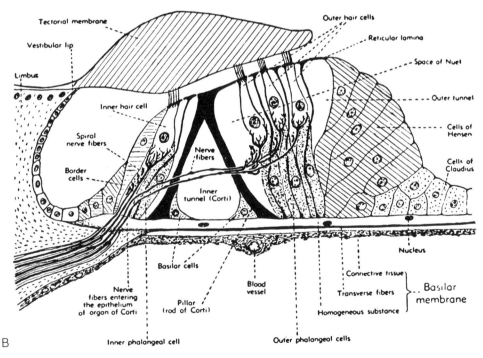

FIG. 9.2. A cross section of the organ of Corti. A: low magnification, and B: higher magnification.

CONDUCTIVE HEARING LOSS

In cases of conductive hearing loss, sound waves are not transmitted effectively to the inner ear because of some interference in the external canal, the eardrum, the ossicular chain, the middle-ear cavity, the oval window, the round window, or the eustachian tube. For example, damage to either the middle ear, which transmits sound energy efficiently, or the eustachian tube, which maintains equal air pressure between the middle ear cavity and the external canal, could result in a mechanical defect in sound transmission. In pure conductive hearing loss, there is no damage to the inner ear or the neural pathway.

Patients diagnosed as having conductive hearing loss have a much better prognosis than those with sensorineural loss, because modern techniques make it possible to cure or at least improve the vast majority of cases in which the damage occurs in the outer or middle ear. Even if they are not improved medically or surgically, these patients stand to benefit greatly from a hearing aid, because what they need most is amplification. They are not bothered by distortion and other hearing abnormalities that may occur in sensorineural losses.

Conductive hearing loss may result from anything that completely blocks the outer ear or interferes with sound transmission through the middle ear. Outer ear problems include birth defects, total occlusion of the external auditory canal by wax, foreign body (such as a piece of cotton swab or ear plug), infection, trauma, or tumor. Large perforations in the tympanic membrane may also cause hearing loss, especially if they surround the malleus. However, relatively small, central perforations usually do not cause a great deal of hearing impairment. If someone with such a perforation has a 30 or 40 dB hearing loss, there is probably also a problem involving the ossicles. Middle ear dysfunction is the most common cause of conductive hearing loss. It may occur in many ways. The middle ear may become filled with fluid because of eustachian tube dysfunction. The fluid restricts free movement of the tympanic membrane and ossicles, thereby producing hearing loss. Middle ear conductive hearing loss may also be caused by ossicular abnormalities. These include fractures, erosion from disease, impingement by tumors, congenital malformations, and other causes. However, otosclerosis is among the most common. This hereditary disease afflicts the stapes and prevents it from moving in its normal pistonlike fashion in the oval window. Hearing loss from otosclerosis can be corrected through stapes surgery, a brief operation under local anesthesia, and it is usually possible to restore hearing.

SENSORINEURAL HEARING LOSS

The word *sensorineural* was introduced to replace the ambiguous terms *perceptive deafness* and *nerve deafness*. It is a more descriptive and more accurate anatomical term. Its dual character suggests that two separate areas may be affected, and this is actually the case. The term *sensory hearing loss* is applied when the damage is localized in the inner ear. Useful synonyms are *cochlear* or *inner-ear hearing loss.* The cochlea has approximately 15,000 hearing nerve endings (hair cells). Those hair cells in the large end of the cochlea respond to very high-pitched sounds, and those in the small end (and throughout much of the rest of the cochlea) respond to low-pitched sounds. Those hair cells, and the nerve that connects them to the brain, are susceptible to damage from a variety of causes. *Neural hearing loss* is the correct term to use when the damage is in the auditory nerve proper, anywhere between its fibers at the base of the hair cells and the auditory nuclei. This range includes the bipolar ganglion of the eighth cranial nerve. Other common names for this type of loss are *nerve deafness* and *retrocochlear hearing loss.* These names are useful if applied appropriately and meaningfully, but too often they are used improperly.

Although at present it is common practice to group together both sensory and neural components, it has become possible in many cases to attribute a predominant part of the damage, if not all of it, to either the inner ear or the nerve. Because of some success in this area and the likelihood that ongoing research will allow us to differentiate between even more cases of sensory and neural hearing loss, we shall divide the terms and describe the distinctive features of each type. This separation is advisable because the prognosis and the treatment of the two kinds of impairment differ. For example, in all cases of unilateral sensorineural hearing loss, it is important to distinguish between a sensory and neural hearing impairment, because the neural type may be due to an acoustic neuroma which could become life-threatening. Those cases which we cannot identify as either sensory or neural and those cases in which there is damage in both regions we shall classify as sensorineural.

There are various and complex causes of sensorineural hearing loss, but certain features are characteristic and basic to all of them. Because the histories obtained from patients are so diverse, they contribute more insight into the etiology than into the classification of a case. Sensorineural hearing loss often involves not only loss of loudness but also loss of clarity. The hair cells in the inner ear are responsible for analyzing auditory input and instantaneously coding it. The auditory nerve is responsible for carrying this complex coded information. Neural defects such as acoustic neuromas (tumors of the auditory nerve) are frequently accompanied by severe difficulties in discriminating words, although the hearing threshold for soft sounds may not be so severely affected. Sensory deficits in the cochlea are often associated with distortion of sound quality, distortion of loudness (loudness recruitment), and distortion of pitch (diplacusis). Diplacusis poses particular problems for musicians because it may make it difficult for them to tell whether they are playing or singing correct pitches. This symptom is also troublesome to conductors. Keyboard players and other musicians whose instruments do not require critical tuning adjustments compensate for this problem better than singers, string players, etc. In addition, sensorineural hearing loss may be accompanied by tinnitus (noises in the ear) and/or vertigo.

Sensorineural hearing loss may be due to a great number of conditions including aging, exposure to ototoxic drugs (including a number of antibiotics, diuretics, and chemotherapy agents), hereditary conditions, systemic diseases, trauma, and noise, among other causes. Most physicians recognize that hearing loss may be associated with a large number of hereditary syndromes (2,3) involving the eyes, kidneys, heart, or any other body system, but many are not aware that hearing loss also accompanies many very common systemic diseases. Naturally, these occur in musicians as well as others; the presence of these systemic illnesses should lead physicians to inquire about hearing and to perform audiometry to screen for hearing loss in selected cases. Problems implicated in hearing impairment include Rh incompatibility, hypoxia, jaundice, rubella, mumps, rubeola, fungal infections, meningitis, tuberculosis, sarcoidosis, Wegener's granulomatosis, vasculitis, histiocytosis X, allergy, hyperlipoproteinemia, syphilis, hypothyroidism, hypoadrenalism, hypopituitarism, renal failure, autoimmune disease, coagulopathies, aneurysms, vascular disease, multiple sclerosis, infestations, diabetes, hypoglycemia, cleft palate and others (2). Prolonged exposure to very loud noise is a common cause of hearing loss in our society. Noise-induced hearing loss is seen most frequently in heavy industry. However, occupational hearing loss caused by musical instruments is a special problem, as discussed below.

Sensorineural hearing loss is one of the most challenging problems in medicine. A large variety of hearing impairments fall in this category. The prognosis for restoring a sensorineural hearing loss with presently available therapy is poor. Although some spontaneous remissions and hearing improvements have occurred with therapy, particularly in cases involving sensory loss, a great need for further research still exists.

MIXED HEARING LOSS

For practical purposes, a "mixed hearing loss" should be understood to mean a conductive hearing loss accompanied by a sensory or a neural (or a sensorineural) loss in the same ear. However, the emphasis is on the conductive hearing loss, because available therapy is so much more effective for this group. Consequently, the otologic surgeon has a special interest in cases of mixed hearing loss in which there is primarily a conductive loss complicated by some sensorineural damage. In a musician, curing the correctable component may be sufficient to convert hearing from unserviceable to satisfactory for performance purposes.

FUNCTIONAL HEARING LOSS

Functional hearing loss occurs as a condition in which the patient does not seem to hear or to respond, yet the handicap is not caused by any organic pathology in the peripheral or central auditory pathways. The hearing difficulty may have an entirely emotional or psychological etiology, or it may be superimposed on some mild organic hearing loss, in which case it is called a functional or a psychogenic overlay. Often, the patient really has normal hearing underlying the functional hearing loss. A careful history usually will reveal some hearing impairment in the patient's family or some reference to deafness which served as the nucleus for the patient's functional hearing loss. The most important challenge in such a case is to classify the condition properly. Functional hearing loss occurs not only in adults, but also in children. This diagnosis should be considered when hearing problems arise in musicians under great pressure regardless of age, including young prodigies.

CENTRAL HEARING LOSS (CENTRAL DYSACOUSIS)

In central hearing loss the damage is situated in the central nervous system at some point between the auditory nuclei (in the medulla oblongata) and the cortex. Formerly, central hearing loss was described as a type of "perceptive deafness," a term now obsolete.

Although information about central hearing loss is accumulating, it remains somewhat a mystery. Physicians know that some patients cannot interpret or understand what is being said, and that the cause of the difficulty is not in the peripheral mechanism but somewhere in the central nervous system. In central hearing loss the problem is not a lowered pure-tone threshold but in the patient's ability to interpret what he hears. Obviously, it is a more complex task to interpret speech than to respond to a pure-tone threshold; consequently, the tests necessary to diagnosis central hearing impairment must be designed to assess a patient's ability to handle complex information.

PSYCHOLOGICAL CONSEQUENCES OF HEARING LOSS

Performing artists are frequently sensitive, somewhat "high-strung" people who depend upon physical perfection in order to practice their crafts and earn their livelihoods. Any physical impairment that threatens their ability to continue as musicians may be greeted with dread, denial, panic, depression, or similar response that may be perceived as "exaggerated," especially by physicians who do not specialize in caring for performers. In the case of hearing loss, such reactions are common even in the general public. Consequently, it is not surprising that psychological concomitants of hearing loss in musicians are seen in nearly all cases.

Many successful performers are communicative and gregarious. Naturally, anything that impairs their ability to interact with the world causes problems similar to those seen in nonmusicians. However, in addition, their vocational hearing demands are much greater than those required in most professions. Therefore, musicians' normal reactions to hearing loss are often amplified by legitimate fears about interruption of their artistic and professional futures through hearing impairment. These concerns are encountered with hearing-impaired musicians regardless of the cause. The problems involved in accurately assessing the disability associated with such impairments are addressed below in the discussion of occupational hearing loss in musicians.

OCCUPATIONAL HEARING LOSS IN MUSICIANS

Because hearing health is so important to musicians, it is especially ironic that music performance can cause hearing impairment. Injury to the ear has been encountered not only among popular musicians, but also those performing exclusively classical music. It is essential that physicians and performers understand the importance of maintaining good hearing, the potential hazard posed by noise exposure, and methods of preventing occupational hearing loss.

For many years, people have been concerned about hearing loss in rock musicians exposed to intense noise from electric instruments, and in audiences who frequently attend concerts of rock music. Hearing loss has been identified in both of these populations. Similar problems have been found more recently in people who listen to music at very high volumes through earphones using portable, personal audio equipment. Because of the obviously high intensity that characterizes rock music, hearing loss in these situations is not surprising. This situation raises serious concerns about prevention that are of compelling relevance to professional rock musicians whose livelihoods depend on their hearing. Clinical observations in the authors' practice suggest that the rock performing environment may be another source of asymmetrical noise-induced hearing loss, a relatively unusual situation since most occupational hearing loss is symmetrical. Rock musicians tend to have slightly greater hearing loss in the ear adjacent to the drum and cymbal, or the side immediately next to a speaker, if it is placed slightly behind the musician. Various methods have been devised to help protect the hearing of rock players. For example, most of them stand beside or behind their speakers, rather than in front of them. In this way, they are not subjected to peak intensities, nor are the patrons in the first rows.

The problem of occupational hearing loss among classical musicians is less obvious, but equally important. In fact, in the United States, this problem has become a matter of great concern and negotiation among unions and management. Various reports have found an increased incidence of high-frequency sensorineural hearing loss among professional orchestra musicians as compared to the general public. Sound levels within orchestras have been measured between 83 dBA and 112 dBA. The size of the orchestra and the rehearsal hall are important factors, as is the position of the individual instrumentalist within the orchestra. Players seated immediately in front of the brass section appear to have particular problems, for example. Individual classical instruments may produce more noise exposure for their players than assumed.

Because many musicians practice or perform 4 to 8 hours a day (sometimes more), such exposure levels may be significant. An interesting review of the literature may be found in the report of a clinical research project on hearing in classical musicians by Axelsson and Lindgren (4). They also found asymmetrical hearing loss in classical musicians, greater in the left ear. This is a common finding, especially among violinists. A brief summary of most of the published works on hearing loss in musicians is presented below.

In the United States, various attempts have been made to solve some of the problems of the orchestra musician, including placement of plexiglass barriers in front of some of the louder brass instruments; alteration in the orchestra formation, such as elevation of sections or rotational seating; changes in spacing and height between players; use of ear protectors; and other measures. These solutions have not been proven effective, and some of them appear impractical and damaging to the performance. The effects of the acoustical environment (concert hall, auditorium, outdoor stage, etc.) on the ability of music to damage hearing have not been studied systematically. Recently, popular musicians have begun to recognize the importance of this problem and to protect themselves and educate their fans. Some performers are wearing ear protectors regularly in rehearsal, and even during performance (5). Considerable additional study is needed to provide proper answers and clinical guidance for this very important occupational problem. In fact, review of the literature on occupational hearing loss reveals that surprisingly little information is available on the entire subject. Moreover, all of it is concerned with instrumentalists, and no similar studies in singers were found.

Study of the existing reports reveals a variety of approaches. Unfortunately, neither the results nor the quality of the studies is consistent. Nevertheless, familiarity with the research already performed provides useful insights into the problem. In 1960, Arnold and Miskolczy-Fodor (6) studied the hearing of 30 pianists. Sound pressure level measurements showed that average levels were approximately 85 dB, although periods of 92 to 96 dB were recorded. The A-weighting network was not used for sound level measurements in this study. No noise-induced hearing loss was identified. The pianists in this study were 60 to 80 years of age; and, in fact, their hearing was better than normal for their age. Flach and Aschoff (7), and later Flach (8), found sensorineural hearing loss in 16% of 506 music students and professional musicians, a higher percentage that could be accounted for by age alone, although none of the cases of hearing loss occurred in students. Hearing loss was most common in musicians playing string instruments. Flach and Aschoff also noticed asymmetrical sensorineural hearing loss worse on the left in ten of eleven cases of bilateral sensorineural hearing loss in musicians. In one case (a flutist), the hearing was worse on the right. In 4% of the professional musicians tested, hearing loss was felt to be causally related to musical noise exposure. Histories and physical examinations were performed on the musicians, and tests were performed in a controlled environment. This study also included interesting measurements of sound levels in a professional orchestra. Unfortunately, they are reported in DIN-PHONS, rather than dBA.

In 1968, Berghoff (9) reported on the hearing of 35 big-band musicians and 30 broadcasting (studio) musicians. Most had performed for 15 to 25 years, although the string players were older as a group and had performed for as much as 35 years. In general, they played approximately 5 hours per day. Hearing loss was found in 40- to 60-year-old musicians at 8,000 Hz and 10,000 Hz. Eight musicians had substantial hearing loss, especially at 4,000 Hz. Five out of sixty-four (8%) cases were felt to be causally related to noise exposure. No difference was found between left and right ears, but hearing loss was most common in musicians who were sitting immediately beside drums, trumpets, or bassoons. Sound level measurements for wind instruments revealed that intensities were greater 1 m away from the instrument than they were at the ear canal. Unfortunately, sound levels were measured in PHONS. Lebo and Oliphant (10) studied the sound levels of a symphony orchestra and two rock-and-roll orchestras. They reported that sound energy for symphony orchestras is fairly evenly distributed from 500 Hz through 4,000 Hz, but most of the energy in rock-and-roll music was found between 250 Hz and 500 Hz. The sound pressure level for the symphony orchestra during loud passages was approximately 90 dBA. For rock-and-roll bands, it reached levels in excess of 110 dBA. Most of the time, music during rock performance was louder than 95 dB in the lower frequencies, while symphony orchestras rarely achieved such levels. However, Lebo and Oliphant made their measurements from the auditorium rather than in immediate proximity to the performers. Consequently, their measurements are more indicative of distant audience noise exposure than that of the musicians or of audience members in the first row.

In 1970, Jerger and Jerger (11) studied temporary threshold shifts in rock-and-roll musicians. They identified temporary threshold shifts greater than 15 dB in at least one frequency between 2,000 and 8,000 Hz in eight of nine musicians studied prior to performance and within one hour after the performance. Speaks (12) and co-workers examined 25 rock musicians for threshold shifts, obtaining measures between 20 and 40 minutes following performance. In this study, shifts of only 7 to 8 dB at 4,000 and 6,000 Hz were identified. Temporary threshold shifts occurred in about half of the musicians studied. Six of the 25 musicians had permanent threshold shifts. Noise measurements were also made on ten rock bands. Speaks, et al. found noise levels from 90 dBA to 110 dBA. Most sessions were less than 4 hours, and actual music time was generally 120 to 150 minutes. The investigators recognized the hazard to hearing posed by this noise exposure. In 1972, Jahto and Hellman (13) studied 63 orchestra musicians playing in contemporary dance bands. Approximately a third of their subjects had measurable hearing loss, and 13% had bilateral high-frequency loss suggestive of noise-induced hearing damage. They also measured peak sound pressure levels of 110 dB (the A scale was not used). They detected potentially damaging levels produced by trumpets, bassoons, saxophones, and percussion. In contrast, in 1974 Buhlert and Kuhl (14) found no noise-induced hearing loss among 17 performers in a radio broadcasting orchestra. The musicians had played for an average of 20 years and were an average of 30 years of age. In a later study, Kuhl (15) studied members of a radio broadcasting dance orchestra over a period of 12 days. The average noise exposure was 82 dBA. He concluded that such symphony orchestras were exposed to safe hearing levels, in disagreement with Jahto and Hellman. Zeleny et al. (16) studied members of a large string orchestra with intensities reaching 104 to 112 dB. Hearing loss greater than 20 dB in at least one frequency occurred in 85 of 118 subjects (72%), usually in the higher frequencies. Speech frequencies were affected in six people (5%).

In 1976, Siroky et al. reported noise levels within a symphony orchestra ranging between 87 and 98 dBA, with a mean value of 92 dBA (17). Audiometric evaluation of 76 members of the orchestra revealed 16 musicians with hearing loss, 13 of them sensorineural. Hearing loss was found in 7.3% of string players, 20% of wind players, and 28% of brass players. All percussionists had some degree of hearing loss. Hearing loss was not found in players who had performed for less than 10 years, but was present in 42% of players who had performed for more than 20 years. This study needs to be reevaluated in consideration of age-matched controls. At least some of the cases reported have hearing loss not causally related to noise (such as those with hearing levels of 100 dB in the higher frequencies). In a companion report, Folprechtova and Miksovska also found sound levels of 92 dBA in a symphony orchestra with a range of 87 to 98 dBA (18). They reported that most of the musicians performed between 4 to 8 hours daily. They reported the sound levels of various instruments as follows:

1. violin   84 - 103 dB(A)
2. cello   84 - 92 dB(A)
3. bass   75 - 83 dB(A)
4. piccolo   95 - 112 dB(A)
5. flute   85 - 111 dB(A)
6. clarinet   92 - 103 dB(A)
7   French horn   90 - 106 dB(A)
8. oboe   80 - 94 dB(A)
9. trombone   85 - 114 dB(A)
10. xylophone   90 - 92 dB(A)

A study by Balazs and Gotze, also in 1976, agreed that classical musicians are exposed to potentially damaging hearing levels (19). The findings of Gryczynska and Czyzewski (20) support the concerns raised by other authors. In 1977, they found bilateral normal hearing in only 16 of 51 symphony orchestra musicians who worked daily at sound levels between 85 and 108 dBA. Five of the musicians had unilateral normal hearing, the rest had bilateral hearing loss.

In 1978, Axelsson and Lindgren (21,22) published an interesting study of 83 pop musicians and noted a surprisingly low incidence of hearing loss. They reanalyzed previous reports investigating a total of 160 pop musicians which identified an incidence of only 5% hearing loss. In their 1978 study, Axelsson and Lindgren tested 69 musicians, 4 disk jockeys, 4 managers and 6 sound engineers. To have hearing loss, a subject had to have at least one pure-tone threshold exceeding 20 dB at any frequency between 3,000 and 8,000 Hz. Thirty-eight musicians were found to have sensorineural hearing loss. In eleven, only the right ear was affected; in five, only the left ear was affected. Thirteen cases were excluded because the hearing loss could be explained by causes other than noise. Thus, 25% of the pop musicians had sensorineural hearing loss probably attributable to noise. Six thousand hertz was the most commonly impaired frequency, and very few ears showed hearing levels worse than 35 dB. After correction for age and other factors, 25 (30%) had hearing loss as defined above. Eleven (13%) had hearing loss defined as a pure-tone audiometric average greater than 20 dB at 3, 4, 6 and 8 kHz in at least one ear. Of these eleven, seven had unilateral hearing loss (8%). In 1981, Westmore and Eversden (23) studied a symphony orchestra and 34 of its musicians. They recorded sound pressure levels for 14.4 hours. Sound levels exceeded 90 dBA for 3.51 hours and equaled or exceeded 110 dBA for 0.02 hours. In addition, there were brief peaks exceeding 120 dBA. They interpreted their audiometric testing as showing noise-induced hearing loss in 23 of 68 ears. Only 4 of the 23 ears had a hearing loss greater than 20 dB at 4,000 Hz. There was a "clear indication" that orchestral musicians may be exposed to damaging noise. However, because of the relatively mild severity, they speculated that "it is unlikely that any musician is going to be prevented from continuing his artistic career." In Axelsson's 1981 study (4), sound level measurements were performed in two theatres, and 139 musicians underwent hearing tests. Sound levels for performances ranged from 83 to 92 dBA. Sound levels were slightly higher in an orchestra pit, although this is contrary to the findings of Westmore (23). Fifty-nine musicians (43%) had pure-tone thresholds worse than expected for their ages. French hornists, trumpeters, trombonists, and bassoonists were found to be at increased risk for sensorineural hearing loss. Asymmetric pure-tone thresholds were common in musicians with hearing loss, and in those still classified as having "normal hearing." The left ear demonstrated greater hearing loss than the right, especially among violinists. Axelsson and Lindgren also found that the loudness comfort level was unusually high among musicians. Acoustic reflexes also were elicited at comparatively high levels, trauma being pathologically increased in approximately 30%. Temporary threshold shifts were also identified, supporting the assertion of noise-related etiology.

In 1983, Karlsson and coworkers published a report with findings and conclusions substantially different from those of Axelsson and others (24). Karlsson investigated 417 musicians, of whom 123 were investigated twice at an interval of 6 years. After excluding 25 musicians who had hearing loss for reasons other than noise, he based his conclusions on the remaining 392 cases. Karlsson et al. concluded that there was no statistical difference between the hearing of symphony orchestra musicians and that of a normal population of similar age and sex. Those data revealed a symmetric dip of 20 dB at 6,000 Hz in flutists, and a 30 dB left high-frequency sloping hearing loss in bass players. Overall, a 5 dB difference between ears was also found at 6,000 and 8,000 Hz, with the left side being worse. Although Karlsson and coworkers conclude that performing in a symphonic orchestra does not involve an increased risk of hearing damage, and that standard criteria for industrial noise exposure are not applicable to symphonic music, their data are similar to previous studies. Only their interpretation varies substantially (24).

Johnson et al. (25) studied the effects of instrument type and orchestral position on the hearing of orchestra musicians. They studied 60 orchestra musicians from 24 to 64 years in age, none of whom had symptomatic hearing problems. The musicians underwent otologic histories and examinations, and pure-tone audiometry from 250 Hz through 20,000 Hz. Unfortunately, this study used previous data from other authors as control data. In addition to the inherent weakness in this design, the comparison data did not include thresholds at 6,000 Hz. There appeared to be a 6,000 Hz dip in the population studied by Johnson et al. (25), but no definitive statement could be made. The authors concluded that the type of instrument played and the position on the orchestra stage had no significant correlation with hearing loss, disagreeing with findings of other investigators. In another paper produced from the same study (26), Johnson reported no difference in the high-frequency thresholds (9,000 Hz to 20,000 Hz) between musicians and nonmusicians. Again, because he examined 60 instrumentalists but used previously published reports for comparison, this study is marred. This shortcoming in experimental design is particularly important in high-frequency testing, during which calibration is particularly difficult and establishment of norms on each individual piece of equipment is advisable.

A particularly interesting review of hearing impairment among orchestra musicians was published by Woolford et al. in 1988 (27). Although this report presents only preliminary data, the authors have put forward a penetrating review of the problem and interesting proposals regarding solutions, including an international comparative study. At this point, they conclude that the presence of hearing loss among classical musicians from various etiologies (including noise) has been established; that some noise induced hearing impairments in musicians are permanent (although usually slight); and that successful efforts to reduce the intensity of noise exposure are possible.

In addition to concern about hearing loss among performers, in recent years there has been growing concern about noise-induced hearing loss among audiences. Those at risk include not only people at rock concerts but also people who enjoy music through stereo systems, especially modern personal headphones. Concern about hearing loss from this source in high school students has appeared in the lay press and elsewhere (28,29). Because young music lovers are all potentially performers, in addition to other reasons, this hazard should be taken seriously and investigated further.

Review of these somewhat confusing and contradictory studies reveals that a great deal of important work remains to be done in order to establish the risk of hearing loss among various types of musicians, the level and pattern of hearing loss that may be sustained, practical methods of preventing hearing loss, and advisable programs for monitoring and early diagnosis. However, a few preliminary conclusions can be drawn. First, the preponderance of evidence indicates that noise-induced hearing loss occurs among both pop and classical musicians and is causally related to exposure to loud music. Second, in most instances, especially among classical musicians, the hearing loss is not severe enough to interfere with speech perception. Third, the effects of mild high-frequency hearing loss on musical performance have not been established. Fourth, it should be possible to devise methods to conserve hearing among performing artists without interfering with performance.

LEGAL ASPECTS OF HEARING LOSS IN MUSICIANS

The problem of hearing loss in musicians raises numerous legal issues, especially the implications of occupational hearing loss; hearing has become an issue in some orchestra contracts. Traditionally, worker's compensation legislation has been based on the theory that workers should be compensated when a work-related injury impairs their ability to earn a living. Ordinarily, occupational hearing loss does not impair earning power (except possibly in the case of musicians and a few others). Consequently, current occupational hearing loss legislation broke new legal ground by providing compensation for interference with quality of life; that is, loss of living power. Therefore, all current standards for defining and compensating occupational hearing loss are based on the communication needs of the average speaker. Since music-induced hearing loss appears to rarely affect the speech frequencies, it is not compensable under most laws. However, although a hearing loss at 3,000, 4,000 or 6,000 Hz with preservation of lower frequencies may not pose a problem for a boilermaker, it may be a serious problem for a violinist. Under certain circumstances, such a hearing loss may even be disabling. Because professional instrumentalists require considerably greater hearing acuity throughout a larger frequency range, we must investigate whether the kinds of hearing loss caused by music are severe enough to impair performance. If so, new criteria must be established for compensation for disabling hearing impairment in musicians, in keeping with the original intent of worker's compensation law.

There may also be unresolved legal issues regarding hearing loss not caused by noise in professional musicians. Like people with other handicaps, there are numerous federal laws protecting the rights of the hearing impaired. In the unhappy situation in which an orchestra must release a hearing-impaired violinist who can no longer play in tune, for example, legal challenges may arise. In such instances, and in many other circumstances, an objective assessment process is in the best interest of performers and management. Objective measures of performance are already being used in selected areas for singers, and they have proven very beneficial in helping the performer to dispassionately assess certain aspects of performance quality and skill development. Such technological advances will probably be used in the future more frequently to supplement traditional subjective assessment of performing artists for musical, scientific, and legal reasons.

TREATMENT OF HEARING LOSS

For a complete discussion of the treatment of hearing loss, the reader is referred to standard otolaryngology texts. In general, conductive hearing loss can be cured medically or surgically. Some causes of sensorineural hearing loss are also amenable to treatment. For example, luetic labyrinthitis (syphilis) responds to medication. So does hypothyroidism. Meniere's disease may also respond to medication or surgery. However, most cases of sensorineural hearing loss produced by aging, hereditary factors, and noise cannot be cured. When they involve the speech frequencies, modern, properly-adjusted hearing aids are usually extremely helpful. However, these devices are rarely satisfactory for musicians during performance. More often, appropriate counseling is sufficient. The musician should be provided with a copy of his or her audiogram and an explanation of its correspondence with the piano keyboard. Unless a hearing loss becomes severe, this information usually permits musicians to make appropriate adjustments. For example, a conductor with an unknown high-frequency hearing loss will call for violins and triangles to be excessively loud. If he or she knows the pattern of hearing loss, this error can be avoided. Musicians with hearing loss (and those without hearing loss) should also routinely be cautioned against avocational loud noise exposure without ear protection (hunting, power tools, motorcycles, etc.) and ototoxic drugs. In addition, they should be educated about the importance of immediate evaluation if a sudden hearing change occurs.

SUMMARY

Good hearing is of great importance to musicians, but the effects on performance of mild high-frequency hearing loss remain uncertain. It is most important to be alert for hearing loss in performers from all causes, to recognize it early, and to treat it or prevent its progression whenever possible. Musical instruments and performance environments are capable of producing damaging noise. Strenuous efforts must be made to define the risks and nature of music-induced hearing loss among musicians, to establish damage/risk criteria, and to implement practical means of reducing noise and hearing conservation.

REFERENCES

1. Sataloff J, Sataloff RT, Vassallo L. *Hearing loss*. Philadelphia, Toronto: JP Lippincott, 1980.
2. Sataloff RT, Sataloff J. *Occupational hearing loss*. New York: Marcel Dekker, 1987.
3. Konigsmark BW, Gorlin RJ. *Genetic and metabolic deafness*. Philadelphia: W.B. Saunders, 1976.
4. Axelsson A, Lindgren F. Hearing in classical musicians. *Acta Otolaryngol* 1981; Suppl. 377:3–74.
5. Toufexis A. A fire hose down the ear canal. *Time* Sept 29, 1989;78.
6. Arnold GE, Miskolczy-Fodor F. Pure-tone thresholds of professional pianists. *Arch Otolaryngol* 1960;71:938–947.
7. Flach M, Aschoff E. Zur frage berufsbedingter schwerhorigkeit beium musiker. *Ztschr Laryngol* 1966;45:595–605.
8. Flach M. Das gehor des musikers aus ohrenarztlicher sicht. *Msch Ohr hk* 1972;9:424–432.
9. Berghoff F. Horleistung und berufsbedingte horschadigung des orchestermusikers mit einem beitrag zur pathophysiologie des larmtraumatischen horschadens. Dissertation. 1968. Cited in: Axelsson A, Lindgren F. Hearing in classical musicians. *Acta Otolaryngol* 1981; Suppl 377;3–74.
10. Lebo CP, Oliphant KP. Music as a source of acoustic trauma. *Laryngoscope* 1968;72(2):1211–1218.
11. Jerger J, Jerger S. Temporary threshold shift in rock-and-roll musicians. *Journal of Speech and Hearing Research* 1970;13:221–224.
12. Speaks C, Nelson D, Ward WD. Hearing loss in rock-and-roll musicians. *Journal of Occupational Medicine* June, 1970;12(6):216–219.
13. Jahto K, Hellmann H. Zur frage des larm—und klangtraumas des orchestermusikers. audiologie und phoniatrie *HNO* 1972;20(Heft 1):21–29.
14. Buhlert P, Kuhl W. Horuntersuchungen im freien schallfeld zum altershorverlust. *Acustica* 1974; 31:168–177.
15. Kuhl W. Keine gehorschadigung durch tanzmusik, simfonische musik und maschinengerausche beim rundfunk. *Kampf dem Larm* 1976;23(Heft 4):105–107.

16. Zeleny M, Navratilova Z, Kamycek Z, et al. Relation of hearing disorders to the acoustic composition of working environment of musicians in a wind orchestra. *Ceskoslovenska Otolaryngologie* 1975;24(5):295–299.
17. Siroky J, Sevcikova L, Folprechtova A, et al. Audiological examination of musicians of a symphonic orchestra in relation to acoustic conditions. *Ceskoslovenska Otolaryngologie* 1976;25(5): 288–294.
18. Folprechtova A, Miksovska O. The acoustic conditions in a symphony orchestra. *Pracov Lek* 1976;28:1–2.
19. Balazs B, Gotze A. Comparative examinations between the hearing of musicians playing on traditional instruments and on those with electrical amplification. *Ful-orr-gegegyogyaszat* 1976;22:116–118.
20. Gryczynska D, Czyzewski I. Damaging effect of music on the hearing organ in musicians. *Otolaryngol* 1977; (Pol) 31(5):527–532.
21. Axelsson A, Lindgren F. Hearing in pop musicians. *Acta Otolaryngol* 1978;85:225–231.
22. Axelsson A, Lindgren F. Horseln hos popmusiker. *Lakartidningen* 1978;75(13):1286–1288.
23. Westmore GA, Eversden ID. Noise-induced hearing loss and orchestral musicians. *Arch Otolaryngol* 1981;107:761–764.
24. Karlsson K, Lundquist PG, Olaussen T. The hearing of symphony orchestra musicians. *Scan Audio* 1983;12:257–264.
25. Johnson DW, Sherman RE, Aldridge J, et al. Effects of instrument type and orchestral position on hearing sensitivity for 0.25 to 20 kHz. in the orchestral musician. *Scan Audio* 1985;14:215–221.
26. Johnson DW, Sherman RE, Aldridge J, et al. Extended high frequency hearing sensitivity: a normative threshold study in musicians. *Ann Otol Rhinol Laryngol* 1986;95:196–201.
27. Woolford DH, Carterette EC, Morgan DE. Hearing impairment among orchestral musicians. *Music Perception* Spring 1988;5(3):261–284.
28. Gallagher G. Hot music, high noise, & hurt ears. *The Hearing Journal* March 1989;42(3):7–11.
29. Lewis DA. A hearing conservation program for high school level students. *The Hearing Journal* March 1989;42(3):19–24.

Textbook of Performing Arts Medicine, edited
by R. T. Sataloff, A. Brandfonbrener, and
R. Lederman. Raven Press, Ltd.,
New York © 1991.

10

Psychiatric Problems of Performing Artists

*Peter Ostwald and †Marc Avery

*Professor of Psychiatry and Medical Director to the Health Program for
Performing Artists, University of California, San Francisco, California 94143
†Assistant Adjunct Professor of Psychiatry, and Psychiatric Consultant to the
Health Program for Performing Artists, University of California,
San Francisco, California 94143

Psychiatry is the branch of medicine which specializes in diagnosis and treatment of emotional problems, personality disorders, and mental illnesses. Like the other medical specialties, it has subfields, including general psychiatry, child psychiatry, geriatric psychiatry, and consultation-liaison psychiatry. Although problems of performing artists have occasionally been described in the psychiatric literature (the conductor Bruno Walter and the composer Gustav Mahler were seen by Freud in Vienna) a specific focus on this group of patients is relatively new.

It has been estimated that up to 50% of the patients seen in general medical clinics are afflicted with mental, emotional, or personality problems, and one might expect that the incidence of psychiatric problems among performers might also be high, considering the high level of stress usually associated with an artist's career. Artists are often considered to be rather special or even peculiar people, sometimes regarded to have eccentric, if not sickly, personalities. This stereotype received emphasis during the nineteenth century, when many scientists believed that unusual creative ability was invariably linked with susceptibility to disease, the so-called mad genius hypothesis (1). While it is true that studies of writers, poets, and novelists show a higher-than-normal incidence of psychiatric illness—specifically depression, alcoholism, and suicide—among these "verbally creative" people (2), no comparable data have ever been presented for musicians, dancers, or other performers whose work involves primarily nonverbal modes of communication. This is clearly a topic for further research. Questions remain about what other factors besides illness (e.g., career frustration, unhappy marriage, poverty, etc.) can produce serious depression. Concerts recently presented in Los Angeles and in Washington, D. C., under the title "Moods and Music," have raised the question of bipolar (manic-depressive) disorder among major composers, including Gustav Mahler, Hector Berlioz, George Frideric Handel, Hugo Wolf, and Robert Schumann

(3). Schumann's case is well-documented (4), but serious questions remain about the other four. One must also consider that among creative individuals, depression and illness itself may serve as a stimulus for superior work (5). History provides many examples: Ludwig van Beethoven's deafness, Marcel Proust's asthma, Robert Schumann's crippled hand.

The current interest in diagnosis and treatment of the ailments of performing artists was stimulated in large measure by the self-revelations of Leon Fleisher and Gary Graffman, two pianists whose careers were jeopardized by crippling physical disabilities. That these and other musicians also suffer emotionally from their handicaps and face serious psychological problems in their rehabilitation, goes without saying. According to some clinicians, all of the musicians seen with nerve entrapment disorders, dystonias, or other physical disabilities have associated psychiatric complaints, usually substantial amounts of anxiety and depression related to the limitations imposed on their playing by the disease and to the uncertainties about outcome of treatment (6). In an arts medicine team that makes a point of attending with equal concern the physical, psychological, and social problems of musicians and dancers, this is not surprising. Separating bodily from mental disease seems artificial and unscientific (7). But what is the true incidence of psychopathology among performers?

THE PSYCHIATRIC COMPLAINTS OF PERFORMING ARTISTS

In trying to obtain a clear picture of what it is that instrumental musicians, singers, actors, dancers, and other performing artists think of as their psychiatric problems, one can find very little reliable information. One useful approach is the recent International Conference of Symphony and Opera Musicians (ICSOM) survey of 48 symphony orchestras (8). Of the 2,212 musicians responding to the questionnaire, 67.5% reported musculoskeletal problems which were located most commonly in the neck and/or back (47.4%); the right arm, elbow, or shoulder (27.6%); the left finger, hand, or wrist (27%); and the left arm, elbow, or shoulder (25.8%). In the category of nonmusculoskeletal problems, an even larger group, 71.2%, registered complaints. *Of the musicians responding, 39% reported themselves to be afflicted with psychological problems.* That appears to be the second highest incidence of disease complaints among the cohort, outstripped only by the complaint of neck and/or back problems (47.4%). Under the category of "psychological problems," stagefright was the most common complaint (24.7%), followed by depression (16.6%), sleep disturbances (14.2%), and acute anxiety (13.2%). Although it seems arbitrary to divide complaints into two categories, musculoskeletal versus nonmusculoskeletal complaints (and there is undoubtedly overlap between them), the ICSOM survey tells us that a significant number of orchestra musicians do attest to having psychiatric problems.

Another way to approach the question of how performers as a group regard themselves psychiatrically is to compare them with other groups. Cohen and Kupersmith (9) have done this by using a standard psychological test, the Symptom Checklist

90 (SCL-90) evaluation, which consists of a list of 90 symptoms referring to the following categories: (1.) somatization, (2.) obsessive-compulsive symptoms, (3.) interpersonal sensitivity, (4.) depression, (5.) anxiety, (6.) hostility, (7.) phobic symptoms, (8.) paranoia, and (9.) psychotic symptoms.

A group of 87 performing artists applying for treatment (psychotherapy) was compared with an unselected group of patients seeking help. This comparison showed *a lower level of symptoms among the artists in all of the nine categories.* The difference was most significant in the categories of interpersonal sensitivity, depression, paranoia, and psychoticism. The investigators felt that performers, perhaps because of their "creativity and often rigorous training," may have stronger defenses against psychological suffering than do other patients. However, as this survey also showed, performing artists requesting psychotherapy have significantly higher symptom ratings in all categories of psychopathology than do people who are not seeking help (i.e., a nonpatient population).

PERFORMING ARTISTS AS PSYCHIATRIC PATIENTS

Patienthood always involves a process of communication between the person who feels unwell and a doctor who offers treatment (10). How psychiatric problems are perceived will thus depend on the patient's view of himself or herself and the sensitivity of the clinician. For example, during the first months of operation of the program in San Francisco, 90 patients requested psychiatric help and/or were referred for consultation to a psychiatrist. This represents approximately a quarter (25%) of our caseload to date (since not everyone who complains of a problem seeks help for it, it is not surprising that our figures vary from the 39% incidence of psychological problems reported by the ICSOM survey) (8). Of our 90 referrals, 44 were men, 46 were women, and the age range was from 18 to 72 years at the time of admission (the mean age was 34). Of the performer-patients, 49 were instrumental musicians, 27 were singers, 4 were actors, 4 were dancers, 5 were active in the graphic arts (filmmaking, scene designing, etc.), and 1 was a singer and actor.

A majority of our patients (65%) identified themselves as professionals; these were fully trained performers who depend on the arts for a livelihood. Most of them were employed when initially seen (nine professional performers were unemployed, and two had retired). The rest of our patients were amateurs (18%) or students (17%).

In terms of the types of disorder afflicting these individuals, their diagnoses are shown in Table 10.1. It should be noted that the total number of diagnoses exceeds the number of patients. That is because a considerable number of our patients carried more than one diagnosis. It is not unusual in psychiatry for patients to have multiple diagnoses. The primary, or Axis I diagnosis, describes the mental disorder itself; the secondary, or Axis II diagnosis, pertains to any concomitant developmental or personality problems; Axis III refers to physical disorders; Axis IV rates the severity of psychosocial stressors; and Axis V describes the highest level of adaptive functioning during the past year (11).

TABLE 10.1. *Psychiatric disorders in performing artists at the health program*

Type of disorder	No.	Percent
Depression (all types)[a]	51	57%
Recurring depressive episodes	18	20%
Bipolar affective disorder	10	11%
Chronic depression	18	20%
Acute agitated depression	3	3%
Atypical depression	1	1%
Anxiety (all types)	25	28%
Performance anxiety	14	16%
Panic disorder	5	6%
Chronic, recurrent anxiety	7	8%
Personality Disorders (all types)	20	22%
Dependent	10	11%
Borderline	5	6%
Histrionic	5	6%
Narcissistic	3	3%
Paranoid	2	2%
Somatoform disorder	13	14%
Psychological factors complicating physical condition	8	9%
Substance abuse disorders	8	9%
Organic mental disorders	4	4%
Psychosexual disorders	4	4%
Schizophrenia[b]	3	3%
Schizo-affective disorder	1	1%
Bulimia/anorexia	2	2%
Sleep apnea	1	1%

[a]Four of these patients were acutely suicidal; one patient had a history of a near-fatal suicide attempt which resulted in a permanent physical disability
[b]One of these patients was acutely self-destructive and had to be hospitalized.

It would require far more space than we have available in this chapter to describe each of the psychiatric syndromes fully and comprehensively. What we will do instead is to focus on those conditions most frequently encountered among performing artists, and to give brief case illustrations in order to demonstrate the most relevant points. There will also be a short, and by no means exhaustive, discussion of treatment for each psychiatric disorder.

AFFECTIVE DISORDERS AMONG PERFORMING ARTISTS

Depression is characterized by a mood of persistent sadness in excess of the normal, everyday feelings of unhappiness which everyone has. Depressed patients feel unwell in a tangible way, and there often is a physical sense of heaviness, sluggishness, or "loss of pep." Other bodily complaints may include tearfulness, poor appetite, indigestion, sleeplessness, and various aches and pains (with every depressed patient it is essential that thorough physical and laboratory examinations be performed to rule out the presence of other diseases which may produce similar symptoms). Psychologically, the individual feels slowed down, unable to think or make decisions as quickly as usual, unable to concentrate, and often plagued with gloomy, pessimistic thoughts. Not infrequently there are self-doubting or self-accusatory preoccupations, feelings of unworthiness, and low self-esteem. If these ideas exceed what can be considered realistic in terms of the patient's true status and accomplishments in life, one must consider that he may be obsessional or even delusional. Very severe, so-called psychotic illnesses are complicated by disturbances in reality testing and plan making, including the development of nihilistic and paranoid delusions, hypochondriacal beliefs, and hallucinations. Self-neglect is a common problem with depression, and suicide is a substantial danger (12).

Depressive disorders can begin suddenly, usually in the context of some specific loss such as separation from or death of a person one has been close to ("mourning reactions"), following a severe disappointment such as losing a competition or a job, or in association with physical illness, a career setback, or other major life stress. It is important to keep in mind that the meaning of an event (i.e., its symbolic significance) may be more important to the patient than the event itself. An example follows.

A 45-year-old violinist became acutely depressed when she lost the opportunity (because of an overuse disorder) to play a concerto. She has had similar problems before. But this particular concerto was written especially for her, and the guilt she felt for not being able to please the composer made her depression so unbearable that she was forced to seek professional help.

Depressive illnesses can also have an insidious onset, with no known or identifiable precipitants. Biological abnormalities in synaptic transmission of norepinephrine and serotonin are suspected to be among the causes of some depressions.

A 28-year-old trombone player has had recurring depressive episodes since adolescence, when he discovered that he is gay. They usually begin rather gradually in the fall, become most severe around the holidays, when he feels exceedingly lonely and vulnerable, and abate in the spring. He had had one manic episode (elation, excitement, unrealistic thinking, poor impulse control) lasting 3 weeks in which he spent a lot of money foolishly, and was nearly arrested for misconduct.

Although most depressions are self-limited and have a benign course, some (20% in our series) become chronic and lead to varying amounts of disability. Other complications include mania, which is an abnormal upswing in mood, as mentioned above, accompanied by overactivity, racing thoughts, and often marked aggressiveness. In the most severe depressions and manias, patients are at risk of losing the ability to judge their condition properly, and may thus believe that neglectful, suicidal, or other maladaptive behavior is acceptable. The long-term consequences may be disastrous for a performer's career.

A depressed 53-year-old virtuoso pianist decided to take his own life with an overdose of barbiturates. Expecting to die, he lay down on the floor with his chin resting on his left hand. When found in a coma 4 days later, the soft tissues of his palm had started to become necrotic. Emergency surgery led to complications, and his hand had been crippled ever since. He is no longer able to perform in public.

Creative artists, composers, designers, playwrights, etc. not infrequently report a mania-like excitement associated with moments of "inspiration" when they become highly productive and may indeed achieve remarkable results. There is a feeling of elation and unquenchable enthusiasm. New ideas come quickly and generously into consciousness. Work seems effortless; sleeping and eating may not seem necessary; there is sometimes an associated hypersexuality. After these creative upswings there often are "letdowns." The artist may feel drained, exhausted, and frankly depressed. A related condition called *postperformance depression* has been described (13). As indicated earlier, whether such cycles of "creative depression" are subclinical variants of bipolar affective disorder is a moot point. It is important for the physician working with performers to be aware of the difference, because artists tend to resent the implication that creative-depressive syndromes, which they enjoy and find socially desirable, constitute psychopathological states.

Treatment of affective disorders always necessitates psychotherapy. Hospitalization may be indicated for the evaluation of severe ("psychotic") states when the patient loses touch with reality and needs protection. Tricyclic antidepressants (e.g., nortriptyline hydrochloride) or monoamine oxidase (MAO) inhibitors (e.g., phenelzine sulfate) are frequently prescribed. For bipolar or manic-depressive disorders, lithium and related medications may be desirable for the control of cyclic mood swings and to prevent recurrence (14). Strict attention must be paid to possible side effects of these medications (such as tremor or dizziness) to prevent hindrance of the patient's functional ability to perform. Chronic depressions may respond well to group therapy, behavior modification, and other approaches. Because patients with affective disorders and anxiety states (see below) constitute such a large proportion of the caseload of most clinical programs, it is often desirable to include nonmedical personnel, clinical psychologists, and clinical social workers in the professional team to assist with the necessary but time-consuming counseling and psychotherapy.

ANXIETY AMONG PERFORMERS

Three forms of anxiety disorder are found among artists. The most common is the sense of unpleasant apprehension or foreboding with the "stagefright" or "performance anxiety" that precedes a public appearance. The symptoms are so well known that it hardly seems necessary to list them here. They include fearsome fantasies about not doing one's best, making mistakes, having memory slips; and various physical symptoms like restlessness, gastrointestinal distress, excess sweating, cold skin, tachycardia, and respiratory discomfort, all evidence of autonomic nervous system hyperarousal (15). Most performers learn to tolerate these symptoms, which are often believed to enhance the excitement of a performance. They may seek relief through hypnosis, meditation, and other methods which do not necessarily involve medical personnel. Patients with performance anxiety who are admitted to our program usually have associated conditions, most frequently depressive disorders or drug abuse problems.

Panic is the most intense form of anxiety and often occurs in the form of acute "attacks" in which the patient is extremely restless, has numerous physical symptoms, and experiences a ghastly fear of catastrophe, not uncommonly including the fear of going mad or dying. There is strong evidence for a genetic factor, and the psychosocial stresses often include fantasies of separation or actual loss of security and acceptance. One of the best descriptions of a panic attack was given by the composer Robert Schumann, at age 23 (16).

> The most terrifying thought suddenly occurred to me, that of "losing my mind." It overwhelmed me so violently, that all consolation and every prayer became ineffective. The anxiety drove me from place to place—my breathing was disrupted by the idea "what would happen if you can no longer think?" In my endlessly terrible excitement, I ran to a doctor, told him everything, that I often seemed to lose my senses, that I didn't know where to turn because of the anxiety, yes, that I could not guarantee whether in such a condition of utter helplessness, I might not raise a hand against my own life

With generalized or chronic anxiety, the symptoms persist and lead to complications such as social withdrawal, agoraphobia, and possibly obsessive-compulsive behavior, not to mention intensification of the physical symptoms mentioned above. Sleep is often disturbed, nightmares are common; and the patient's life is restricted in many unpleasant ways. The possibility that chronic or recurring anxiety states are associated with a history of trauma or abuse must always be considered, as in the following case of a performer who had a posttraumatic stress disorder.

Perspiration literally dripped from the hands of this 19-year-old violinist whenever he played his instrument. A victim of war in Asia, he grew up under conditions of extreme danger and insecurity. Escaping from his homeland as a child, he nearly drowned. After his father became disabled following a stroke 4 years ago, the patient developed insomnia, irritability, and many recurring fears. He is chronically restless, has difficulty making friends, feels overambitious yet pessimistic, and cannot concentrate.

Psychotherapy, behavior modification, and desensitization techniques are effective in the treatment of anxiety (17). Patients must learn to tolerate their distress and gain insight into those factors which precipitate or worsen the symptoms. Benzodiazepines [e.g., alprazolam (Xanax)] produce effective relief but may lead to habituation. Beta-blockers [e.g., propranolol (Inderal)] taken in small doses (10 to 30 mg 1 hour before going on stage) can ameliorate many of the undesirable symptoms of performance anxiety. Antidepressants can also be useful in treating panic states by reducing severity and frequency of attacks (18). It should be emphasized that the taking of medication is hazardous unless properly supervised by a physician. All drugs have side effects, and performers who use them should be aware of the risks.

PERSONALITY STYLES AND PERSONALITY DISORDERS OF PERFORMING ARTISTS

Because all psychiatric disorders express themselves through the personality, and because certain illnesses such as chronic schizophrenia, severe obsessive-compulsive disorder, and long-term depression may actually deform the personality in significant ways, it is essential to focus on the personality style of every performer who seeks medical help. This can be done best by exploring the patient's daily activities, especially those pertaining to his involvement with music, dancing, acting, etc.; his growth and personality development as an artist; and his relationships with people both within and outside his work. Each phase of the life cycle brings with it certain coping tasks and responsibilities which can lead to successes or failures (19).

Infancy and Childhood

Interest in sound and movement usually begins to develop during infancy as a natural consequence of the rhythmic and tonal experiences a child has while being rocked, sung to, played with, or punished. The baby depends upon older people for protection, nourishment, comfort, and love; and thorugh its own psychobiological responses—crying, sucking, cooing, smiling, tensing, relaxing, etc.—provides satisfaction as well as frustration to these caregivers. A range of basic emotions, including pleasure, pain, fear, anger, sadness, and surprise is thus elaborated through the network of reciprocal soundmaking, movements, gestures, and other so-called nonverbal communications. Parents who enjoy singing, dancing, etc. will find it easy to reinforce the innate rhythmicality and soundmaking of their children (20). Speech, language, and verbal communication are added to this early repertoire after the second year of life, and will be strongly emphasized once the child enters school. At this point the individual is expected to socialize, to conform to the expectations of teachers, and to establish loyalties and collaborations with peers.

Musical training often begins during this critical early phase of psychological development; thus lending certain distinctive qualities to the personality which may result in feelings of differentness or specialness when the child compares himself to others who are not similarly involved in an art form. Parental support is of great importance in helping the child to cope with these feelings (21). Another distinguishing feature of the artistic personality is its intense involvement with the medium of expression, as with the musical instrument or the technique of dancing. Some children make choices on their own regarding an art form or an instrument after observing with admiration and wonder their parents, older siblings, neighbors, or public figures in concerts, movies, or television. Such a child, upon choosing participation in artistic education, then has a willing, self-motivated quality that may enhance his identification with, and closeness (real or imagined) to, these external models. Other children are brought to an artistic medium under some duress from parents and teachers. Thus, the patterns of attachment to and dependence upon those to whom he is already tied biologically and socially are modified by virtue of the artistic behavior.

If a parent is at the same time the teacher of music or dance, as not infrequently happens in families that encourage artistic expression, the child's sense of autonomy and individuality, which is part of personality development, will also be affected. We have seen complicated problems arise from this configuration, which can lead to great artistic success, but also considerable skewing in personality development.

A 22-year-old virtuoso cellist is afflicted with recurring panic attacks in which she precipitates crises that affect her career. For example, she will fail to appear at scheduled concerts, or create confusion in her friends and colleagues by suddenly disappearing, making demands that are unfulfillable, or behaving in a histrionic and sexually provocative manner, even though she has never been physically intimate and fears closeness. The background history shows that her father was an alcoholic businessman who married a cellist after his divorce. The new wife became the patient's teacher. Every attachment to a music teacher since then has been fraught with conflict and ambivalence.

Adolescence is a time of rapid physical growth, sexual maturation, and identity formation. Peer relationships become more influential as parental input fades. However, in the case of performing artists this pattern is often modified by the presence of a music or dance teacher who exerts control and provides direction, thus instilling moral standards and ethical attitudes which can continue to influence the development of personality in lasting ways. This is especially noticeable when a child is gifted and triumphs early, with the result that he or she leaves the family circle prematurely. The teacher then becomes an extension of parental authority, a sort of "transitional object" significantly influencing the adolescent's developing attitudes in regard to education, career choice, friendships, and even sexual identity.

A 30-year-old pianist, in psychotherapy for recurring depression and a deep-seated sense of insecurity, manifested what can best be described as a "dependent" personality style. She needs constant reassurance about her playing which was of a very high calibre, and has enormous difficulty making decisions on her own. Pertinent in her background is the fact that she had a close, loving family but was the only child interested in music and thus became "special" at an early age, when her father pushed her to perform while her mother, preferring that she become "a normal child," tried to hold her back. During a critical phase of her adolescence, she was "adopted" by a music teacher who insisted on physical intimacy. Although she is now happily married, she retains some dysphoric sexual memories of this relationship, and resists her own as well as her husband's interest in having children.

Choosing an Instrument

An important factor which seems to impact on personality style, and perhaps even has some effect on symptom formation, is the kind of instrument a child chooses or accepts in order to express his musical impulses. The piano, for example, is often seen as part of the furnishing of a household, and even when acquired for the specific purpose of bringing up musical children, is often regarded as something of value for the entire family. This is in contrast to clarinets, trumpets, violins, or other musical instruments which the child may bring home from school, is able to carry to a friend's house, or can play outdoors with a band. Keyboard instruments in general tend to encourage solitude; one can perform entire works on them without needing an accompanist or coperformer. Organs arc often associated with the capacity for filling up large spaces, churches, and auditoriums with sound, and many organists enjoy the feeling of power felt in playing this instrument. On the other hand, guitars, violins, and other string instruments tend to enhance socialization, since the performer has to seek out other musicians for chamber music and orchestral playing. Even the size of an instrument can have a significant effect on personality development.

A thirty-five-year-old double bass player has serious overuse problems and complains about the lack of satisfaction with his career as a professional musician. He was a fearful, lonely person, "narcissistic" in the sense of needing always to be told how well he plays and preoccupied with his own success to the detriment of developing empathy for others. His father was a very busy man who seldom had time to play with his children. His mother was unusually neat and resented having children because they were too "messy." As the youngest and smallest member of the family, the patient deliberately chose to play the double bass because he felt that it might help him to compensate for his small stature. But he has remained small, and has had serious technical difficulty with this instrument, which he cannot give up or exchange for something that can be played more comfortably.

Competitiveness

Even before performers reach adulthood, competitiveness looms as a major factor in their personality development. A biological component seems to be of significance here, since competition may already exist among twins before they are born (22), and it is known that temperamental differences in regard to vigor and alertness are discernible at birth (23). Sibling rivalry can serve to enhance competitiveness in some children, but may inhibit it in others. Schools tend to encourage competition by grading the work students do, and there are many music teachers who encourage competitiveness by having their students perform and "show off" to each other. The "juries" system in music conservatories is supposed to promote the survival of the fittest and best students, and considering the reality of life in the performing arts, where success in competitions and auditions is often essential to one's career, all of this may be desirable. Competitiveness may also be a factor in strengthening the quest for technical perfection. But serious criticism has been leveled against extreme competitiveness because of its emphasis on success at the expense of artistry. It may even be that the highly competitive environment of music conservatories and dance schools fosters an unhealthy atmosphere of overwork ("workaholism"), or produces one-sided, constricted personalities among performers (24).

A flutist in her early 20s calls regularly to request renewal of her medication (propranolol) for performance anxiety. She has been precociously successful since the age of 8, when a schoolteacher gave her a flute and said, "It will be a challenge for you to be outstanding." Throughout her years at a leading music conservatory, she was pushed by a demanding instructor, and it gave her great pride to do better than the other students. Since graduation she has supported herself by playing in professional orchestras, and she regularly enters auditions for better positions and seeks additional work. A complication is that she usually misses out on "normal" life activities such as dating, vacations, or "just taking it easy for a while."

The Adult Performing Artist

Adulthood calls for the consolidation of personality resources and the making of commitments which have long-range effects on a performer's career. Decisions regarding marriage and parenthood, for example, can pose enormous challenges for artists who must be constantly on the go, traveling from city to city, meeting contractual obligations, or submitting to the demands of a string quartet, ballet company, or other structured system incompatible with a "normal" life style. The denial of psychobiological needs for intimacy, privacy, and family life can only go so far. Sooner or later every artist must face the fact that he is a human being. This recognition may even enhance his artistry.

The 29-year-old son of a distinguished physicist has excelled on the violin since early childhood, won scholarships, had the best teachers, but never succeeded as a virtuoso. In his late teens he became interested in chamber music and formed a professional string quartet. But with the loss of one of the members, his quartet disbanded, and the patient was forced to accept an orchestral "job" that he found less than fully satisfying.

He presented with symptoms of depression, indecisiveness, and anxiety about the future, coupled with a sense that he was not doing as well as his father. Offers to play in leading orchestras were rejected. Finally, it was his wife's pregnancy and the arrival of a healthy baby which allowed him to see that he can be the equal of his father. Thereafter he accepted regular employment in a studio orchestra.

The mid-life period forces into consciousness a recognition of unfulfilled goals and irremediable career disappointments. Professional "burnout" may then become a problem for the artist, just as for other highly trained and strongly motivated individuals. Some personalities cope with this stress by developing new interests; others fall into dejection and apathy. For the superstar there is the danger of losing ground, of being supplanted in the fickle eye of the public by younger and more glamorous artists. Along with these psychosocial dilemmas often come the first signs of loss of physical competence or actual disability. Not to be performing is one of the most serious stresses for an artist who has been on stage since childhood, and whose self-esteem depends heavily on public acclaim. Dancers are more vulnerable in this respect than musicians since, like an athletic career, dancing, especially for men, usually cannot continue effectively past the fourth decade.

A 43-year-old dancer is struggling to compete as a choreographer, but with little success. His main love in life is the ballet. Having had numerous love affairs, he now finds himself with no permanent mate, and is losing physical attractiveness, which adds to his depression. Alcohol binges make matters worse, and he tries to shore up his flagging morale by using cocaine. His angry, defensive, "paranoid" personality style leads him to blame others for his own weaknesses, and undermines whatever opportunities come along for him to work as a teacher.

Different patterns of aging can be observed among artists. Some great personalities like Arthur Rubinstein or Alexsandra Danilova, seem ageless and continue to do their work as performers or teachers until physical disability intervenes. Retirement poses a threat because of the loss of accustomed patterns of daily activity. The fear of growing old may be a factor among those artists who have had lifelong insecurities. Interestingly, it is the orchestral musician who often faces retirement most gracefully, feeling relieved to be able to move out of the ritualized grind of daily rehearsals and concerts into less demanding modes of living (25). Economic factors are obviously important, since it is easier for a performer to retire when there is security through savings, investments, or pension programs. But psychosocial conflicts may make this difficult.

A 65-year-old professional singer seeks help because he is afraid he may have cancer of the larynx, despite numerous consultations with otolaryngologists who can detect no structural abnormality. His voice sounds tearful, and a recent episode of the voice "breaking" makes him reluctant to continue to sing in public. Further discussion reveals that he has had lifelong problems with competition, and that he is especially worried about an excellent younger singer who is waiting to take his place as soloist in the church choir where both of them work. The patient could easily retire on his savings, but while his wife wants to travel and spend more time with their children, he prefers to go on singing.

Psychotherapy is the treatment of choice for problems that involve the performer's personality and psychological development. Crisis intervention may suffice with immediate, acute difficulties that can be resolved through counseling and by giving advice. For more persistent disorders, it is necessary to plan a sequence of interviews over periods of time ranging from weeks to months. Psychoanalysis on a daily basis, or psychoanalytic psychotherapy twice a week usually go more deeply into developmental issues, and, depending on the therapist's philosophy and training, may include the unraveling of unconscious dynamics and restructuring of the personality. Successful artists tend to avoid so intense and costly a form of treatment, while less successful ones usually cannot afford it (26). Essential for psychotherapy to proceed is the development of trust and empathy between patient and therapist. Participants in psychotherapy must be self-revealing, emotionally honest, and willing to come to grips with the vast differences between reality and fantasy in the psyche. Support, reassurance, explanation, and interpretation are the tools of the psychotherapist's trade, and it is always important to focus on relevant issues (27). For this reason, familiarity with the performing arts is helpful.

SOMATOFORM DISORDERS

Many performers who seek help from arts medicine programs have physical complaints, most commonly pain, fatigue, weakness, or functional disabilities related to singing, playing an instrument, or dancing. The responsibility of the physician is first of all to locate the causes and identify the pathological processes involved. If neither the symptoms nor the findings resemble a medical condition, and when there is no plausible explanation for the physical complaints, diagnoses like somatization disorder, conversion disorder, somatoform pain disorder, or hypochondriasis may be justified. However, such a diagnosis cannot be made with conviction unless a psychodynamic formulation based on understanding of the personality, motivations, conflicts, and primary as well as secondary gains emerges from discussion with the patient and his family, friends, or coworkers. Primary gain means that the patient obtains relief from anxiety, depression, or other intolerable emotions by virtue of having physical symptoms. Secondary gain refers to social benefits (e.g., relief from unwanted obligations) and economic rewards (e.g., disability payments) associated with being an invalid.

A 41-year-old trombone player who looks considerably younger and appears in robust health complains of "asthma," "epilepsy," and "a blockage to my brain and heart." Repeated physical evaluations, laboratory tests, and CT scans at major medical centers have confirmed none of these conditions, nor any other physical diseases. The developmental history shows that his father was abusive toward the children, his mother abandoned them, and the patient himself has never formed an emotional attachment to a man or a woman. He learned to play trombone in a school band, and after graduating from high school, worked professionally until age 28, when he decided to go to college. Unable to graduate, he has never returned to music. After working for a while as a cab driver, he decided to apply for disability because "my mouth is too dry for me to play my instrument, and nobody can find the right glasses for me to read the notes."

Treatment of somatoform disorders usually calls for a team approach, with physicians and physical therapists working to help the patient achieve better understanding of normal versus pathological body functions, while psychotherapists attend to the patient's emotional needs. Unfortunately, when there are marked secondary gains and the patient is not motivated to abandon the role of a sick person, little can be done to reverse these conditions (28). They are not infrequently associated with severe personality disorders or other major psychiatric illnesses.

SCHIZOPHRENIC DISORDERS AMONG PERFORMING ARTISTS

Schizophrenia refers to a group of mental disorders characterized by primary disturbances in thinking and social adaptation. Depending on the diagnostic criteria used, these illnesses afflict 1% to 2% of the general population. The presenting symptoms (thought disorganization, delusions, hallucinations, and inappropriate behavior) may show up acutely and subside quickly.

A 17-year-old cello student is brought to the emergency room after midnight with a fractured femur resulting from a bicycle accident. Voices have been telling him to drive as fast as possible, without lights. Two years ago he was hospitalized after becoming mute and socially withdrawn, isolating himself in a cave without food, and talking about "shooting" someone with his hunting rifle. Throughout his course on the orthopedic ward, he was delusional, believed himself to be a special messenger of God, heard voices, showed odd behavior, and required neuroleptic medication.

Schizophrenia may also have a gradual, insidious onset, and a tendency to chronicity. Adolescence and early adulthood seem to be times of high risk for the development of this disease (hence the older term *dementia praecox*). The famous dancer Vaslav Nijinsky is often thought to have been schizophrenic, but recent research shows that his diagnosis was actually "catatonia," an illness which nowadays is usually considered to be a form of bipolar affective disorder (29). Pianist John Ogdon's career was mercilessly undermined by a type of schizophrenic disorder (30). Patients who manifest symptoms of both schizophrenia and affective disorder are usually diagnosed as suffering from "schizo-affective" disorder. The cause of these illnesses is not known, but a genetic predisposition has long been suspected; excessive dopamine secretion may be a significant contributing factor; psychosocial stressors seem important in precipitating and/or prolonging the illness; and neurodegenerative changes have been found in chronic cases (31). Due to the need for maintaining a generally outgoing personality and an effective social adaptation in order to pursue a career as a performer, schizophrenia can be one of the most disabling conditions among musicians, actors, and dancers.

A 45-year-old violinist requests help because "my vibrato is unsteady." His background shows extensive musical training by outstanding teachers and a very supportive, musical family. But extreme social awkwardness and delusional thinking in adolescence required the interruption of his studies. He has been hospitalized several times. When asked to demonstrate the problem with his violin playing, he "forgot" to bring his shoulder pad, manifested great clumsiness in unpacking his instrument, and played beautifully, except for noticeable stiffness in his bow arm. He harbors a delusion of emitting pungent and disturbing odors, hence can barely socialize and makes music only with his mother, who plays the piano.

Treatment of schizophrenia is both behavioral and pharmacological. Neuroleptic medication (e.g., haloperidol) is effective in reducing the hallucinations and delusions, but poses problems in long-term management because of the risk of neuromuscular side effects (such as tardive dyskinesia) which are extremely undesirable for performers. Beta-blockers (e.g., propranolol) can be very helpful in controlling the severe anxiety experienced by many schizophrenic patients. Lithium carbonate and tricyclic antidepressants help to suppress symptoms in those illnesses which have a prominent affective component. Social support is absolutely essential to help these patients in regulating their daily lives, hence the need for flexible hospital facilities, day-care centers, etc. (Nijinsky and Ogdon both married strong, managerial wives who undoubtedly helped them to live better lives). Individual psychotherapy requires a high degree of tolerance for social deviance, as well as great sensitivity in judging the patient's emotional rapport (32).

OTHER CONDITIONS NECESSITATING PSYCHIATRIC CARE FOR PERFORMERS

Bulimia/anorexia is a disorder seen more frequently among dancers than other performers, and will therefore be discussed in the appropriate chapter of this book. Less serious appetite disorders, however—overeating, fad dieting, unrealistic concern with weight, and worry about physical appearance—are not infrequently associated with many of the illnesses described above. For this reason, a dietician is part of our team and helps those singers, instrumentalists, and dancers who are troubled in this area. Group therapy is a useful adjuvant in long-term treatment, and a number of our patients have found weight-control organizations to be beneficial.

Substance abuse disorders, too, constitute a serious difficulty for which we rely on community resources such as Alcoholics Anonymous, ALANON, and drug counseling centers. Unfortunately, some of the more severely addicted performers, especially in the rock-and-roll world, persist in taking street drugs and repeatedly endanger their lives. Two earlier drug-related fatalities in San Francisco (Janis Joplin and Michael Bloomfield) received wide publicity through news media, which was a factor in setting up specialized drug programs for rock musicians, and undoubtedly helped to spark interest in the concept of the "Health Program for Performing Artists" in our community. A specialized treatment program for treatment of the alcohol- or drug-dependent person may require years of professional care.

A 38-year-old percussionist, Juilliard-trained, began abusing amphetamines, marijuana, LSD, and other readily available drugs in his 20s and was hospitalized for six months, after which he gave up music for 10 years. Return to his career, and employment in a symphony orchestra brought back severe performance anxiety. He started to drink heavily, passed out during a rehearsal, and failed to show up for a concert. His rehabilitation required supportive psychotherapy, abstinence from alcohol, strict control of unprescribed medication, and the use of beta-blockers and benzodiazepines for control of severe anxiety. After becoming a father, he decided to quit playing professionally for a while and go into business.

Homosexuality is no longer considered a psychiatric disease, and for this reason will be discussed only very briefly here. Four of our patients were sufficiently disturbed about their sexual orientation to include this among their reasons for seeking professional help. One of them, a gay activist actor, is severely depressed because he has not been able to form a satisfactory attachment and, before the AIDS epidemic, persisted in being wildly promiscuous, often with drug abuse complicating his behavior. Another gay man, a woodwind player, has been seeing many doctors because of "overuse" disorder. In our program he disclosed for the first time an agonizing conflict between separating from his AIDS- disabled lover of 5 years and continuing to care for this man in a supportive and affectionate manner. Another patient, a female brass player, sought help because of her recurring problem of falling in love with women, getting overly attached to them, then pulling out of the relationship and suffering intense separation anxiety. The fourth patient, a very prominent performer, saw himself trapped in a lamentable conflict between wishing to marry the woman he loved and his desire to have casual homosexual encounters.

Problems associated with organic brain disease can be particularly frightening and disabling for performing artists, who since childhood have perfected their bodily equipment in pursuit of artistic goals. One patient, a well-known pianist, had a sudden stroke at age 65 and lost control of his left hand. A conductor with early Alzheimer's disease could no longer remember his scores or give proper directions to the orchestra; he had to consider retirement.

Having access to the diagnostic and therapeutic resources of a major medical center is obviously of great benefit when arts medicine programs assume the responsibility of caring for performers. For example, a symphony violist complained of feeling drowsy and nodding off during rehearsals. With medical evaluation he was found to be afflicted with sleep apnea, a condition which had never been properly treated in the past.

SUMMARY AND CONCLUSION

Psychiatric disorders constitute a significant portion of the medical problems of performing artists. The conditions of primary concern are depression and anxiety. However, patients can present with a variety of other syndromes, including bipolar disorder, schizophrenia, and somatoform disease. For this reason, it is essential that specialists in this field be part of the performing arts medicine team, to provide adequate consultation and specific treatment.

Little is presently known about the effects of psychotropic medication upon musicians, dancers, and actors in terms of their emotional experiences before, during, and after performances. There also is a need for carefully designed research into the developmental aspects of musical behavior, and the possible connections between personality style and susceptibility to psychiatric disease among performers.

REFERENCES

1. Becker G. *The mad genius controversy: a study in the sociology of deviance*. Beverly Hills: Sage Publications, 1978.
2. Andreasen NC. Creativity and mental illness: prevalence rates in writers and their first-degree relatives. *American Journal of Psychiatry* 1987; 144(12):1288–1292.
3. See also Jamison KR. Manic-depressive illness and accomplishment: creativity, leadership, and social class. In: Goodwin FK, Jamison KR, eds. *Manic-depressive illness*. New York: Oxford University Press (in press).
4. Ostwald P. *Schumann, the inner voices of a musical genius*. Boston: Northeastern, 1985.
5. Pickering G. *Creative malady*. London: Oxford University Press, 1974.

6. Charness M. Personal communication.
7. Ruesch J. *Knowledge in action.* New York: Aronson, 1975.
8. Middlestadt SE, Fishbein M. Health and occupational correlates of perceived occupational stress in symphony orchestra musicians. *Journal of Occupational Medicine* 1988;3(9):687–692.
9. Cohen BJ, Kupersmith JRF. A study of SCL-90 scores of 87 performing artists seeking psychotherapy. *Med Probl Perform Art* 1986;1:140–142.
10. Ostwald P. How the patient communicates about disease with the doctor. In: *Approaches to semiotics*, Sebeok TA, Hayes AS, Bateson MC, eds. The Hague: Mouton, 1964:11–34.
11. American Psychiatric Association, *Diagnostic and Statistical Manual of Mental Disorders*, 3rd ed., revised. Washington, D.C.: American Psychiatric Association Press, 1987.
12. Mann JJ, ed. *The phenomenology of depression.* New York: Human Sciences Press, 1988.
13. Robson BE, Gillies E. Post-performance depression in arts students. *Med Probl Perform Art* 1987;2:137–141.
14. Consensus developmental panel, mood disorders; pharmacologic prevention of recurrences. *American Journal of Psychiatry* 1985;142:469.
15. Aronson T, Logue C. Phenomenology of panic attacks; a descriptive study of panic disorder. *Journal of Clinical Psychiatry* 1988; 49(1):8–13.
16. Ostwald P. *Schumann*, p.401.
17. Lehrer PM. Finding a way to manage performance anxiety: the problems and promises of science. Private publications based on a paper given at the International Society for the Study of Tension in Performance, 1983.
18. Lydiard R, et al. Recent advances in the psychopharmacological treatment of anxiety disorders. *Hospital and Community Psychiatry* 1988; 39(11):1157–1166.
19. Erikson EH. *Identity and the life cycle.* New York: Norton, 1980.
20. Ostwald PF, Morrison D. Music in the organization of childhood experience. In: Morrison DC, ed. *Organizing early experience; imagination and cognition in childhood.* Amityville, New York: Baywood, 1988;54–73.
21. Robson B. Paper presented at the Seventh Annual Symposium on Medical Problems of Musicians and Dancers, Snowmass, Colorado, 1989.
22. Ostwald P, Freedman DG, Kurtz JH. Vocalization of infant twins. In: Ostwald P, ed. *The semiotics of human sound.* The Hague: Mouton, 1973;313–324.
23. Thomas A, Chess S. *Temperament and development.* New York: Brunner/Mazel, 1977.
24. Gelber G. Psychological development of the conservatory student. In: eds. Roehman FL, Wilson FR, *The biology of music making.* Proceedings of the 1984 Denver conference, 1988; 3–15.
25. Smith DWE. *Aging and the careers of symphony orchestra musicians. Med Prob Perform Art* 1989; 4:81–85.
26. Gedo JE. Some differences in creativity in performers and other artists. *Med Probl Perform Art.* 1989; 4:15–19.
27. Greenson RR. *The technique and practice of psychoanalysis.* New York: International Universities Press, 1967.
28. Ford CV. *The somatizing disorders: illness as a way of life.* New York: Elsevier, 1983.
29. Ostwald P. *Vaslav Nijinsky: dancer and madman.* New York: Lyle Stuart, in press.
30. Longworth RC. When titans crumble; John Ogdon's agonizing battle to recover a dream. *Chicago Tribune* April 30, 1989.
31. Stafanis CN, Rabavilas AD. *Schizophrenia: recent biosocial developments.* New York: Human Sciences Press, 1988.
32. McGlashan TH, Keats CJ. *Schizophrenia: treatment process and outcome.* Washington, D.C.: American Psychiatric Press, 1989.

Textbook of Performing Arts Medicine, edited by R. T. Sataloff, A. Brandfonbrener, and R. Lederman. Raven Press, Ltd., New York © 1991.

11

Psychological Aspects of the Development of Exceptional Young Performers and Prodigies

Kyle D. Pruett

Clinical Professor of Psychiatry, Yale Child Study Center, Yale University, New Haven, Connecticut 06510

The expression of exceptional ability in the performing arts in the early years inspires wonder, excitement, and not a little envy. Precocious specialness of any kind has marked children for elevation, exploitation, and scrutiny for centuries. Slowly, we have come to realize that, although such talent may dazzle early on, there is no guarantee it will not flicker, sputter, change course, or simply expire over time. The problem is that exceptional talent, whether or not it is prodigious, is but one piece of a whole life that is being carried down the swift moving currents of maturation and development. There is more myth and folklore about this specialness than there is science, although a better balance is coming. There has been some reluctance to study this circumstance, lest it somehow be muted or knocked off course by the mere act of examining it. As Stephen Hawking (1) explains, the problem of shining a probative light on something is that it moves when illuminated. Nevertheless, such reluctance is slowly yielding to another more nurturing, less worshipful impulse to assist children, families, and educators to support, instead of control, the healthy evolution of remarkable talent so that it remains in concert with life, not vice versa.

In this chapter we will examine suppositions and data regarding psychological development and what psychological vulnerabilities and risks there may be in the expression of exceptional performing arts ability in young children and prodigies. Those problems that do seem to be real and present will then be reviewed in the context of strategies for prevention and intervention.

Before examining some of the suppositions and prejudices that lace this topic, a word about lumping prodigies and exceptional young performers together for discussion, even though they may not, and indeed probably do not, share many vicissitudes as groups. What they *do* share is the fact that they are almost never self-proclaimed as either, but instead are so depicted by highly subjective social criteria.

The criteria are a group of expectations that define *what* these children are doing and *that* they are doing it (sometimes in itself a wonder) much earlier than expected. This is both fascinating and troubling. The *Oxford English Dictionary* reveals to us our own hopes and fears about this phenomenon in the myriad meanings given by the editors for the word *prodigy*. First: "an amazing, marvelous thing, especially something out of the ordinary course of nature; something abnormal or monstrous." Second: "anything that causes wonder, astonishment." Third: "a person endowed with some quality which excites wonder, especially a child of precocious genius." Fourth (and this is what is so inauspicious for the child): "something extraordinary from which omens are drawn; a portent." Finally, it is worth noting that "prodigy" and "prodigal" share the same root. This apposition hints at the cost to the child and family of the often extravagant expenditure of assets of all kinds.

Although prodigies are rare, they share certain psychological and developmental vicissitudes with young talented performers. Because the latter group is larger, its members are more likely to be seen by clinicians for whatever reasons, and I have subsequently grouped the two categories together for discussion. I will distinguish them as groups when appropriate to do so.

Here is a brief catalog of the common assumptions about the young talented performer's susceptibility to psychological trouble (sooner or later) because of, or in spite of, his talent. First, the child's talent renders him an alien in his generation, designated as different, driving him to be a loner, albeit an exquisite one. Second, social skills suffer a disuse atrophy because of the exclusive focus on developing the performing art. Third, the child's "sensitivity" renders him vulnerable to conflict and frustration in other spheres of his life. Fourth, the dazzling talent stems from an intense inner reservoir of unique perception and passion that leads to an overall lack of stability and personality structure, growth, and development. Fifth, this talent is part of a wider aura of exceptional value and ability, boosting other functions, such as cognition, to higher ability as well. Sixth, his talent is the hothouse propagation of overinvolved parents, struggling to bring to fruition some unfinished aspect of themselves by fostering the hypertrophy of this one aspect of their child's developmental repertoire. This obviously requires the child's collusion at some point.

Many of these assumptions about the psychological characteristics of musical aptitude, in particular, are rooted in the attempt early in this century to study the development of musical genius. The Pannenborgs (2), Feis (3), and Kretschmer (4), in conducting individual retrospective studies of talent, concluded that musicians, as a group, were emotional, often mentally unstable, and given to hysteria and immature behaviors. These studies, as well as other "reflections" on the development of musical talent, as seen in personal narratives and autobiographies, while occasionally illuminating, tend to generate more heat than light. They make highly interesting psychohistorical reading, but the tyranny of the unconscious, failed and fulfilled wishes, the sometimes startling omissions of events and facts all combine to shape a *remembered* life. This remembered life is subject to selective memory, emotional trauma and idealization, leading to a list of distractions which is endless. Such descriptions may be quite intriguing, but they are *not* the actual story of the evolution of a child's giftedness. Many such historical analyses leave us with the frequent impression that a musician's creative life begins at or after puberty and that, with the exception of a musical parent here or there and a serendipitous choice of instrument, not many other forces are at work.

As to the first assumption, the issue of feeling outside one's own group, for the very young child this could mean his family, and there are a variety of contributors who share this observation. Ostwald (5) and, to a much larger extent, Pollock (6) observe as clinicians that the artist is, by dint of his talent alone, set apart from his friends and family, and that with this outsiderness comes, *parri passu*, a burden of vulnerability.

Vulnerability may be present, but the outside world will never learn about it unless it interacts with some environmental factor which then turns that vulnerability into a risk—environmental factors such as unsupportive parental or educator attitudes toward the child's talent or an actively hostile social response to the child's talent from classmates or siblings. Then the vulnerability becomes a risk factor which may require remediation of some sort for the child's special ability to remain free enough of conflict for it to enjoy fruition.

As for the elicitation of particular performing arts psychological profiles that look at issues such as "sensitivity" or "social isolation," we know almost nothing about children. As for adults, Cohen and Kupersmith (7) conclude, in their study of 87 performing artists who requested psychological services at a performing arts clinic, that they differed from nonperforming psychotherapy outpatients in that the overall severity of their symptoms was less. As a group, they tended to have comparatively strong defenses: "Their creativity and often rigorous training may be the basis of the relative intensification of ego strengths." For adolescents, there is some data to suggest that general (not necessarily exceptional) musicianship may actually be related to superior, not deficient, social skills and adjustment (8,9). It is wise to resist the temptation to extend these findings retrospectively to the evolution of specialness in children. It simply is not valid.

As to the relationship between exceptional talent and other forms of excellence, we have merely to look at the curious relationship between measured intelligence and musical aptitude (not necessarily exceptional skill). Gordon (10) summarizes his own research, along with that of Colwel (11) and Moore (12), by concluding that verbal and nonverbal general intelligence scores were found to be almost identical in musical and nonmusical students:

> It is possible to interpret the foregoing research as indicating that intelligent persons are not musical but that musical persons are intelligent. It must be remembered, however, that the correlation between measures of general intelligence and general creativity (not necessarily musical creativity) has been found to be not so high as anticipated by early researchers and lay persons.

As to the final assumption about the relationship between parental misuse of a child's promise as a performer and that child's psychological risk, we have only anecdotal data. Much of those data are often strong and compelling in individual cases. The process of such misuse is amply documented in retrospective case studies in Alice Miller's *The Drama of the Gifted Child* (13), and outlines the child's talent as a mechanism to guarantee an existential, secure relationship with a psychologically disabled nurturing object who can provide it in no other way. In a related conceptualization, Babikian (14) concludes from his own psychoanalytic treatment experience with 14 performing adult musicians that the superego (or conscience) of the young artist plays a major role in the training of the performing artist. The conscience, derived as it is from early parent–child interaction, can assist in the development of talent through its imposition of discipline and expectations. It extracts a heavy toll on the emotional life of the performer throughout the life cycle, however. Intriguing and erudite as these observations are, there is no clue as to how widespread such entanglements, per se, are and how often they are brought to bear in seminal ways to influence the development of exceptional performing abilities, as opposed to other types of compensation.

Having reviewed what little substance there is to many of these assumptions, I should like to turn to more substantive contributions to our understanding of the development of exceptional young performers and prodigies, beginning with some distinguishing features of prodigies in the few cases where we seem to have data.

Howard Gardner (15,16), unlike Terman (17) and Hollingsworth (18), draws a signficant distinction between the kind of intelligence that drives performing arts talent and that which drives more cognitive gifts. Unique processing of auditory and rhythmic stimuli and idiosyncratic syntheses of a variety of symbolic representations seem to make musical form and content especially pleasurable and facile in such minds. He reports relatively little overlap between the various "frames of intelligence." He sees certain traits as important for sustaining talent over time:

> An individual who would be great needs to be daring, able to take risks, confront the unknown. . . . The individual must also display staying power: he must have the fiber to transcend an early triumph or disaster and continue to deepen. The presence of sensitive models and teachers, the existence of an audience to appreciate his inventions, and a healthy injection of luck all these are at a premium (p. 199).

Feldman's (19) prospective work on a small group of prodigies is unique in its usefulness in understanding the forces at work on the prodigy. Based on his observations, he concludes that prodigies are not a special subspecies unto themselves but instead are individuals who move through certain domains at a fast rate, completing particularly narrow developmental progressions very swiftly. How does this come about, and what are its psychological implications? He believes that prodigiousness is due to a set of events that he termed *coincidence* (19):

> Early prodigious achievement is the occurrence in time and space of a remarkable preorganized human being, born and educated during perhaps the optimal period, and in a manner perhaps most likely to engage the child's interest in commitment to the mastery of a highly evolved field of knowledge. A "coincidence" occurs more remarkable even than the awesome talents which make it possible. This subtle delicate coordination of elements of human potential and cultural tradition is even more dazzling than the abilities characteristically attributed to these children.

Interestingly, Feldman's subjects typically are totally absorbed in their work, rarely lose their balance, love performing, and appreciate congratulations. Furthermore, they seem relatively tracked. Prodigiousness seems to wear a groove, or develop in one, rarely cutting across domains. Sosniak (20) makes a very careful distinction between young adults who demonstrate exceptional talent from those who begin their musical life as prodigies. Her conclusions, based on the study of the 21 concert pianists who participated in the Development of Talent research project (21), are summarized as follows. The development of musical talent in demonstrably gifted adult performers takes a long time, and it is a process which is essentially one of qualitative change. It involves a continual and perhaps systematic reorientation and transformation—both of an individual and of the activity of learning. She also concludes that talent development involves many people working for the achievement of just one. These artists are distinguished from prodigies, who develop their musical talent often apart from the long-term successful learning and gradual development of commitment. Unlike prodigies, the pianists studied by Sosniak (21):

> developed a deep interest in and involvement with music making before they were expected to do the work required for mastering the technical skills of the art. It was important for the pianists in our study that they could appreciate small signs of growth and that their parents and teachers could do the same. It was important further that the pianists in our study were willing to take chances—to work at skills and understandings that were beyond their grasp at the moment without becoming overwhelmed or discouraged by lack of immediate success. Prodigies are unlikely to have these sorts of experiences.

Interestingly, Feldman, Gardner, and Sosniak all agree that at adolescence the exceptionally talented young performer and prodigy both face a crisis, that is, a dangerous opportunity. All three researchers focus on the psychological processes that Bamberger (22), for somewhat different reasons, defined as the "midlife crisis" of the talented young performing artist. This is a time when his talent—and the individual's relationship to his talent—is at the greatest risk of trouble in relating to the ownership of his art. Gardner (15) summarizes their interest: "Why am I doing this? Is it for me or for other people? Is it worthwhile? Those who cannot fashion a satisfactory answer often cease their creative efforts at this point in their life."

Bamberger (22), in her laboratory study of six 7-to-10-year-olds who are musically talented, argues that young performers undergo significant changes in the internal representation of musical structures themselves. The multiple dimensions of perception, synthesis, audiation, and affect all begin to come apart spontaneously around adolescence, threatening the previously well-functioning overall reciprocity. They have to coordinate these now separate dimensions and their underlying mental representations consciously. When successful, the remarkable but nonreflective performance of the prodigy is transformed into the more adult, thoughtful but spontaneous artist's performance. Schnitt (23) has examined this "midlife crisis" in the lives of talented young dancers, calling the third of his six stages in the psychological evolution of the dancer the phase of "maximal conflict." "The arrival of puberty, the psychologically normal testing of authority, and the preoccupation with body shape and size all collide with the need to compete for a few coveted roles and the approval and adoration of the dance master and the fact that success no longer comes naturally can lead to a real 'combustion' which some talent survives and some doesn't"—prodigious or not, it seems to matter little.

A special example of a psychological vulnerability which is receiving increasing attention is the problem of the exceptionally gifted performer's postperformance depression. It is a paradigm for the old saw that our strengths and our weaknesses are each other's shadow. This, too, appears to be a risk for both prodigy and exceptional young performers. Robson (24) describes it thus:

> Post-performance depression is characterized by sadness, crying bouts, anxiety and panic attacks in some individuals, anhedonia or lack of interest, lethargy, fatigue, excessive sleeping, truancy or failure to attend class or coaching, failure to complete homework assignments, suicidal ideation and in some instances, attempts.

Robson also cites several predisposing factors which may make a performer unusually vulnerable to this psychological problem. Several that she cites are: (1.) the stress of repeated auditions and competition with hundreds of others for one or two positions, leading to insidious erosion of self-esteem; (2.) the isolation of traveling and touring students makes them feel particularly distant from family and friends; (3.) the tendency toward developing a unidimensional lifestyle among friends, acquaintances, and roommates, even spouses (who are likely to be performers themselves) decreases the probability of having someone other than a performer to talk to about the postperformance crash. Many performers, and especially dancers also report that no one "warned" them of the tremendous physical demands or fatigue.

As for the direct usage and usefulness of psychological treatment, prodigious talent is no stranger. Robert Schumann, Anton Bruckner, Rachmaninoff, and Nijinsky are but a few whom psychiatric treatment assisted at critical points in their lives. Are the young talented musicians likely to need psychological assistance more than their nonperforming peers? Interestingly, Ostwald (5), citing his experience as codirector of the health program for performing artists in San Francisco, concludes:

> Performing artists do appear to be at risk for the development of psychiatric disorders that are amenable to psychotherapy. However, the risk seems to be somewhat lower than for the general population. . . . It may well be that performing artist patients have developed personality patterns and coping styles that are significantly different from those of nonperforming artist patients. These differences may account for some of the special vulnerabilities as well as the special resistance to psychiatric disorders that has been observed among performers.

Caution should be employed to resist the extrapolation backward to the experience of the young performer, as there are so many additional factors to be weighed in assessing the need for psychotherapeutic intervention.

The Development of Talent research project by Bloom and Sosniak may be of assistance here, despite the significant limitations of its retrospective perspective.

Although the study protocol did not include prodigies, it did follow the stories of especially accomplished musicians. What is notable about the themes reported at various life stages is that they could serve as models for normal child development in their basic outlines. The initial phase (the first decade of life) was characterized by "tinkering and playing *with* music," gentle support, and encouragement of music as a "good thing." Instruction was provided by "nice people," and achievement was relatively subjective. Although music is the medium, the tasks are typical developmental tasks in a typical nurturing domain of the first decade of life.

Sosniak's middle phase, 10 to 13 years, is one of increasing precision and time spent on details. Technique and vocabulary become the focus, and teachers intensify their demands. The relationship with the student is carried well beyond that of weekly lessons. Here again, these are the normal developmental tasks of the latency and early adolescent phases. The subject could be soccer or viola.

The third phase, of less interest to us here, begins at age 16 and ends at 20 years, where the emphasis shifts from the disciplined mastery of specific skills to a broader, more personal, self-reflective understanding and commitment to music. This is characterized by attempts to bring more of the artist's own self (now that he has one) to the experience of making music. These findings, retrospective though they are, highlight a sense that, for the exceptional young performer (remembered from his own adult years), talent need not distort the basic business of growing up.

In an interview with Cho-Liang Lin reported by Brandfonbrener (25), we hear this highly talented performer reporting that his introduction to the violin was truly accidental, encountering it in a neighbor/friend's home. He describes his parents as:

> feeding me all those books to read about music. Violin wasn't really the priority, even though I practiced every day. They thought a balanced life was important. I played baseball, basketball and I bicycled. There was no sort of child prodigy burden that was pushed onto me and there was no pressure to play concerts. I played a little kiddy performance when I was seven, and I didn't really step on the stage until I was nine. Even then I didn't consider myself in any way outstanding.

This is hardly the stuff of a *heldenleben*.

My own research into the psychological aspects of exceptional young performers has focused on children's views of their own developing talents (26,27) (Pruett). I chose to use a certain good fortune of having a number of promising young musicians in my own circle of performers. This is a nonclinical population and, consequently, I knew them musically. As child psychiatrists and child developmentalists painfully relearn, an accurate view of one's own childhood experiences cannot be found in conversation with grownups about their growing up. My own research has attempted to focus on the musically talented child's experience of his own giftedness *as* it is developing. It allows the data to be more firmly rooted in the canons of developmental psychology as it is emerging. I have discovered repeatedly that what children think of their own giftedness is often quite different from what grownups may think of it.

As a musician myself, I have had an abiding interest in the evolution of musical skill and giftedness. I have had an opportunity to talk to many young children about their ongoing experiences over time.

There are so few longitudinal studies of musical giftedness because of the difficulty in identifying the gifted child early. By the time talent is established and expressed, much of the child's critical early developmental history is long since gone. Because of my own involvement in the musical community where I live, I have had the rare opportunity to be involved with a number of artistic and musical children and their families as a fellow performer, family friend, and occasional confidante over a protracted period of time. The operatic, oratorio, small vocal ensemble, and recital repertoire have served as a stage and backdrop for some of these conversations.

In summarizing my two longitudinal reports to date (26,27), there are several general conclusions. First, most of the interviews I conducted with children contained references to the *necessity* to make music, not merely the wish. They would sometimes describe a euphoria, born of the capacity to concentrate intensely on something of great pleasure. The normal sense of time and self were sometimes lost.

Next, many of the children whose talent was considerable found themselves sometimes saddled with a sense of pressure, an almost obligatory quality to expand their talent from their own inner drive, not exteriorly imposed. Greenacre (28) commented on the power of this pressure, "The creative activity of the artist seems to me highly aggressive, but the aggression is allocated as a special growth promoting development." It is my own hunch that there may be a predispositional factor responsible for this drive to make music, and it exists somewhat independent of a musical environment. The capacity to make music in a talented and gifted way is frequently seen by children as a "love gift" more characteristically prior to the onset of adolescence. After adolescence, what was previously a pleasure sometimes begins to feel more like an obligation to delight people.

Third, I saw a capacity demonstrated in these children to hear and feel something in music which they could not articulate verbally and apparently experienced nowhere else, but which they occasionally appear addicted to repeating and re-experiencing.

Fourth, all of the children articulated the negative aspects of owning a musical talent and sometimes wished that they were rid of it. Fifth, most exceptional young performers do not initially see themselves as especially valuable human beings. They are just doing what they need to do—no big deal. Finally, a sense of what is aesthetic in music seems to arrive at around 9 or 10 years of age. The difference between what is *artistic* in a thing and what is merely pleasing begins to dog them and their creative explorations.

I have also focused my attention on the aspects of public exhibitionism in the exceptional young performer. We see the public musical stage presence running the gamut from painfully egotistical and exhibitionistic all the way to people who must avoid eye contact with the audience. The natural public ease and exhibitionism of the primary grade musician is well known, underlined by the fact that medications to combat anxiety are rarely requested by kindergarten children. Center stage is as natural a habitat for them as the living room. The closer one gets to adolescence, however, the more that looking relaxed becomes almost more important than being relaxed. This new awareness can be immensely powerful and a source of conflict for the young musician. Privately he may be feeling very much in love with his music in a very intimate, often vulnerable way. On the outside, however, he must appear cool and totally in control, almost invincible.

The young musician who chooses an anxiety-binding pattern of grandiosity and omnipotence risks his self-esteem. That self-esteem can become anchored in the possession of certain *qualities*, such as musical talent and success, instead of the more sustaining authenticity of one's own perceptions. He can become increasingly dependent upon adulation and admiration. This path is not chosen consciously, but can be a result of a deeply troubled entanglement of poor early nurturing experiences.

The adolescent who decides to join up with his buddies, work through the battle over the ownership of his own musical talent, and honestly embrace the notion that his music is his to nurture or abandon and is not a publicly held property, discovers that he is frequently not the first performing artist to struggle with significant anxiety. Furthermore, he can develop an artistic autonomy without having to attack the important intimate relationships in his life, developing a healthier form of narcissism.

Having scoured the relevant literature together, it must by now be clear that, given the current state of knowledge (and/or ignorance), there is nothing inherently risky psychologically about being exceptionally talented, even prodigious. That is not to say that there are not risks or vulnerabilities galore, but the very presence of talent does not doom to psychological trouble. Developmental issues seem to be the same intrinsic ones shared by the rest of the species.

To date, we must conclude that there seems to be no common factor which is suggestive of personality traits or characteristics of exceptional young performers or prodigies which place them by sheer dint of talent at psychological risk. Problems, of course, arise, but the problems appear to evolve more in the realm of the development of talent than in the maturation of talent. [Development is defined as the interaction of maturation (the orderly biological unfolding of constitutional endowment) and environment (everything that the child experiences outside himself)]. Most clinicians appear to agree that it is the environment, whether historic or heuristic, that is the culprit more often than not when trouble arises.

You have undoubtedly noticed that performance anxiety, per se, has not been singled out as a special psychological aspect of the development of exceptional young performers and prodigies. That is because, as a phenomenon, it is dealt with elsewhere in the text, and also it is hardly unique to this population. Most studies of its incidence rank its prevalence as nearly universal in some form. It is also highly debatable as to whether or not it should be classified as a psychopathological phenomenon. Lockwood (29) reminds us that a certain amount of stress and anxiety focus attention and are part and parcel of optimal performance. Experience, per se, does not always reduce anxiety. Severe somatic symptomatology obviously requires intervention in any performer who can't perform, whether the talent is prodigious or not. Of course, the potential for trouble in the psychological domain of the exceptional young performer is probably as great as his talents promise. The threshold for trouble is so low, however, because the expression of existing talent requires both aptitude and an environment that facilitates in an abiding way. It is also not so much that the psychological issues bearing down on the performer are so different. Plaut (30) concludes that, in the special circumstance of performance anxiety, the unconscious issues underlying anxiety about exposure in public are mostly identical for the performer and nonperformer. It's just that, when the pecking order of the most important realm of your life is determined almost exclusively by demonstrable *skill*, regardless of age, the pressure seems never to end.

A number of environmental risk factors can make certain psychological vulnerabilities blossom forth into real trouble in the psychological life of the young performer. Parental facilitation of exceptional talent can turn negative from positive if, for specific psychodynamic reasons having to do with the adult's emotional needs, parental appreciation of the child's talent turns into exploitation, throwing the ownership of that talent into contention. Similarly, the teacher as sycophant can parasitize young talent like a tapeworm, taking nourishment from the young talent instead of the reverse.

Another risk factor is the exaggeration of the delicacy of the musical gift. My own experience is that talent, when it occurs in the matrix of otherwise healthy development, is anything but delicate. The intensity, aggression, and power that many children demonstrate toward their music is anything but fragile, not that its fabric cannot be torn by negative life experiences, pain, substance abuse and the like. Truly prodigious talent and genius may not be destroyed easily. Enormous genius, as in the case of Mozart, appears so vigorous as to be essentially indestructible.

So what can we do to make use of our limited understanding to ameliorate psychological stress and distress in the development of exceptional talent in the performing arts? Most of the following suggestions fall under the categories of prevention, of not making things worse, or attempting to help the student and his family not make things worse for themselves. First among adult charges is to encourage children to avoid the sense of the unfinished life, the asymmetric or misshapen self. Over and over again we hear from children that adults need to sponsor opportunities for them to have varied experiences which encourage them to reflect upon their *whole* life, rich in the humanities and a sense of well-being to inspire a reverence for one's whole imagination. The most enduring artistic achievements involve the whole person, not just his rotator cuff or vocal cords. The single monocular focus and the exclusion of everything but talent promote a transformation from prodigy to prima donna in the most pejorative sense.

Second, as adults, we must guard against overinvolvement with, and overunderstanding of, the exceptional young performer's talent. Prodigies fascinate us middle-aged musicians, audiences, and researchers for many reasons. They can be at risk even in our most empathic hands. We must encourage the child to follow his own intentions with regard to his music, regardless of outside influences or purported understandings. I have my doubts about the value of understanding or even explicating such intentions, however, for children. In the end it may be the *instinctive* that counts more in the conveyance of music. What matters more than what the musician intends to say is what is being said through him, or even in spite of him. Overemphasizing mental discipline and intentionality can lead to a mental overuse syndrome, analogous to the overuse syndromes experienced by many muscle groups in instrumental performers. Psychological mechanisms can burn out just as easily as a teres minor.

Our third critical job is to help the young talent pace itself. Lifelong careers are the goal here, unlike basketball or football. Even dancers can find extraordinarily productive and satisfying adaptations of their art after their bodies no longer cooperate. Gedo (31) reminds us that "Creative success tends to be extremely stimulating over long periods of time—probably more so than competitive or sexual triumphs, the effects of which tend to wear off relatively quickly. In order to avoid overstimulation the individual must have at his disposal effective means to reduce tension." One way to help a child learn to pace himself is to emphasize that, for most of his performing life, he will always feel that he could have done better. He should be helped to understand from very early in his life that he will and must make mistakes—it is part of his obligation to himself as an artist. We must make room in our current educational programs for encouraging students to appreciate and learn from their less-than-successful experiences. Discouragement is not an indication for psychotherapy. Incidentally, psychotherapy, when it is not indicated for remediation of psychological difficulties, is not an innocent procedure and can lead to its own problematic sequelae.

Fourth, our musical institutions, both public and private, must encourage young performers to immerse themselves in their support systems, outside of the musical domain as well as inside. Help for the midlife crisis of the musician is available in a variety of ways, not the least of which is parental or teachers' encouragement of artistic children to form groups of peers outside of the musical domain to help them when their disillusionment about their art takes hold in early adolescence.

Robson encourages similar remediation to guard against the postperformance depressive phenomenon. She encourages the development of an ensemble or group that can support students and performers by enabling them to share experiences and express their feelings to one another to counteract isolation. Students should be encouraged to resume regular routines as soon as possible after performance with regularly scheduled meals and sleep patterns. Excessive sleep is to be avoided. And positive plans for pleasurable activities soon after the curtain goes down, not necessarily related to art, are a very wise idea. This overall respect for one's whole self can also take the form of encouraging children early not to push themselves through injuries or pain. As Robson points out, directors who keep everyone at rehearsal far into the night are to be shunned, not adored.

Finally, there are a number of things that can be done to prepare the exceptionally talented child for the crucible known as public performance. The guiding principle should be the preservation of self-esteem, not the layering of armor. Children can be encouraged to think about the people in the audience, not as enemies, but as supportive, expectant colleagues and friends. Critics, like umpires, are part of the game. Nervousness in performance should be talked about and anticipated. This helps young children understand that they are involved in a commonality of experience, not unique to their own situation or deficiencies. They can be helped to understand that facing the unknown is about as well known as any other feeling known to the species. We can teach them how to get on and off the stage, how to use relaxation techniques, what to do about the audience. Later on we can talk with them about reviews and what they say and do not say about their musicianship and their complete irrelevance to their innate worth as human beings. We can prepare them for the difference between what they appreciate in their performance and what the audience appreciates. We can help them make use of videotapes in constructive, rather than destructive, ways, beginning by never showing a videotape immediately after a performance when defenses are down and vulnerability is up.

Of course, in the end, we all lose our performing careers one way or another. Learning early that our psychological vulnerabilities are among our most enduring and endearing human characteristics can endlessly enrich our appreciation of the performing arts. It helps to know, earlier rather than later, that the pursuit of perfection is always done while riding on a hobbled horse.

REFERENCES

1. Hawking S. *A brief history of time*. New York: Bantam, 1988.
2. Pannenborg HJ, Pannenborg WA. Die psychologie des musikers. *Zeitschrift fur Psychologie* 1915;73:91–136.
3. Feis O. *Studien zur genealogie und psychologie der musik*. Wiesbaden: JF Bergman, 1910.
4. Kretschmer E. *The psychology of men of genius*. New York: Harcourt Brace, 1931.
5. Ostwald PF. Psychotherapeutic strategies in the treatment of performing artists. *Med Probl Perform Art* December, 1987;131–136.
6. Pollock GH. The mourning liberation process and creativity. In: *The annual of psychoanalysis*. New York: International Universities Press, 1978.
7. Cohen BJ, Kupersmith JR. A study of SCL-90 scores of 87 performing artists seeking psychotherapy. *Medical Problems of the Performing Artist* 1986;1:140–142.
8. Gardner CE. Characteristics of outstanding high school musicians. *Journal of Research in Music Education* 1955;3:11–20.
9. Lehman C. A comparative study of instrumental musicians on the basis of the Otis Intelligence Test and the Minnesota Multiphasic Personality Inventory. *Journal of Educational Research* 1950;64:57–61.
10. Gordon EE. *The nature, description, measurement and evaluation of music aptitudes*. Chicago: GIA Publications, Inc, 1987.
11. Colwel R. An investigation of musical achievement among public school students. *Journal of Educational Research* 1964;57:355–359.
12. Moore R. The relationship of intelligence to creativity. *Journal of Research in Music Education* 1966;14:243–253.
13. Miller A. *The drama of the gifted child*. New York: Basic Books, 1981.
14. Babikian HM. The psychoanalytic treatment of the performing artist: Superego aspects. *Journal of the American Academy of Psychoanalysis* 1985;13(1):139–148.

15. Gardner H. *Frames of mind: The theory of multiple intelligences.* New York: Basic Books, 1983.
16. Gardner H. *Art, mind and brain: A cognitive approach to creativity.* New York: Basic Books, 1982.
17. Terman LM, Oden MH. *The gifted group at mid-life: A 35-year follow-up of the superior child.* Stanford, CA: Stanford University Press, 1957.
18. Hollingsworth L. Musical sensitivity of children who score above 135 IQ. *Journal of Educational Psychology* 1926;17:95–109.
19. Feldman D. *Beyond universals in cognitive development.* Norwood, NJ: Ablex Publishers, 1980.
20. Sosniak LA. A long term commitment to learning. In: Bloom BS, ed. *Developing talent in young people.* New York: Ballentine Books, 1985;477–506.
21. Bloom BS. *Developing talent in young people.* New York: Ballentine Books, 1985.
22. Bamberger J. The mind behind the musical ear. Paper presented at the Biology of Music Making Conference, Denver, CO: June, 1987.
23. Schnitt J, Schnitt D. Psychological dimensions of a dancer's career. Paper presented at the Fifth Annual Symposium on Medical Problems of Musicians and Dancers, Aspen, CO: July, 1987.
24. Robson BE. Post-performance depression in arts students. *Med Probl Perform Art* December, 1987;137–141.
25. Brandfonbrener A. Interview with Cho-Liang Lin. *Medical Problems of the Performing Artist* March, 1989;3–8.
26. Pruett K. A longitudinal view of the musical gift. *Medical Problems of the Performing Artist* March, 1987;31–38.
27. Pruett K. Young Narcissus at the music stand: Developmental perspectives from embarrassment to exhibitionism. *Med Probl Perform Art* June, 1988;69–75.
28. Greenacre P. The childhood of the artist: Libidinal phase development and giftedness. In: Greenacre P, ed. *Emotional growth,* vol 2. New York: International Universities Press, 1971;479–504.
29. Lockwood A. Medical problems of musicians. *New England journal of medicine* 1989;320:221–227.
30. Plaut EA. Psychotherapy of performance anxiety. *Med Probl Perform Art* September, 1988;113–118.
31. Gedo J. *Portraits of the artist.* New York: Guilford Press, 1983.

Textbook of Performing Arts Medicine, edited by R. T. Sataloff, A. Brandfonbrener, and R. Lederman. Raven Press, Ltd., New York © 1991.

12

Psychological Issues in the Clinical Approach to Dancers

*Jerome M. Schnitt and †Diana Schnitt

*Associate Clinical Professor of Psychiatry, Yale University School of Medicine,
New Haven, Connecticut 06510
†Chairman of the Dance Department, Connecticut College,
New London, Connecticut 06032

Although stereotypes of dancers' personalities abound, in reality, little is known scientifically about the personalities of dancers, or of their propensities toward any particular psychiatric disorders. Formal study has until recently been quite limited. According to Medline, psychological abstracts, and BRS computer searches, between 1945 and mid-1989 there were less than 100 articles in English directly relevant to the psychology of dance in refereed journals. The majority of these either were naturalistic studies, or they used groups of "dancers" (essentially any group that could be considered to be dancing) as comparison groups. The more scientific papers among them center primarily on the question of ballet dancers' possible susceptibility to eating and menstrual disorders.

Accordingly, much of what can be said about the clinical approach to the individual dancer is impressionistic, anecdotal, and limited by insufficient data. This is not to say that the literature on the psychology of dance is small. There are available an increasing number of "how-to" and autobiographical books for dancers, usually based on the experiences of the author, and consequently often idiosyncratic, although frequently deeply personal and sometimes quite astute.

This chapter focuses on a general clinical approach to dancers for physicians or other medical personnel. Relevant literature is presented along with clinical data about psychiatric disorders for which dancers may be especially at risk. Emphasis is placed on how the clinician's attitudes about the dancer-patient may have a significant influence on outcome.

One crucial caveat is to recognize that the range of individuals calling themselves "dancers" is quite broad. While it is tempting to think of the professional performer as the appropriate representative of the term *dancer*; professional ballet, modern, jazz, tap, and ethnic dancers make up only a small percentage of the population of

Americans who think of themselves as dancers. The largest population is the vast group of students, ranging from the college level down to elementary school.

Members of a group this size have little in common other than the willingness to attend dance classes and to explore a highly personalized fantasy of what a dancer is and does. Thus it seems unduly speculative to assume anything about common personality features at this level. The clinician seeing a dancer-patient for the first time will do well not to presume too much about the individual.

LITERATURE AND CLINICAL REVIEW

The following is a brief summary of clinically relevant research on the psychology of dance from refereed journals through mid-1989, with a concurrent commentary on clinical applications. The relatively sparse literature on the psychology of dance to 1985 has been reviewed in detail elsewhere (1).

Researchers typically have found data to support the contention that dance is good for us all. Taking dance classes seems to help everything from self-esteem (2,3) to anxiety (4). This is a satisfying finding, consistent with intuition and general observation and consistent with findings on well-being and self-esteem in athletics (5). However, such satisfying conclusions are not always correct.

Contrary findings include those of Bakker (6), who reports finding lowered self-esteem in 11- to 12-year-old ballet students, when compared to nondancing agemates. This finding was supported when 15- to 16-year-old ballet students, who had been at the school several years more, were compared to nondancing agemates; that is, even if students entered ballet with disruptions of self-esteem, the picture worsened over several years of study. Puretz (7), while finding significant improvement in body image for subjects taking a 15-week physical conditioning course, found no change in body image of subjects taking a modern dance or ballet course.

Overinterpretation (or misinterpretation) of data in this research area may occur easily if one is not wary. This is partly because of differing definitions of "dancer," and partly because of the inherent risks in experimental research. For example, Dyer & Crouch (8) found that dance students showed real improvements in measures of tension, depression, anger, vigor, fatigue and confusion within a semester of beginning classes; these improvements compared favorably with those achieved by runners over the same time frame. The findings cannot be generalized to all forms of dance, in part because they are based on volunteer college students participating in a thrice weekly "dance aerobics" class. Both the class and the students might be quite different from students taking a ballet class. Also, the sample was mixed and stilted: the aerobic dancers included both beginners and more advanced returnees, and 2/3 of the subjects either withdrew from class or failed to return questionnaires prior to the end of the study! None of the reports cited in the paper investigated subjects who appeared not to benefit from the classes, or to find out why those who dropped out did so.

Eating Disorders

Obesity is more typical among beginning than advanced dancers; body image distortions can occur in either of these populations (9). However, professional or career-directed dancers (e.g., college dance majors) may be perceived as "overweight" when still below the average expected body weight for nondancers (10). An example is quoted by Ryan and Stephens (11) of a "slightly overweight" ballet dancer who fractured her right big toe while performing *en pointe*. Her pointe work was seen to have progressively worsened as she gained weight. Loss of 8 pounds and realignment exercises resolved her discomfort.

More frequently, one encounters the beginning student who hopes to use dance to help become more graceful and/or to lose weight. We are aware of unpublished anecdotal cases of obese students who wished for their weight not to be seen as an issue in classes, and who did well with classes until the aesthetic and/or physical limitations brought about by their weight were confronted either by a serious critique of their performance or by poor audience response. Disruptions of self-esteem followed, in one case manifest by withdrawal from class. In the second case the student became angry at her critics, expecting them to overlook the real limits of her performance and to focus only on her intent. In retrospect it would appear that neither individual was helped by having the obesity ignored by the teacher until the last minute.

Anorexia nervosa and bulimia may be more frequent in dancers than in the general public. One study found 6.5% of a dance sample had unequivocal cases of anorexia nervosa (12). A recent large study of female undergrad UCLA students compared eating attitudes and eating disorder symptoms of several campus subgroups. The Eating Disorders Inventory revealed a study-wide current prevalence of eating disorders of 2.1% (lifetime prevalence of 4.8%). The most abnormal subgroups were from the primary health care clinic and dance majors; the most normal were athletes. In between were those from the women's health clinic, sororities, and psychology class attendees (13). This is consistent with the existing literature on dancers. Joseph et al. (14) compared the eating attitudes of dance, drama, English and physical education majors; they found dance and drama majors had the most abnormal attitudes, while physical education majors were the most normal.

Research in this area for a decade focused on separating the issues of thinness, abnormal eating attitudes, and eating disorders. First, pressures for thinness in dancers can be extreme, especially in settings where competition is high for performance slots or for teacher approval.

One group of nearly 200 female, teenage, serious ballet students was found to average just under 87% of expected body weight (12). Another group of 62 female, college-age, serious modern dance students averaged 88% of expected body weight (15). Both studies agreed that there were intense pressures for thinness, some teacher-driven, some peer-driven, and some self-driven. In attempting to understand these forces, relevant factors included high performance expectations, perfectionism, and focusing on development of one's body control in preference to (and sometimes even to the exclusion of) other life tasks (16,17).

The successful achievement of thinness did not necessarily correlate with abnormal eating attitudes (e.g., 75% of the modern dance sample cited above demonstrated normal eating attitudes on the Eating Attitudes Test). Caution was advised; the dance teacher or clinician could not make the diagnosis of anorexia nervosa based solely on body weight and eating attitudes. Adaptation to the dance subculture might account for thinness; psychopathology and disease might have little to do with the presentation of a thin, amenorrheic, intense young dancer. Szmuckler et al. (18) support this observation; at 1-year follow-up, ballet students who previously had displayed symptoms of anorexia nervosa improved spontaneously.

Compounding the difficulty of diagnosing eating disorders in dancers, it appears that menstrual differences may be highly affected by the dancer's environment. A recent careful study reviewed delayed menarche in 350 mid-adolescent girls and their mothers, comparing girls who attended competitive national company dance schools with a demographically matched group of nondancers from private schools (19). The mothers had comparable ages of menarche; the genetic loading was similar. The dancers were significantly later in menarcheal age.

Within the subgroups of dancers, comparison of possible contributing factors (using multiple regression analysis) found that for dancers, body mass was the only significant variable in predicting age of menarche. The dancers' eating attitudes and number of hours dancing were not predictive, nor were the dancers' mothers' variables of maternal education, age, or menarcheal age. However, for the comparison group of nondancer private school girls, maternal menarcheal age was the most predictive variable, followed by body mass; nonpredictive for these girls was participation in a varsity athletic pursuit. Thus the authors concluded that environmental effects may have significant impact on menarcheal age, able to outweigh genetic predisposition. Despite their finding that amount of exercise did not relate to menarcheal age, the one longitudinal study in this area (20) reports that the delay of menarche in adolescent dancers was more likely to occur during injury- or vacation-induced periods of inactivity, rather than periods of active exertion.

A further twist in the problem of deciding if a thin dancer is at risk for eating disorder comes from a 2- and 4-year prospective study of ballet students. Garner & Garfinkel's group (21) evaluated and conducted follow-up interviews and retested 32 midteen student ballerinas on the Eating Disorders Inventory (EDI). At followup, 25.7% met criteria for anorexia nervosa, and 14.2% either had bulimia nervosa or a partial syndrome.

The school suffered a high dropout rate during the study: 23 of the initial 55 subjects had left school, including 7 of the 9 who had anorexia nervosa at first testing. This may be an important finding: adolescents who have dropped out of intensive dance training may require evaluation or intervention just as much as those who stay in dance.

Of the 15 students who originally had high scores on the "drive for thinness" subscale, six dropped out of school and seven had eating disorders at follow-up. Of the eight who were postmenarcheal at first testing, four left school and three had anorexia nervosa at retesting. These students had significantly higher than average "body dissatisfaction" scores. In the intervening years, some of the anorectic girls had gained weight as they matured. However, the fact that many of those picked up on initial testing continued to suffer significant symptoms consistent with eating disorders several years later was viewed as an important new finding. Two to four years of abnormal eating and of symptoms of eating disorders were not viewed as benign adaptations to the ballet subculture; rather they seemed to be signs of illness or grave risk of illness.

The authors concluded that clinically useful data could be achieved in mass screenings, using the EDI's "drive for thinness" and "body dissatisfaction" subscales; they suggested that these could reliably and economically predict who needed follow-up clinical evaluation in at-risk populations.

Males appear to suffer eating disorders less frequently than females, at least in the general population. In the 10 years following 1970, only 107 male cases of anorexia nervosa were reported in the medical literature (22). In a large later sample, 10% were male, with anorexia nervosa, bulimia, or partial symptom pictures. Males differed in that prior to symptom emergence, most had been slightly obese and dieting. They also tended to have a narrower range of severity: more toward the extremes than did females (23). A small sample of bulimic athletes demonstrated a possibly significant issue for male dancers: a quarter of the sample developed symptoms trying to meet athletic weight standards (24). Another report found males with eating disorders often were seeking better muscle definition rather than thinness (25). A further study also found histories of dieting and preoccupation with appearance in males with eating disorders (26). There are no published data to suggest sexual preference is a factor in the development of eating disorders in males or in females.

Substance Abuse

Substance abuse has been anecdotally reported in dancers, but as yet there is no formal study. In a performing arts clinic, cocaine and alcohol were the leading drugs abused among dance performers (27). The authors expressed concerns about the dangers of opiates, benzodiazepines, amphetamines, barbiturates, and beta-blockers among this population, with the assumption that most drugs were taken by their dancer-clients to reduce stress. Two studies of ballet schools done a decade ago found that adolescent students were more likely to abuse laxatives (to lose weight) than other drugs, including diuretics and amphetamines (16,28). These studies found little prevalence of other drugs of abuse, either by self-report, observation, or teacher observation. Anecdotally, nicotine addiction is frequently seen in this adolescent group, though the rationalizations of "neutral addiction" and "personal preference" are occasionally still heard.

Beta-blockers, which block the autonomic manifestations of anxiety without decreasing the anxiety itself, have been used increasingly to minimize the impact of performance anxiety in instrumentalists, singers, and actors (29). The popularity of beta-blockers in these populations appears not to have made a complete transition into the world of dance, but a number of anecdotal reports have occurred. Typically, the individual takes a single dose of the available beta-blocker an hour before performing, with the goal of decreasing anxiety, increasing focus and performance, and having the effect fade out once the performance has ended. Risks are several. Adverse reactions tend to appear more in chronic use, especially in a cardiac- and pulmonary-compromised population, but since a single dose of a beta-blocker will impair the ability of the heart to increase its rate, acute use in dancers can have negative effects on the dancer's athletic performance capacity. A single dose can also provoke an acute attack of bronchial asthma, rendering performance impossible. Chronic use tends to develop when the medication is deemed effective in a single use (whether the effect is pharmacological or largely placebo), and the individual decides it should be used whenever anxiety occurs. The performer thus may come to feel the normal anxiety of performing as a dangerous anxiety, to be avoided by always taking the pill. Pharmacologically-induced sleep disturbance, depression, or, more rarely, hallucinations are also possible. Although beta-blockers are not physically addicting, there is a strong potential for psychological dependence when the performer sees the medicine as a necessary precursor to successful performance. This type of self-reinforcing use can lead to higher or more regular dosing, with inherent risks of abrupt discontinuance if the supply is terminated or if guilt feelings cause the person to suddenly stop.

For similar situational reasons, benzodiazepines may become drugs of abuse unless prescribed carefully. Despite one incorrect reference in the dance literature which states there are no withdrawal symptoms (11), chronic use has a definite danger for tolerance, addiction, and withdrawal. Benzodiazepines should be reserved for the treatment of specific disorders, with education as to their potential dangers, and careful longitudinal follow-up. Many of those who request relief from performance anxiety would be able to benefit from psychotherapeutic interventions either concurrent with or instead of medications. Where benzodiazepines are necessary because of a generalized anxiety disorder, or a panic or phobic disorder, the use of clonazepam may be superior to other drugs of the class. As a longer-acting drug (half-life of 18 to 44 hours), it often avoids the roller-coaster effect of its shorter-acting relatives (profound relief followed by loss of efficacy over brief periods, leading to a sense of need for the next dose: especially problematic with medications requiring three to four doses per day. Clonazepam also appears to promote tolerance (and subsequent addiction) less than its relatives, and does not produce a euphoric or intoxicated feeling (30).

Multiple factors may predispose the dancer to substance abuse. Stress reduction, antianxiety or temporary antidepressant effects, recreation, combatting boredom, increasing the illusion of self-control by controlling a state change toward intoxication are all psychological forces which may play a role. Social forces often include peer pressure, imitating and experimenting with "adult" behavior, and group acting out. When subcultural forces are clear, it is easy to overlook the biological vulnerability to abuse of certain substances. There is now clear-cut evidence that increased susceptibility to alcohol abuse can be genetically passed (31). Similarly, higher than average vulnerability to cross-tolerance and cross-addiction among alcohol, benzodiazepines, and opiates may be inherited.

Performance Anxiety

Regardless of the degree of technical skill or artistry a dancer may command, inability to perform at one's best for an audience can be devastating. The term *performance anxiety*, widely used in the arts and athletics, covers the whole range of psychological and physiological phenomena which interfere with optimum performance. Performance anxiety is universal, and usually does not require therapy (29). However, if expected levels of nervousness increase to panic proportions, inhibiting adequate performance, professional intervention is useful (27).

According to one round table discussion about performance anxiety among musicians, music teachers and physicians use many different approaches in addressing "stress" and performance anxiety (32). Some avoid discussion unless a student brings it up; others address it obliquely. Still others create a "paradoxical intention:" this is a therapeutic and teaching intervention which involves an almost playful exaggeration of the student's fears to the extreme, and then exaggerating this worst-case scenario until it becomes humorously ridiculous to the student. Auditions, juries, and recitals all tend to increase the sense of tension and the apprehension of failure.

The psychoanalytic view of performance anxiety suggests that the cause may be quite individual, with some common elements (33). Most important are the notions of unconscious mental activity, unconscious conflict, and anxiety as a conscious awareness that some unclear thing is wrong. For example, a 12-year-old dancer knows she is the best in her class, but is aware that many older girls are more accomplished. She is auditioning for a company school, and wishes with all her heart to be accepted so she can fulfill her dream of one day becoming a prima ballerina. For the past 7 years she has sacrificed most of her childhood play time for dance; strong encouragement has helped her to ignore the losses of friends, of playtime, and of the opportunity to develop other interests. At the audition, she becomes overwhelmed with feelings of anxiety, and executes poorly a piece she knows fully and performed superbly in the same studio in rehearsal only the day before. Her inner conflict is clear: she has already given up her childhood; entering the company school may pit her against better dancers, and she will have to give up more. This is an impossible bind: if she realizes the bind consciously she must choose between the dance she loves and having a more normal adolescence. She must become aware of how the time and effort she has invested already in dance have replaced a more "normal" childhood. Rather than consciously see this bind, she freezes, gives a poor performance, and does not qualify.

This dancer's problem could be helped by psychotherapy; over time, exploration of her own feelings and preferences might enable her to choose more clearly which life she wants.

Looking at performance anxiety from a different perspective, the field of sports psychology has devoted considerable energy to helping athletes shape positive and competitive attitudes, and to minimize the distractions of personal emotional issues or current stressors. Early this century, researchers found that an optimum degree of tension provided the best task performance; too little arousal could be as detrimental as too much (34). By the mid-1960s, a range of performance-enhancing "mental" techniques had been applied to athletes, ranging from hypnotic suggestion (35) to mental imagery (36). Later, Jencks and Krenz (37) used hypnosis to suggest anxiety reduction, mental imagery, and mental rehearsal. Autogenic training, the use of self-hypnosis and relaxation, has become more popular in recent years. One such method, "modified autogenic training," which involves self-hypnosis, relaxation exercises, and dissociation techniques, has been tried with a small group of ballet dancers (38). The intent is "to relax the body but keep the mind active and aware so that special instructions can be inserted." In the author's globally-described case study, training was provided to eleven members of a professional *corps de ballet* who felt themselves unable to advance because of feelings of excessive stress and anxiety and difficulties concentrating. Instructors found "marked improvement" in concentration and performance. More impressively, five of the eleven subsequently moved up to solo or principal roles.

Other Major Psychiatric Disorders

Published scientific data on affective disorders in dancers are sparse. Horosko and Kupersmith (27) report 84% of performers answering a questionnaire said that in the last year they had experienced feelings of depression. At least one group believes in a strong link between depression and the chronic pain often suffered by injury-prone but stoic dancers (39). To the surprise of the authors, a sample of 65 modern dancers showed no trace of depression on the Beck depression test; a subset of 30 also had normal Minnesota Multiphasic Personality Inventory (MMPI) depression scales (40). Clearly, further data need to be gathered.

There is no evidence for a link between bipolar (manic-depressive) disorder and dancing, though one retrospective study finds a high incidence of bipolar disorder in famous writers, with little familial and almost no personal schizophrenia (41).

Although Nijinsky was labeled schizophrenic when institutionalized, raising the question of the prevalence of schizophrenia among dancers, there are no data to suggest such a linkage.

Officially, homosexual behavior or preference has not been considered evidence of psychopathology for the past decade, but has been considered a personal preference issue, an early life developmental issue, or a genetic issue. Societal changes have weakened the old stereotype of the male dancer as necessarily homosexual.

This type of subject often has been dropped from public discussion. There is no published demographic evidence for the percentage of gay dancers, male or female.

AIDS

AIDS, the recent epidemic in world health, has not spared the smaller world of performers. AIDS is caused by HIV, which usually is acquired by sexual or blood-borne transmission. One initially publicized high-risk population for AIDS was made up of gay males, with higher risk for those engaging in anal intercourse with multiple partners. Given the stereotype of the male dancer population as incorporating a significant number of gay men, the high visibility of deaths among young male dancers in recent years has served to reinforce this public image. Recent evidence reveals that the HIV transmits readily between heterosexual partners, vastly broadening the at-risk population. The psychological impact is profound.

The Dancer's Personality

As noted in the opening paragraph, there is no "dancer's personality." No large systematic study of dancers' personality styles has been published in the scientific literature. Three limited refereed papers are available: a survey from a performing arts psychiatric clinic (27), a controlled study of personality differences between dancers and nondancers (6), and a test-based personality profile report of modern dance students (1,40). There is little additional literature on the transition out of dance, consisting of a brief report of a Performing Arts Center for Health (PACH) career-counseling center (42), a description of the work of the Dance Transition Centre of Canada (43), and a description of a career-transition counseling model (44). These are reviewed below.

The psychiatric paper is a demographic survey of the performer-patients of the clinic established by the PACH in Manhattan (27). Of the 93 patients participating in the survey, mean age was 26, two thirds were female, almost all were white. Apparently a symptom survey, the report notes more than two thirds with complaints of depression, loneliness, or inadequate diets (for nonfinancial reasons). More than half claimed severe anxiety or sleep problems. More than a third stated family problems, employment problems, or divorce or breakup of relationships. A sixth had suffered the death of a significant other. The staff of the clinic found a common difficulty with emotional expressivity: their clients were more comfortable talking about their injuries and eating disorders than they were about their feelings. The authors conclude that "the kind of illness experienced by performers is no different from that of the general population."

The comparison study used girls attending a Dutch ballet school, in 11- to 12-year-old and 15- to 16-year-old groups (6). These girls studied classical and modern ballet 15 hours per week and had a modified academic schedule in the school. They were compared wth public school students on a number of measures, to look specifically at several psychological and behavioral factors. In terms of behavior, the interests and leisure activities of the dancers did not differ appreciably in quantity or quality from the nondancers, except that the dancers had significantly less interest in sports (participating in, reading about, or observing athletics). They had as many hobbies and other outside interests, but the dancers had a higher interest not only in dance but also in the arts in general.

In terms of attitudes and traits, the dancers, contrary to expectations, had less favorable self-attitudes and self-esteem than their peers. The author speculates that this results from the demanding nature of the professional school, with its critical attitude about physical abilities and performance. The dancers also scored high on emotionality scales, low on thrill- and adventure-seeking and impulsivity. The author speculates that this might account for part of their low self-esteem: having been encouraged toward emotional expressivity in a judgmental environment, they might simply be more able than their peers to express the negatives. This seems to run counter to the observation in American ballet schools that the students were not especially emotionally communicative in their private lives; rather, they withdrew from emotionally- and cognitively-based activities in favor of those which were kinesthetically based (16,28). It also differs from the above-reported psychiatric clinic experience (27).

The 15- to 16-year-old dancers were more achievement-motivated than their non-dancing agemates. This might be due either to the environment or to self-selection of motivated students; the data for 11- to 12-year-olds were not statistically significant. Both groups of dancers were more introverted than were their nondancing peers. Their anxiety scores were slightly higher but not significantly so. The author concludes that self-selection may be the most important factor, since he subscribes to Eysenck's contention (45) that both emotionality and extroversion are biologically based.

The test-based personality profile report is a preliminary, skewed-sample finding from 62 modern dance students attending a national summer modern dance festival. The subjects were studied demographically and given a battery of psychological tests (1,15,46). Demographically, they were a somewhat homogeneous population made up largely of college-attending 18- to 23-year-olds usually majoring in dance; they averaged a decade of serious dance study. Three quarters saw dance as their primary life commitment. Two thirds saw themselves primarily as performers, averaging 30 hours in the studio per week.

The group averaged 88% of expected body mass, with a third reporting menstrual abnormalities (as opposed to the 87% expected body mass and 75% abnormal menses reported by Garner and Garfinkel (12) in their study of adolescent ballet students). Their thinness did not necessarily correlate with eating attitudes: 75% had normal eating attitudes but were as thin as the 25% with abnormal attitudes.

Half of the group took the MMPI, a well-documented, reliable personality inventory which looks at various traits, patterns of style, and symptoms. The MMPI also controls for lying, distortion, random guessing, and skipping answers. On the MMPI, the 30 subjects were rather normal. Most scales were within the normal range, with small variances. The exceptions were the very low scores for symptomatology on the schizophrenia, hypochondriasis and psychasthenia scales, where the means were just over a standard deviation lower than the mean for the general population. The control scales were normal (no lying or random answering). The depression scores were normal. The entire group also took the Beck depression test, which resulted in normal scores with little variance. Thus the sample demonstrated little psychopathology.

The modern dancer's locus of control was studied in two ways. Internal locus of control implies belief that the person internally controls his or her own destiny and fate. External locus implies belief that external forces beyond one's immediate control are more relevant (47). First, in a test of locus of control in general, the mean score for the group was in the external range with little variance. This finding would tend to support the image of the dance student who is compliant, sees adult authority as inevitable, and tends toward fatalism. However, the second test of locus of control on the same subjects bore significantly different results.

Measuring health locus of control, one finds whether the subjects believe that their health is determined by what they themselves do (e.g., diet, careful exercise), by powerful others' recommendations (e.g., nutritionists, teachers, doctors), or by chance (bad luck, accidents) (48). Given the findings that the modern dance students had a strong extenal locus of control over their lives in general, the authors expected the same finding with regard to the students' health locus of control. Surprisingly, the opposite occurred. The group mean score (with small variance) was the highest internal health locus of control score for any group yet reported.

To interpret this score the authors assumed that the subjects felt that they could have little influence on the many external forces in their lives; however, they could and did control their bodies. This assumption is consistent with the hypotheses of groups that anecdotally have described the individual and group dynamics of ballet students attending national schools (16,28). The validity of this interpretation remains unproven.

Little has been published about the transition out of dance. Pickman (42) reported briefly on career counseling with professional dancers considering new careers. His union-funded clinic's dancer-clients were typically in their mid-30s, self-referred after screening by the union. At the time of the writing, 20 professional dancers had entered career counseling. The first task usually was exploration of the individual's readiness to stop dancing. Loss of prestige, of prowess, of friends, of structure, and even of self-identity, were forces typically relevant. Anger, frustration, depression, substance abuse, and eating disorders were reported. Some of the subjects had little experience with other nondance interests; their focus for decades was almost exclusively on technique. Others had long-standing or long-dormant interests which could be stimulated. His overall impression of the significant differences in coping styles among his clients reminds us not to assume all dancers are alike, even at the end of their careers.

The Dancer Transition Centre of Canada has assisted over 150 dancers in psychological, legal, financial, and career counseling services. The Centre's purpose is to confront the issues facing professional dancers who have no model for ending their careers or for making the transition into new work. The specific types of counseling are supplemented by a broad educational program, a newsletter, and a limited amount of financial aid for re-education and training (43).

A concrete approach to counseling dancers who are moving out of dance is presented by Wolofsky (44), employing a narrowly constructed developmental model to support the individual's self-perceptions during the transition. It uses the inherent stresses of such a transition to address both the interpersonal and the internal psychological issues of the individual. While its theoretical structure may narrow the appeal of this approach, it does provide counseling clinicians with a model of how one might conceptualize the transition out of dance.

There is a theoretical schema of the typical psychological developmental stages of dancers (40). Although a summary of the schema would be beyond the scope of this chapter, some of its salient features are outlined below. The driving principle is that formal dance study, like any other structured activity, can have profound influence on the child who takes lessons. When carried out over more than a decade with increasing intensity, such study can have pervasive influence on development of personality. Given the most popular dance alternatives of ballet, modern, and jazz, those who stay in dance study and those who choose to study more intensively one of these alternatives will all be better suited to and more influenced by the subculture of that field of dance as time goes on. However, many students leave dance after a briefer time, and may have more subtle effects from their experience. Personality and behavior are multidetermined, so even a stereotypical dancer will have many personality variables not essentially determined or significantly affected by dance training.

Clinical Approach to the Dancer

Since there is no specific dancer's personality, there is no one correct approach to a dancer-patient. Specific risks have been discussed as they apply to various disorders. In addition, however, there are a number of factors which may "make or break" the working relationship with the dancer-patient and so profoundly affect the complexity of arriving at a diagnosis, choice of treatment, and chance of full compliance.

Given a special population, clinician attitude may be the most important factor in determining outcome. Myers notes that "many dancers have developed fear and frustration with the efficacy of the medical art in relation to dance" (49). Many dancers instead (or additionally) have turned to alternative systems such as chiropractic, acupuncture, and nutritional therapies. These have tended to look beyond the specific problem and address the individual more holistically, or at least weigh more heavily the individual's desire or need to remain active in dance as much as possible during diagnosis and treatment.

For the dancer, there may be considerable frustration with slow or unsuccessful medical interventions; conservative approaches which require avoidance of dance will seem as abhorrent to the dancer as would suspension of practice for a physician. A given dancer-patient may have difficulty with a physician's style, whether authoritarian, paternal, or collegial; most, however complain about the former approaches and not the latter. The frustration of dealing with real uncertainties explained by a medical doctor who describes the various possibly effective treatments for severe back pain may stand in marked contrast to the promise of success from a simple-sounding approach (e.g., megavitamin therapy or spinal manipulation) to address that same back pain.

There also may be a more fundamental dislike or avoidance of physicians. This may be based on the expense of medical care (many postadolescent dancers are uninsured); on aesthetics or anti-establishment feelings (doctors are seen as impersonal, high-tech and materialistic); on the worry that treatment may lead to permanent complications and be career-impairing or career-ending; or on the fear that medical modalities may be as difficult to tolerate as the pain of all but the most severe injuries, and bring with them the loss of control over the dancer's body.

This last factor may be, for some, the most difficult hurdle. Clinicians are familiar with the fear of loss of control over one's body, seeing it often in nondancers. It may represent loss of control over one's life, fears of disability or even of death. For the dancer, whose focus may be almost exclusively on keeping the body in perfect condition, illness and injury may imply a personal failure. Giving up control to someone else is difficult enough. It may seem intolerable to give up control to a doctor who may appear to be too busy to listen or, even worse, to be insensitive to the fears the dancer brings to the situation.

Accordingly, the clinician's capacity to be aware of these needs and preferences and to tolerate them without taking them personally, without feeling the need to challenge them to assert correctness, wisdom, or authority, are crucial to the successful negotiation of medical care for the dancer-patient. In dance medicine, rapport may be the single most important factor in determining outcome.

REFERENCES

1. Schnitt JM, Schnitt D. Psychological aspects of dance. In: Clarkson P, Skrinar M, eds. *The science of dance training*. Champaign, IL: Human Kinetics Press, 1988;239–267.
2. Puretz SL. A comparison of the effects of dance and physical education on the self-concept of selected disadvantaged girls. In: Priddle RE, ed. *Psychological perspectives on dance*. New York: Congress on Research in Dance, 1978.
3. Gurley V, Neuringer A, Massee J. Dance and sports compared: effects on psychological well-being. *Journal of Sports Medicine* 1984;24:58–68.
4. Leste A, Rust J. Effects of dance on anxiety. *Perceptual and Motor Skills* 1984;58:767–772.
5. Folkins CH, Sime WE. Physical fitness training and mental health. *American Psychologist* 1981; 36:373–389.
6. Bakker FC. Personality differences between young dancers and non-dancers. *Personality and Individual Differences* 1988;9(1):121–131.

7. Puretz SL. Modern dance's effect on the body image. *International Journal of Sport Psychology* 1982;13:176–186.
8. Dyer JB III, Crouch JG. Effects of running and other activities on mood. *Perceptual and Motor Skills* 1988;67:43–50.
9. Wadden TA, Stunkard AJ. Social and psychological consequences of obesity. *Annals of Internal Medicine* 1985;103:1062–1067.
10. Maloney MJ. Anorexia nervosa and bulimia in dancers: accurate diagnosis and treatment planning. *Clinics in Sports Medicine* 1983;2:549–555.
11. Ryan AJ, Stephens RE. *The dancer's complete guide to healthcare & a long career.* Princeton NJ: Princeton Books, 1988;118–119.
12. Garner DM, Garfinkel PE. Socio-cultural factors in the development of anorexia nervosa. *Psychological Medicine* 1980;10:647–656.
13. Kurtzman FD, Yager J, Landsverk J, Wiesmeier KE, Bodurka DC. Eating disorders among selected female student populations at UCLA. *Journal of the American Dietetic Association* 1989;89(1):45–53.
14. Joseph A, Wood IK, Goldberg SC. Determining populations at risk for developing anorexia nervosa based on selection of college major. *Psychiatric Research* 1982;7:53–58.
15. Schnitt JM, Schnitt D, Del A'une W. Anorexia nervosa vs. "thinness" in modern dance students: comparison with ballet students. *Annals of Sports Medicine* 1986;3(1):9–13.
16. Druss RG, Silverman JA. Body image and perfectionism of ballerinas: comparison and contrast with anorexia nervosa. *General Hospital Psychiatry* 1979;1:115–121.
17. Schnitt JM, Schnitt D. Eating disorders in dancers. *Med Probl Perform Art* 1986;1(2):39–44.
18. Szmukler GI, Eisler I, Gillies C, Hayward ME. The implications of anorexia nervosa in a ballet school. *Journal of Psychiatric Research* 1985;19:177–181.
19. Brooks-Gunn J, Warren MP. Mother-daughter differences in menarcheal age in adolescent girls attending national dance company schools and non-dancers. *Annals of Human Biology* 1988;15(1):35–44.
20. Warren MP. The effects of exercise on pubertal progression and reproductive function in girls. *Journal Clinical Endocrinology and Metabolism* 1980;51:1150–1157.
21. Garner DM, Garfinkel PE, Rockert W, Olmsted MP. A prospective study of eating disturbances in the ballet. *Psychotherapy & Psychosomatics* 1987;48:170–175.
22. Vandereycken W, Van den Broucke S. Anorexia nervosa in males: a comparative study of 107 cases reported in the literature (1970 to 1980). *Acta Psychiatr Scand* 1984;447–454.
23. Anderson AE, Mickalide AD. Anorexia nervosa and bulimia: their differential diagnosis in 24 males referred to an eating and weight disorders clinic. *Bull Menninger Clin* 1985;49:227–235.
24. Mitchell JE, Goff G. Bulimia in male patients. *Psychosomatics* 1984;25:909–913.
25. Anderson AE. Anorexia nervosa and bulimia in adolescent males. *Pediat Ann* 1984;13:901–907.
26. Hall A, Delahunt JW, Ellis PM. Anorexia nervosa in the male: clinical features and follow-up of nine patients. *J Psychiat Res* 1985;19:315–321.
27. Horosko M, Kupersmith JRF. *The dancer's survival manual.* New York: Harper & Row, 1987.
28. Lowenkaupf EL, Vincent LM. The student ballet dancer and anorexia. *Hillside Journal of Clinical Psychiatry* 1982;4:53–64.
29. Nies AS. Clinical pharmacology of beta-adrenergic blockers. *Med Probl Perform Art* 1986;1(1):5–29.
30. Cohen LS, Rosenbaum JE. Clonazepam: new uses and potential problems. *Journal of Clinical Psychiatry* 1987;48 (Suppl 10):50–55.
31. Goodwin DW, Schulsinger F, Hermansen L, Guze SB, and Winokur G. Alcohol problems in adoptees. *Archives General Psychiatry* 1973;28:238–243.
32. Brandfonbrener AG, Brantigan CO, DeGaetani J, DeLay D, DeNelsky GY, Dichter M, Nagel J, Proctor MR, Weisblatt S, Zlotkin LF. Coping with stress. *Med Probl Perform Art* 1986;1(1):12–16.
33. Weisblatt S. A psychoanalytic view of performance anxiety. *Med Probl Perform Art* 1986;1(2):64–67.
34. Yerkes RM, Dodson JD. The relation of strength of stimulus to rapidity of habit formation. *Journal of Comparative Neurology and Psychology* 1908;18:459–482.
35. Naruse G. Hypnosis Treatment of Stage Fright in Champion Athletes. *Psychologia* 1972;1(3–4):199–205.
36. Pulos L. Hypnosis and Think Training with Athletes. Abstract. Annual Meeting, American Society of Clinical Hypnosis, San Francisco, 1969.

37. Jencks B, Krenz E. Hypnosis in sports. In: Smith AH, Wester WD, eds. *Comprehensive clinical hypnosis*. Philadelphia: Lippincott, 1984.
38. Krenz EW. Improving competitive performance with hypnotic suggestions and modified autogenic training: Case reports. *American Journal of Clinical Hypnosis* 1984;27(1):58–63.
39. Horosko M. Depression: is it normal? *Dance Magazine* February, 1985;78–79.
40. Schnitt JM, Schnitt D. Psychological issues in a dancer's career. In: Ryan AJ, Stephens RE, eds. Dance medicine: a comprehensive guide. Chicago: Pluribus Press & The Physician in Sportsmedicine, 1987;334–349.
41. Andreason N. Creativity and mental illness: prevalence rates in writers and their first-degree relatives. *American Journal of Psychiatry* 1987;144(10):1288–1292.
42. Pickman AJ. Career transitions for dancers: a counselor's perspective. *Journal of Counseling and Development* 1987;66:200–201.
43. Greben SE. The dancer transition centre of Canada: addressing the stress of giving up professional dancing. *Med Probl Perform Art* 1989;4(3):128–130.
44. Wolofsky Z. The constructive-developmental model in counselling career transition dancers. *Med Probs Perf Artists* 1989;4(3):122–127.
45. Eysenck HJ. *A model for personality*. New York: Springer, 1981.
46. Schnitt JM, Schnitt D, Del A'une W. *Health Locus of Control in Modern Dancers*. Unpublished manuscript, 1989.
47. Rotter JB. Generalized expectancies for internal versus external control of reinforcement. *Psychological Monographs 80* 1966;1(609 whole).
48. Wallston KA, Wallston BS. Development of the multidimensional health locus of control (MHLC) Scales. *Health Education Monographs* 1978;6:160–170.
49. Myers M. What dance medicine and science mean to the dancer. In: Clarkson PM, Skrinar M, eds. *The science of dance training*. Champaign, IL: Human Kinetics Press, 1988;3–15.

Textbook of Performing Arts Medicine, edited
by R. T. Sataloff, A. Brandfonbrener, and
R. Lederman. Raven Press, Ltd.,
New York © 1991.

13

Foot and Ankle in Dance

G. James Sammarco

*Director, Center for the Performing Arts; Clinical Professor of
Orthopaedic Surgery at the University of Cincinnati, Cincinnati, Ohio 45219*

Ballet dancers are extraordinary athletes. They place great demands upon their feet and ankles. Consequently, it is not surprising that foot and ankle injuries are common in dancers. In many cases, they can be prevented by proper training and equipment, especially appropriate shoes and dancing surfaces. When injuries do occur, it is important to understand the special consequences for the professional dancer of both the injury and its treatment. The orthopaedist caring for foot and ankle injuries in professional dancers should be acquainted with the demands and language of dance.

DANCE POSITIONS

The three "balance points" of the foot are: (1.) ¼ pointe—the weight is not over the metatarsal arch (this is used by males in staging many poses); (2.) ½ pointe— the weight is over the metatarsal arch (this is used in pirouettes and *relevé* for females when a full pointe is not being utilized, and it is used extensively by males; (3.) ¾ pointe—the body rises as high as possible on the foot (this is desirable for all quick footwork because it lends lightness and speed rarely attained or made in pirouettes or in a holding pose). Dancing *sur les pointes*, on the tips of the toes, requires good coordination of the whole body, with each part holding its place and moving to new positions correctly and without strain (Fig. 13.1). Pointe dancing before the dancer is ready (3 years of training and at least age 11 years) may result in several problems. If the ankle has not attained full "extension" (plantar flexion) and the foot is stiff, lateral ankle strain results. Balance must then be controlled by the calf muscles, with the hips and knees flexed (1). The lumbar spine compensates by hyperextending (lordosis) rather than being erect. This poor posture causes an unaesthetic style, overdevelopment and fatigue of calf muscles, and in later years symptomatic arthritis of the spine. If the arch of the foot is not developed, the toes

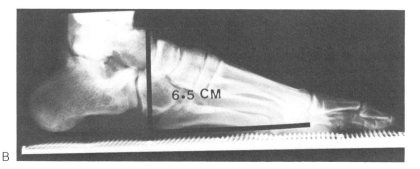

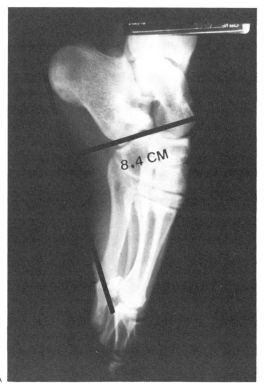

FIG. 13.1. X-rays of a dancer standing flat-footed and *A*: *sur la pointe. B*: This dancer is able to support his or her weight without the support of a ballet pointe shoe. Note how the height of the arch increases when on pointe.

tend to "clutch," "curl," or "knuckle over;" that is, they hyperflex in the pointe shoe (Fig. l3.2). No amount of lamb's wool padding in the pointe shoe substitutes for a well-developed arch and adequate ankle motion. Treatment consists of discontinuing dancing *sur les pointes* until such time as the child has been adequately prepared.

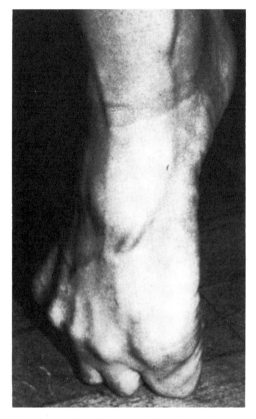

FIG. 13.2. "Clutching," "curling," or "knuckling over." The dancer is bearing full weight, demonstrating what happens within the ballet pointe shoe when a dancer is permitted to dance *en pointe* prior to being physically able to do so.

DEVELOPING THE ARCH

A high arch, long considered desirable for the dancer, gives an aesthetic appearance to the entire leg. Suppleness of the foot combines with the arch, enabling the dancer to perform quick and difficult steps in a graceful manner. An important goal of early training is the development of both the intrinsic and extrinsic foot muscles in order to raise the arch. A student with flexible pes planus can develop this actively supported arch within 6 months. If it is not developed sufficiently, dancing may become painful, and the student will discontinue his or her studies. Males usually begin dance training later than females. Their tarsal joints tend to be stiff, and this can cause "rolling in" as the dancer attempts to increase his turnout. A result of such chronic strain is acquired hallux valgus.

CONGENITAL ABNORMALITIES

The desire for achievement in art often overcomes a physical handicap. In modern dance, where asymmetric positions are common, steps may be developed by a dancer to hide a physical deformity. The great seventeenth-century dancer Bournonville perfected ballon to conceal his own foot deformity. Children with pes planus or a congenital or acquired foot deformity should not be discouraged from dance (2). If they are discouraged, they will feel as though they have been cheated; they must therefore find out for themselves whether they are able to dance. For minor deformities, cotton or wool padding in the ballet and pointe shoe is recommended. A forefoot prosthesis, however, causes loss of the proprioceptive feedback needed from foot contact with the floor and is not recommended.

THE DANCER'S NORMAL FOOT

There is no ideal shape for the dancer's foot. If the second toe is longer than the hallux, flexion of the distal interphalangeal joint occurs. Floor contact occurs through the hallux and the flexed distal interphalangeal joint of the second toe. The foot with toes in a "falling away" shape (that is, with each of the lateral four toes shorter than its medially adjacent neighbor) is not commonly found in toe dancers. Here floor contact occurs through the tip of the hallux while dancing on pointe. Load concentration is too high and thus painful. The average area of contact between the floor and the shoe is about 4 cm^2 (3).

BUNIONS

Bunions are common in dancers (4). An important factor in female dancers is that static deforming forces in the pointe shoe hold the metatarsal heads together and force the great toe into valgus. The lateral toes are forced into adduction, with the weight line passing through the first and second toes (Fig. 13.3) (5, 6). Associated mallet of the second toe or a hammertoe may accompany this. Such deformities may be seen by the age of 18 if the dancer has been dancing on point since the age of 11. Symptoms of pain over the medial first metatarsal commonly occur after rehearsing *en pointe* and abate within a few hours, although this may be associated with bursitis. Pain in the second toe at the medial aspect of the proximal interphalangeal joint is caused by hallux pressure.

Males may develop hallux valgus by improper training to improve turnout through performance of a forced grand plié. During a grand plié, the dancer rolls forward, putting stress on the medial aspect of the first metatarsophalangeal joint. This stretches the medial ligaments. If not corrected, severe hallux valgus may develop.

Treatment of minor foot pains includes elevation after dancing for 2 hours, with the feet elevated above the slightly bent knees. Active motion and elevation provide

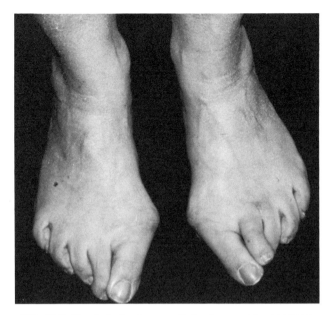

FIG. 13.3. The feet of a dancer with bunions and hammertoes.

"milking action" to the foot, reducing stiffness and possible edema. Classes need not be interrupted, but a longer "warm-up" and flexibility program are prescribed.

HAMMER TOE

The closed space of the pointe shoe forcibly shortens the toes and contributes to hammertoe formation. Dancers spend much of their time on the "balance points" with the metatarsophalangeal joints extended and the proximal interphalangeal joints flexed. Flexible hammertoe deformity develops early and may become fixed in the older dancer (Fig. 13.3) (5). Soft tissue changes include callus and soft corns over the proximal interphalangeal joint. Callosities at the terminal tuft and beneath the metatarsal head of the respective toe are usually not symptomatic.

SPLAYFOOT

The ballet shoe is made of soft, lightweight leather and cannot restrict metatarsal spread. The intermetatarsal ligaments stretch with time. The long flexor tendons may slip between the metatarsal heads, and the dancer bears weight directly on the metatarsal heads without the flexor tendons for cushioning. The foot appears narrow when non-weight-bearing, but spreads when weight-bearing. In younger dancers, the feet are asymptomatic. However, older dancers, particularly males in their fourth and fifth decades, develop painful forefeet when standing for long periods.

The medial longitudinal arch is retained, but bunions and hammertoes can develop in spite of the splaying.

In the older dancer, a full-insole molded arch support with an elevated medial longitudinal arch and a metatarsal pad 5 mm high is prescribed. This is worn during class as well as in street shoes. Dancers do not wear orthoses during performances because they decrease the sensitivity and proprioceptive feedback in the foot.

HALLUX RIGIDUS

While dancing *en pointe*, increased loads crossing the hallucal metatarsophalangeal joint can hasten the onset of arthritis. Acute flexion injury to the metatarsophalangeal joint can injure the dorsal joint capsule and lead to the formation of osteophytes. Standing in $^1/_2$ pointe strains the ligaments and increases loads at the joint. Since full dorsiflexion of the metatarsophalangeal joint is most important while dancing in the *demi pointe* position, the position in which a dancer spends much performing time, limitation of this motion, particularly if it is painful, causes alteration in dancing style (5,7,8).

Osteophytes, joint space narrowing, and restricted motion make it difficult to dance (Fig. 13.4). Going from the *demi pointe* position to pointe position is uncomfortable, and may predispose to further injury. The dancer attempts to dance until stiffness and pain have significantly caused a change in style. Treatment is based on the amount of pain and limitation of motion. The occurrence of osteophytes at the joint will not preclude fitting a pointe shoe. Appropriate padding can be made if this is painful but most of the pain occurs with motion of the toe, not with pressure over osteophytes.

Cheilectomy of the metatarsophalangeal joint through a medial incision should be performed only after appropriate counseling of the dancer as to alternatives, including cessation of a career or performing dances that do not require such forced dorsiflexion. If cheilectomy is performed, a full 90 degrees range of dorsiflexion should be obtained at the time of surgery. Cheilectomy should not be expected to increase motion significantly but rather decrease pain. Silastic prosthetic replacement of proximal hallucal phalanx has been performed rarely and is not recommended. Arthrodesis of the joint precludes motion and therefore is also not recommended for dancers.

Dancers tend to be self-motivated, goal-oriented individuals and tolerate a considerable amount of discomfort. A full range of motion in the hallux is required for the dancer. Most procedures for bunion correction require 6 to 12 months for recovery and may result in the termination of a dance career. No procedure for splayfoot hallux rigidus or bunion correction has yet been devised that will allow consistently good results without the risk of disaster. If surgery is to be considered, it should be discussed in detail and with full recognition of the potential necessity to choose alternative career goals, e.g., teaching or choreography.

A hammertoe tends to be flexible and minimally symptomatic during the period of a professional dancer's career. Procedures that shorten or stiffen toes in order to

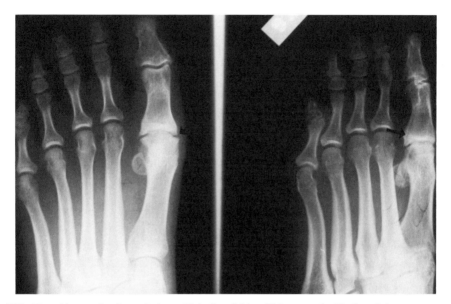

FIG. 13.4. X-rays of a dancer's feet with hallux rigidus. This caused stiffening of the great toe (*arrows*).

"align" them often lead to permanent loss of motion and painful joints. There is no indication for correction of the mallet deformity of the second toe in the pointe dancer since this is a common normal variant, i.e., the second toe is longer than the first.

X-RAY CHARACTERISTICS

The Ankle and Foot

Roentgenograms of the dancer's ankle may show osteophytes on the anterior lip of the tibia and the superior portion of the talar neck. This is seen in individuals in other professions that require forced dorsiflexion of the ankle, e.g., baseball catchers (9). Calcification within the medial and lateral ankle ligaments is not common without a history of previous ankle injury. Osteochondritis dissecans can be confused with an osteochondral fracture but is usually asymptomatic.

Characteristics of the tarsal bones in dancers can be divided into two categories, those in dancers who began ballet training before cessation of bone growth, and those in dancers who began training when or after growth of the foot is completed. Those who begin training at a younger age have the grooves for tendons and areas of attachment of intrinsic foot muscles prominent, whereas arthritic changes characterized by osteophyte formation and ossification within ligaments occur in those who begin training at an older age (Fig. 13.5) (10–13). The arch of the ballet dancer, particularly females, is elevated, but pes planus also occurs in dancers.

The diaphysis of the second and occasionally the third metatarsal has thickened cortex (Fig. 13.5). Although this may occur in females as a result of dancing *sur la pointe* or as a sequela to a healing fatigue fracture (13,14), it is common in asymptomatic dancers of both ballet and modern dance. Cortical hypertrophy secondary to chronic stress on the forefoot through the most rigid portion of the foot is the cause. (2).

Increased density in the subchondral bone of the metatarsophalangeal and interphalangeal joints of the hallux and along the lateral cortex of the first metatarsal is also common.

The tarsal navicular is somewhat flatter and shorter than normal in dancers. The dorsoplantar angle of inclination of the talar neck is slightly less than 90° when compared with that in nondancers (10).

FATIGUE FRACTURE

The "Dreaded Black Line"

Common areas for stress fractures in dancers include the base of the second metatarsal (5,15), navicular (16), cuneiform, calcaneus, sesamoid (17) phalanges and in the cuboid (18). They may be either intra- or extra-articular. Insidious onset

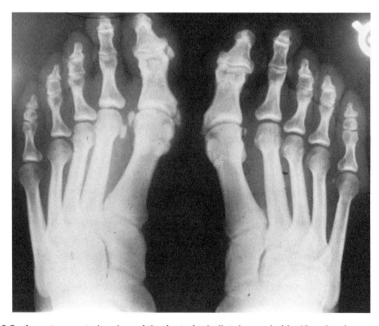

FIG. 13.5. An anteroposterior view of the feet of a ballet dancer in his 40s, showing extensive ligament calcification and osteophyte formation. Also note increased cortical thickening of the second metatarsophalangeal due to increased loading on the forefoot. (From Sammarco GS, ref. 12, with permission).

is the rule, but the dancer may complain of acute onset of pain only after a stress fracture has become complete.

In dance, the foot and ankle are commonly stressed beyond their limits of repair. Some floor surfaces on which dancers are forced to perform are made of concrete or of linoleum on concrete or wood. The recommended floor is one of hardwood that rests on springs or hardwood on wood rafters anchored directly to the walls without support beneath the center floor (19,20). Wood floors absorb the energy of foot-floor reactive forces more than other more rigid surfaces, which require the foot and body to absorb almost all of the force (21).

When the microfractures that occur with everyday dancing do not have time to heal before the next day's class, a stress fracture may begin to develop. Symptoms may precede x-ray findings by several months. An area of tenderness about the fracture is present. The pain becomes pinpointed over the fracture or remains diffuse, causing confusion of the diagnosis with chronic muscle fatigue, tendinitis, ligament strain, or periostitis. A sudden sharp pain is felt after several weeks of "ache" at the particular site (22). Roentgenographic evidence of a fracture may be lacking, even at this stage. A bone scan is useful to localize such fractures, as well as a CT scan, but even these may be negative within the first few weeks.

Fibular fatigue fracture usually occurs 10 cm above the lateral malleolus (Fig. 13.6) (23). A second common area is in the proximal fibular shaft. The fracture

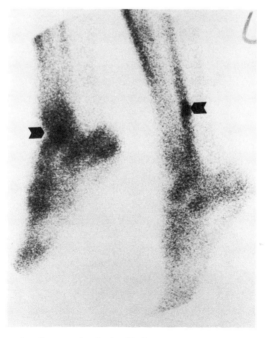

FIG. 13.6. Bone scan showing reaction in the fibular cortex 10 cm above the lateral malleolus (*right arrow*) secondary to fatigue fracture. Increased uptake in the opposite ankle (*left arrow*) indicated increased use of that ankle.

may recur within several months of complete healing if training is accelerated too rapidly. Fractures of the tibia occur most commonly in the shaft and may be multiple and bilateral (16). Fatigue fractures of the distal tibial metaphysis and plafond but can occur in the posterior malleolus. Recommended treatment is limited weight-bearing on crutches for at least 4 weeks. A rehabilitation program and water barre are then recommended.

High loads are transmitted through the second metatarsal. A fatigue fracture may occur in any portion including the neck, shaft, and base. Diagnosis may be difficult even in the presence of marked symptoms (Fig. 13.7). Close scrutiny of the anteroposterior and oblique roentgenograms, bone scan, and CT scan may be necessary to determine if a suspected fracture enters Lisfranc's joint.

A short weight-bearing leg cast is prescribed for 4 weeks. The use of an elastic adhesive dressing and crutches is offered as an alternative. After cast removal, rehabilitation is necessary. During this time, the patient may complain of symptoms similar to those noted earlier. Unrestricted routine is not permitted until there is roentgenographic evidence of bony union. Remodeling at the fracture site or periosteal reaction may remain on x-rays for some time and should not prevent return to a full dance routine.

A fracture at the base of the fifth metatarsal, unlike most acute fractures, may be the completion of a stress fracture (24). It occurs in an area where symptoms of pain were previously present. A sudden inversion step causes acute increase in pain. Often this occurs when landing from a leap. An x-ray prior to complete fracture may reveal "the dreaded black line," an incomplete fracture. Because of difficulty in healing, cessation of dance is necessary until union is evident on roentgenograms and symptoms have abated. If union is not complete within 3 months, repair of the nonunion with bone graft may be indicated. The bone graft is taken from the anterior medial distal tibial metaphysis through a small incision.

Fatigue fractures of the phalanges also occur. Taping of the fractured toe to the

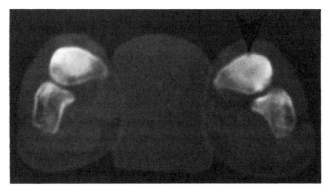

FIG. 13.7. Bone scan showing navicular stress fracture (*arrow*) treated for 3 months as tendinitis. CT scan revealed a fracture. From Sammarco GJ, ref. 23, with permission.

adjacent toe with placement of a cotton pad in the web space for 3 weeks will suffice. The tape is changed daily, and dancing *sur la pointe* is restricted until symptoms abate. The toe of the ballet or pointe shoe is padded with lamb's wool to relieve pressure.

FRACTURE OF THE FIFTH METATARSAL

Fracture of Fifth Metatarsal Styloid

The avulsion of the peroneus brevis tendon with a bony fragment from its insertion at the styloid process of the fifth metatarsal occurs when the foot is abruptly inverted. Pain and swelling are present over the styloid process of the fifth metatarsal. Passive inversion is quite painful. Roentgenograms reveal the characteristic fracture, which includes the styloid process and often a portion of the tarsometatarsal joint surface (Fig. 13.8). A fracture through the base of the fifth metatarsal often indicates the completion of a stress fracture. Treatment of styloid fracture is application of an elastic adhesive dressing for 3 weeks, followed by a slow return to active exercises at the barre. Recovery of full range of motion and strength may be expected in 2 months.

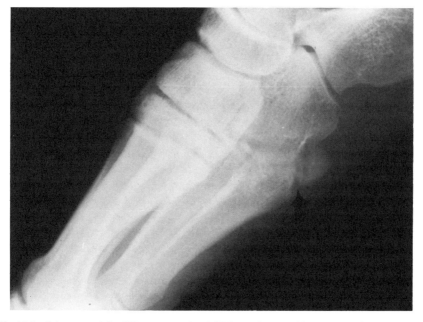

FIG. 13.8. A fracture of the fifth metatarsal styloid (*arrow*) caused by landing off balance and attempting to compensate by forceful contracture of the peroneus brevis muscle. Note fracture is distinct from the apophyseal growth plate.

In skeletally immature dancers, partial avulsion of the peroneus brevis tendon from its insertion may present with similar symptoms. In these patients, there is usually no roentgenographic evidence of a fracture. Confusion with an ossifying styloid apophysis is eliminated by comparison views of the opposite foot. Treatment includes application of an elastic adhesive dressing for 2 weeks, followed by barre and warm-up exercises on the exercise board (Fig. 13.9).

Fracture of the Fifth Metatarsal Neck and Shaft

Fracture of the fifth metatarsal occurs in the distal shaft or neck region of the bone as a result of inversion (Fig. 13.10). Significant displacement or angulation of the fracture is not uncommon. Such a fracture may take 5 months to heal with simple immobilization. The reasons for this are unclear, but constitutional factors such as

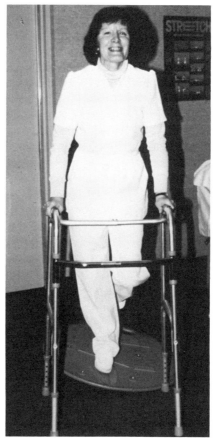

FIG. 13.9. Photograph of the foot and ankle exercise board, also known as a "wobble board" (Baps Board).

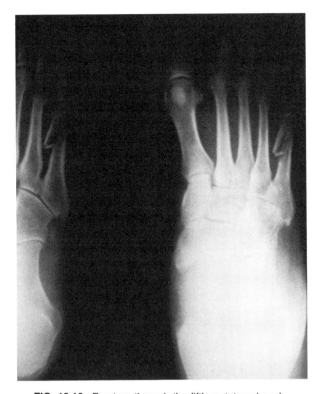

FIG. 13.10. Fracture through the fifth metatarsal neck.

low body weight and poor nutrition have been implicated. If alignment is not anatomic, an open reduction may be necessary. The fracture requires no longer to heal with open reduction and internal fixation than if treated by the closed method with cast immobilization. Cast immobilization for 6 weeks following surgery is recommended. A rehabilitation program is then instituted. Full use of the foot should not be permitted until there is roentgenographic evidence of bony union.

LIGAMENT AND MUSCLE INJURY

Stressing the midfoot may cause acute ligament strain at the intertarsal joints. Tenderness is usually localized over the specific area of strain, such as the lateral tarsometatarsal joints. Holding the heel firmly and gently manipulating the forefoot helps to localize the area. Roentgenograms may reveal evidence of a chip fracture. Treatment includes elevation, analgesics, and elastic taping of the foot while dancing. There are periods of exacerbation and remission.

Muscle spasm may be quite disabling. Spasm of the abductor hallucis muscle is characterized by medial longitudinal arch pain associated with stiffness of the hallux. Such acute problem respond to massage and gentle passive stretching of the toes. In summer or in tropical climates, electrolyte balance is of great importance. Rehearsals and classes must include periods of rest. Since lumbar spine disease is common among dancers, unilateral cramping of the foot may indicate a herniated disc. Persistent symptoms may be caused by a stress fracture, and a bone scan is recommended if treatment is unsuccessful.

NERVE INJURY

Dorsal Cutaneous Neuritis

The medial cutaneous branches of the deep peroneal nerve may be injured as they cross the ankle and the tarsometatarsal joints. Direct trauma is caused by repetitive sitting on the inverted dorsum of the bare foot, as required within certain modern dance steps. Stretching while dancing *en pointe* or simply pointing the foot can also cause this injury. Chronic irritation from the elastic strap that crosses the dorsum of the foot and holds the ballet shoe and/or shoe ribbons is infrequently the cause. A positive Tinel's sign confirms the diagnosis, with characteristic paresthesia. Treatment consists of application of porous paper adhesive tape across the tender area to decrease skin friction or use of a thin, foam rubber pad over the dorsal midfoot. Moving the elastic strap of the ballet shoe away from the involved area may also correct the problem.

Interdigital Neuroma

The symptoms of interdigital neuroma begin insidiously. Characteristically this malady occurs in the third and fourth web space and much less commonly in the second and third. The symptoms include metatarsalgia associated with paresthesias of the affected toes on the adjacent side of the web space. Treatment includes lamb's wool placed behind the metatarsal head in the ballet shoe or a felt pad taped to the sole. However, in modern dance or other barefoot dancing this is impractical. A good flexibility program is important, as well as nonsteroidal antiinflammatory drugs (NSAIDS). If symptoms persist, excision of the neuroma through a dorsally placed 3 cm incision is indicated. Meticulous care is taken to protect the neurocirculatory structures with magnification used to properly visualize the neuroma. Postoperative treatment includes refraining from dance until the wound heals, followed by a rehabilitation program including flexibility exercises, whirlpool, and use of a foot and ankle exerciser board.

AVASCULAR NECROSIS OF THE METATARSAL HEAD

Symptoms of metatarsalgia and joint stiffness limited to a single metatarsophalangeal joint, the second or third in particular, should alert one to the possibility of an infraction of the articular cortex. The *demi pointe* position exacerbates pain and stiffness at the joint (Fig. 13.11). Roentgenograms may not show the

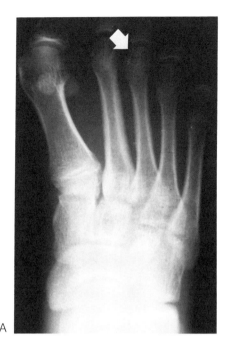
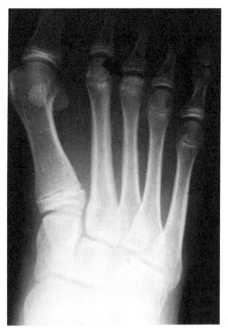
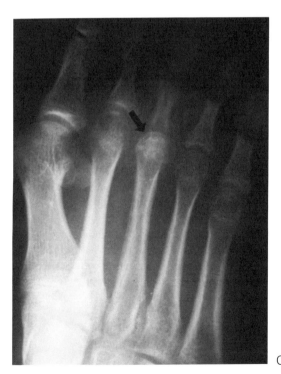

FIG. 13.11. X-rays of a dancer with avascular necrosis of the head of the third metatarsal (*arrows*). Progressive insidious pain and stiffness may precede x-ray changes by several months. (*A*) as symptoms began, (*B*) 3 months later, (*C*) after resection of the proximal 20% of the proximal phalanx.

characteristic subchondral lysis with collapse of the head and osteophytes for up to 3 months. Treatment in the early stages includes NSAIDS and a flexibility program. If symptoms persist, an arthroplasty of the metatarsophalangeal joint through a dorsal approach is indicated. The dancer is counseled before surgery. Excision of the proximal 20% of the proximal phalanx is recommended with cheilectomy of the metatarsal head (16,18). A smooth axial .045 Kirschner wire is used to immobilize the joint through the phalanges, skewering the flexor digitorum longus tendon which has been brought into the wound at the metatarsophalangeal joint. This holds the plantar plate and soft tissues in place until healing has occurred. The wire is removed in 4 weeks and a rehabilitation program begun. The dancer is permitted to return to class when symptoms permit. A prosthesis and simple cheilectomy are not recommended, since they do not relieve stiffness or pain.

SUBLUXING TOE

An unusual cause of metatarsalgia occurs when the dancer stands in the *demi pointe* position. It is associated with laxity, and synovitis involving the metatarsophalangeal joint of the second or third toe also occur (6,18,25). This is the area through which highest stresses pass in that position. Although the etiology is unknown, a laxity is present in the collateral ligaments and plantar plate. Symptoms begin insidiously over a period of several weeks, occasionally with a history of trauma. A history of previous surgery may be present prior to dancers seeking treatment for this new problem. Diagnosis is made by grasping the proximal phalanx in one hand while stabilizing the forefoot with the other, and moving the toe dorsally and plantarward to demonstrate motion. The metatarsophalangeal joint feels lax and characteristic pain is produced. The differential diagnosis includes avascular necrosis of the head of the metatarsal, stress fracture and acute synovitis from any cause, including infection or a transfer lesion from previous surgery. Treatment includes NSAIDS and buddy taping to the adjacent toe as well as using lamb's wool to pad around the tender joint on the plantar surface. If these measures fail and if symptoms significantly alter the dancer's performance, excision of the proximal 20% of the proximal phalanx may be considered. The dancer should be counseled accordingly, especially regarding time off.

Surgical technique is as for avascular necrosis except that cheilectomy is not necessary. The pin is removed at 4 weeks and gentle active range of motion with a flexibility program is begun. The dancer is permitted to return to pointe dancing as symptoms warrant after 6 weeks.

CYSTS

Cysts of the metatarsophalangeal joint occur as a result of trauma, commonly in the second and third days. The mass develops in 10 days. The dancer notices metatarsalgia associated with a mass between the metatarsal heads which is cystic and tender. MRI, CT scan, and soft tissue roentgenograms are all helpful in determining the nature of the cyst (Fig. 13.12). The shape may be dumbbell-like (18). It is recommended that excision of the cyst be performed since aspiration may lead to recurrence. A compression dressing is applied following surgery. Active range of motion and a rehabilitation program are begun within 7 days. Injection with corticoid steroids is not recommended.

PLANTAR FASCIITIS

Acute plantar fasciitis causes plantar pain on passive extension of the hallux and direct tenderness over the plantar fascia. This usually occurs following a period of abstention from dance. Tenderness is noted at the insertion of the plantar aponeurosis into the plantar calcaneal tuberosity. No nodules are palpable. The dancer is restricted from rehearsal for 2 to 3 days until acute symptoms subside. A stiff wooden clog is recommended along with elevation of the foot, analgesics, and NSAIDS. A foot and ankle exercise program (26) is performed for 10 minutes during warm-up before class. This condition may progress to chronic fasciitis. Steroid injections and surgery are infrequently indicated.

THE HALLUX

Fracture

Fracture of the proximal phalanx is uncommon in ballet. Certain movements of folk dance, such as the Spanish flamenco, in which the toe is forcibly and rapidly

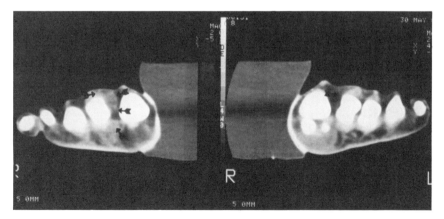

FIG. 13.12. Axial CT scan of the right and left forefoot showing a dumbbell-shaped cyst (*arrows*) between the right first and second metatarsal heads. Simple excision through a dorsal incision is recommended. (From Sammarco GJ, Chapter 49 in *The Foot*. Helal B & Wilson D (eds) Churchill Livingston, London, 1988).

driven against the floor, have caused fatigue fractures in the proximal phalanx, particularly in the adult student. The hallux is normally not subjected to such trauma. To minimize the risk of such injuries, dance study must proceed at a prudent rate to allow bone hypertrophy. Treatment consists of taping the hallux to the second toe and wearing a stiff-soled shoe for 3 weeks. Recovery may require 3 months and is associated with metatarsophalangeal stiffness that may remain for several months.

Injury to the Sesamoids

Sesamoiditis occurs in dancers whose routine requires rapid slapping of the forefoot and frequent leaps. Certain ethnic dance, such as Javanese dance, requires such slapping steps. The ball of the foot becomes tender shortly after the routine is begun. Within 1 month, it is quite painful beneath the medial sesamoid. Extension of the hallux allows the area of tenderness to advance, owing to the phalangeal insertion of the flexor hallucis brevis tendons. The sesamoid view on roentgenogram reveals a compression fracture of the tibial fibular sesamoid (Fig. 13.13). Bone scan and CT scan are helpful in differentiating this condition from stress fracture. Treatment consists of shaping a $^3/_8$-inch felt pad beneath the tender area of the sesamoid for relief. Since symptoms require as much as 6 months to subside, a foot orthosis placed beneath the first metatarsal head is helpful to provide relief when wearing street shoes. Prognosis is good.

Fracture of the sesamoid occurs from landing after a leap, such as *tour en l'air*. Treatment consists of placing a felt pad, 1 cm thick and shaped to relieve beneath the area of the sesamoids at the first metatarsal head. This treatment is also effective for stress fracture. Dancing is restricted until the pain subsides, usually 3 weeks.

ACUTE FLEXION INJURY

A common injury among dancers, more frequently in males, is acute hyperflexion injury of the metatarsophalangeal joint of the hallux. This injury is caused by tripping or "falling over" the foot during quick steps, as in glissade. The hallux is forcibly flexed as the tip of the toe is caught. The body weight falls on the flexed joint, causing the dorsal portion of the capsule to stretch or to tear. Pain is immediate and disabling. Tenderness over the dorsal aspect of the joint and pain on active flexion of the toe are present. Stability, however, is not lost. Roentgenograms are helpful only in excluding fracture. Treatment consists of elastic adhesive strapping of the great toe and forefoot. Splints are not required, but a stiff-soled street shoe and crutches are helpful. After 10 days, gentle and passive motion is begun. Full motion should return within 4 weeks. Hyperextension with abduction of the hallux is uncommon in dancers. This condition is known as "turf toe."

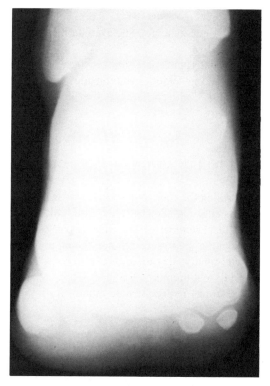

FIG. 13.13. Compression fracture of the fibular sesamoid. This occurs as a result of slapping steps that are performed in modern dance and ethnic dance.

Injury to the Interphalangeal Joint

Acute strain of the interphalangeal joint of the hallux is seen in the ballet student using pointe shoes that no longer have sufficient stiffness in the toebox. The student may not have the strength to support herself. Pain and swelling accompanied by inability to dance *sur les pointes* follow. Diagnosis is made by gently rotating the distal phalanx of the hallux while holding the metatarsophalangeal joint. This elicits pain over the dorsum and sides of the joint. No instability is present. Dancing *sur les pointes* is restricted for several days. Obtaining new, properly fitted pointe shoes and knowing when to change shoes are important factors in preventing recurrence.

Chronic hyperflexion of the interphalangeal joint of the hallux in children may result from allowing the student to dance *en pointe* before her ability, training, balance, and maturity dictate. This also occurs with knuckling down where all toes are flexed in the pointe shoe. The distal phalanx bears weight over the dorsum and nail in the pointe shoes. The result of such overzealous advancement by teachers or parents may delay development of the dancer's art. For both knuckling down and interphalangeal flexion, pointe dancing is delayed until the child is properly developed physically and mentally.

Hyperextension of the interphalangeal joint of the hallux is not uncommon. It develops in toe dancers and is seldom symptomatic. If symptoms occur, padding with lamb's wool is helpful. Surgery, especially arthrodesis to permanently stiffen the joint, is contraindicated.

DISLOCATION OF THE TOES

Accidents such as striking the foot against scenery can cause fracture dislocation of interphalangeal or metatarsophalangeal joints (Fig. 13.14). This is immediately incapacitating. Dorsal displacement of the phalanx causes an obvious deformity. Treatment is closed reduction by hyperextending the joint, applying traction to pull the phalanx distally, and finally, flexing of the toe to reduce the deformity. The toe is buddy taped to the adjacent uninjured toe for 3 weeks. Water barre exercises are begun during this time. It may require several months for full motion to return.

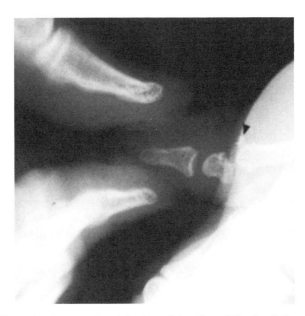

FIG. 13.14. X-ray showing unreduced fracture dislocation of the fourth toe proximal interphalangeal joint (*arrow*), preventing any efforts at dance. Reduction and arthrodesis of the joint effected a permanent cure.

CALLUSES AND CORNS

The pointe shoe is designed to distribute the weight of the dancer across the entire forefoot, gradually concentrating it on the hallux and second toe. It is then transmitted through the pointe shoe to the floor.

Callus formation over the medial interphalangeal joint of the hallux and the dorsal portions of the proximal interphalangeal joints is normal in the toe dancer, as is callus formation over the lateral aspects of the fourth and fifth toes (Fig. 13.15). These are asymptomatic when toughened by daily classes *en pointe*. If painful, recommended treatment includes porous paper (Micropore) and adhesive tape wrapped about the toe to decrease friction.

The design of the ballet and pointe shoe is such that there is no right or left, simply a general form which shapes the forefoot and also allows the forefoot to shape it. This results in medial compression of the forefoot. The areas between the toes, particularly the skin medial and lateral to the proximal interphalangeal joints of the second, third, and fourth toes, as well as that of the medial aspect of the fifth

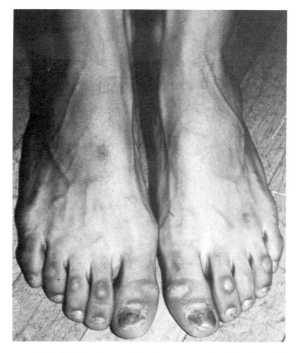

FIG. 13.15. The normal feet of a dancer showing areas of callus formation, padding over areas of tenderness, onycholysis, and, in particular, heavy callus formation over the first and second toes.

toe, may macerate if not allowed to dry. Soft corns form, which may become infected. Chronic pressure on the sides of the interphalangeal joints leads to osteophyte formation and contributes to localized pain and ulcer formation. Maceration of skin due to web space moisture may lead to abscess formation. The abscess is located deep within the web space. This develops over a period of months and may be accompanied by intermittent drainage. An MRI shows dense scar and sinogram demonstrates the sinus tract and abscess.

Painful soft corns are best treated with a felt or foam rubber "U"-shaped pad made from material that is 5 mm thick. These must be individually fashioned so that the base of the "U" of the pad lies distal to the corn and the legs extend dorsal and plantar to the painful area. The pad is taped between the toes.

Treatment of abscess formation is surgical incision and drainage through the dorsal web space, with excision of the sinus tract. Sutures are removed after 10 days. This is followed by barre exercises. Cultures are taken intraoperatively, and appropriate antibiotics administered. Surgical excision of osteophytes is not recommended unless conservative measures have failed. If this is necessary, however, a short longitudinal incision is made through the corn without excision of skin, the osteophyte is removed with a needle-nosed rongeur. Since the basic cause of ulcerations remains, that is, the design of the ballet and pointe shoes, the use of "U"-shaped pads or "donut" pads is mandatory to prevent recurrence after dancing is resumed.

PROBLEMS OF THE NAILS

Paronychia

Complaints about nails are common among dancers. Paronychia occurs frequently in the hallux, medially or laterally. Treatment of the mild condition includes soaking, elevation of the foot after class or rehearsal, and appropriate antibiotics. Padding the pointe shoe with lamb's wool is helpful. Surgical incision and drainage may require removal of a 5 mm portion of nail adjacent to the infected area, leaving the remaining nail to protect the hallux. The nail should not be removed entirely, since it is needed for protection of the hallux and may require a year to regrow. Destruction of the germinal area of the nail is likewise condemned, since the empty nail bed remains tender. After total removal of the nails, dancing *en pointe* may be impossible because of pain.

"Black Toe"

Chronic minor trauma to the hallux while in a shoe may lead to subungual hematoma. This is asymptomatic, but due to its chronic nature it appears quite dark beneath the nail. It requires no treatment.

Onycholysis

Onycholysis occurs transversely. The body weight is placed axially on the tuft of the hallux in the pointe shoe, bending the distal nail upward. This also causes the nail to delaminate. Dancers commonly lose portions of all their nails, with occasional subungual hematoma. Although not aesthetically pleasant in appearance, it is usually painless. Protection of the nail with several applications of clear nail polish helps limit cracking. The dancer should be cautioned against removing the nail.

Onychomycosis

Onychomycosis is difficult to treat. Oral griseofulvin for 1 year, a change of all footwear and stockings, and sterilizing bath facilities may fail to eradicate the infection. It can be controlled locally with clotrimazole (Lotrimin). All dancers should be taught good pedicure. Although this condition is annoying, it should not affect dancing.

THE ANKLE

Tendon Problems

Tendo Achilles

Dancers are particularly prone to develop tendinitis and tears of the tendo Achilles. Tendinitis occurs 3 cm above the insertion of the Achilles tendon into the calcaneus. This happens when beginning a new or different exercise or when returning to dancing after laying off. It occurs in both males and females, and is not causally associated with the ribbons of the ballet toe shoes which are wrapped about the ankle (27, 28).

Pain is noted on landing. Tenderness is present over a 5 cm section of the tendon, and may be associated with swelling and redness. A "leather bottle" crepitus may be present on palpation. Treatment consists of elevation, application of heat over the affected area, and nonsteroidal antiinflammatory medication. A 1-inch heel lift may be worn in street shoes. A warm-up period of active and passive stretching for 10 minutes is necessary. Tendinitis may represent microruptures of the tendon; one should look for a possible tendo Achilles rupture.

Pain at the insertion of the tendo Achilles occurs more commonly in dancers who have not yet completed their growth. The pain occurs during plié and on landing from a leap. This is due to partial avulsion of the tendo Achilles from the calcaneus. Roentgenograms are negative since the tendon inserts into the cartilaginous calcaneal apophysis. Tenderness on palpation at the Achilles insertion confirms the diagnosis, although this may also be associated with retrocalcaneal bursitis. Treatment is the same as for tendinitis.

Partial rupture at the medial musculotendinous junction of the gastrocnemius muscle occurs in the skeletally mature dancer. Symptoms are a sharp pain in the midposterior calf following a leap, with or without a palpable defect on palpation of the muscle. Dancing should cease for a week. The leg is splinted with the ankle plantar flexed. A 1-inch heel lift is used after splint removal. A rehabilitation program should be instituted as symptoms subside.

Complete rupture of the tendo Achilles may signal the end of a professional dancer's career. The injury is more common in males. The diagnosis is obvious with a palpable defect about 10 cm above the tendon insertion. Treatment consists of surgical repair by one of several methods (29–32). Cast immobilization for 6 weeks is required postoperatively, followed by a rehabilitation program. Prognosis is guarded for return of a principal dancer to the roles danced prior to injury. However, return to major roles following complete rupture of the Achilles tendon can occur. The self-motivation of such a performing artist should never be underestimated (6).

Medial Compartment Tendons

Tendinitis of the Tibialis Posterior and Flexor Hallucis Longus

Tendinitis of the long flexor tendons at the medial aspect of the ankle is common. It occurs most frequently in the flexor hallucis longus tendon (33–35). The primary symptom is posteromedial pain while *en pointe*, which may be exacerbated by attempts to raise the arch of the foot. Diagnosis of acute tendinitis of the tibialis posterior is made by palpating the tendon just behind the medial malleolus of the ankle and following the tibialis posterior tendon proximally while the dancer plantar flexes the ankle and inverts the foot. Tenderness is noted in a 5 cm area of tendon adjacent to the ankle. Treatment is symptomatic, with elevation, application of heat, and antiinflammatory medication.

The diagnosis of flexor hallucis longus tendinitis is made by palpating deeply 2 cm posterior to the medial malleolus just proximal to the tendo Achilles. As the dancer moves the ankle and hallux through a range of motion, pain is noted as the tendon slides beneath the palpating finger. Crepitus is common. Gradually increasing symptoms may be present for several weeks. Treatment consists of elevation and application of hot packs before dancing during periods of acute symptoms. Warm-up periods of 15 minutes to prevent further injury are indicated and NSAIDS are helpful.

Partial Rupture of the Flexor Hallucis Longus Tendon

"Trigger Toe." When a dancer begins to show triggering of the hallux, partial rupture of the flexor hallucis longus tendon should be suspected (16,36). It is characterized by the following: When the foot is in neutral position, the hallux can be

flexed at the metatarsophalangeal and interphalangeal joints with ease. As the foot is brought into plantar flexion, the ability to flex the toe is lost. In this position, the toe can be flexed passively, but not actively, by contraction of the flexor hallucis longus; a snap is noted in the posteromedial ankle when the toe finally flexes. The dancer is then unable to extend the interphalangeal and metatarsophalangeal joints of the hallux. Now, when the ankle is passively brought back to a neutral position, clawing of the hallux is apparent, caused by the tenodesis effect of the tethered flexor hallucis longus tendon in its tendon sheath (Fig. 13.16). Passive extension of the interphalangeal joint of the hallux produces a snap in the posteromedial region of the ankle, again with subsequent freeing of motion in the great toe.

If the tendon is palpated in the posteromedial compartment of the ankle 2 cm posterior to the medial malleolus and 1 cm above the calcaneus during the periods of flexion and extension of the hallux, a snapping sensation is felt.

At surgery, through a posteromedial curvilinear incision 6 cm in length, the neurocirculatory structures of the posteromedial compartment of the ankle are retracted anteriorly. The flexor hallucis longus tendon is identified by its muscle fibers lying deep and anterior to the tendo Achilles. A fusiform thickening in the tendon is observed in the portion distal to the retinaculum as it passes beneath the calcaneus. A longitudinal rent from 2 cm to 5 cm is usually found in the tendon (Fig. 13.17). The central fibers of the tendon rupture and contract, causing a thickening in the region of the contracted fibers and a narrowing just proximal to this fusiform enlargement. The retinaculum is divided, the thickening reduced by sciving the tendon down, and the tear of the tendon is repaired using 5-0 braided polyester suture. This allows the tendon to move freely. A splint is applied postoperatively, which is removed and active range of motion begun 2 weeks postoperatively. The dancer is permitted to return to dancing *en pointe* 3 months postoperatively, when strength has returned and pain abated.

Complete rupture of the flexor hallucis longus tendon has not been seen in the dancers. The nature of the partial tears in such that direct repair is preferred over tendon graft. The length of the flexor hallucis longus is not compromised by lengthening in partial tears. The nature of the tear is longitudinal, not transverse, indicating a degenerative disruption of tendon fascicles in continuity. Retraction and contracture of the muscle have not been observed.

Lateral Compartment Tendons

Tendinitis of the Peroneus Brevis and Peroneus Longus

Peroneal tendinitis is common among dancers. Tenderness is noted just behind the lateral malleolus and may extend several centimeters proximally in the lateral compartment. Occasionally, swelling is noted behind the lateral malleolus. Steps such as *relevé* cause aching. Inadequate warm-up and abnormal postures such as "rolling in" the foot contribute to the condition. Peroneus brevis tendinitis gives

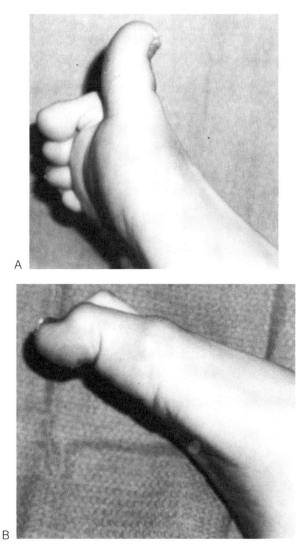

FIG. 13.16. A: Lateral view of the forefoot showing the great toe locked in extension with the foot pointed. B: Note the flexion at the interphalangeal joint when the foot and ankle are brought to neutral position. From Sammarco GJ, Miller EH, ref. 36, with permission.

symptoms along the tendon at and distal to the lateral malleolus. Partial rupture of this tendon is rare in dancers and is associated with chronic instability of the ankle (25). Treatment includes elevation of the feet and NSAIDS. There should be an extended warm-up period daily. Rehabilitation of the calf muscles to increase control of the ankle is aided with the use of the foot and ankle flexibility board or exercise board (Fig. 13.9). This is a roughly circular platform with hemispherical

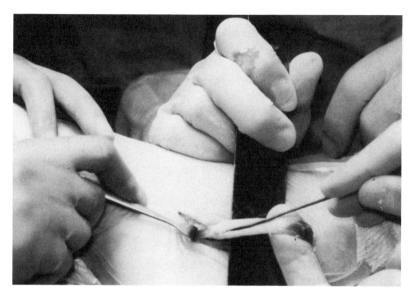

FIG. 13.17. The flexor hallucis longus is exposed in another dancer with a trigger toe. (The toes are to the left.) A probe has been passed into the longitudinal rent in the tendon, which may measure as long as 3 cm.

knobs of varying sizes in the center of the underside. It is placed on the floor and the dancer stands at the barre. The affected foot is placed in the center of the platform, and the dancer slowly rotates the foot from side to side and fore and aft, causing the platform to rise and fall in the desired direction.

Tendinitis of the peroneus longus occurs where the tendon turns beneath the cuboid bone. Pain may be exacerbated by *ronde de jambe*. There is tenderness at the lateral plantar border of the cuboid. X-rays are of no help and may cause confusion with a fracture if an os peronei is present in the tendon, or if the apophysis of the fifth metatarsal styloid is not closed. The differential diagnosis includes partial avulsion of the peroneus brevis tendon at its insertion onto fifth metatarsal, which also causes tenderness over the styloid process of the fifth metatarsal. A stress fracture of the cuboid should be ruled out by a bone scan. Treatment of peroneus longus tendinitis is similar to that of peroneus brevis tendinitis. Injection of corticosteroid preparation is mentioned only to be condemned.

Dislocation of the peroneal tendons at the lateral malleolus occurs during *relevè sur les pointes* and less commonly during *demi plié* or *grand plié*. Symptoms consist of a snap with a feeling of giving way at the lateral malleolus. Palpation during *relevé* confirms the diagnosis. Periosteal reaction may be present on x-ray over the lateral fibula.

Chronic recurrent dislocation requires surgical repair. The recommended procedure is through a posterolateral curved incision, avoiding the prominence of the lateral malleolus. The sural nerve is protected. The superior peroneal retinaculum is elevated from its attachment to the posterior fibula. The groove for the peroneal tendon is often shallow and is deepened with a gouge or burr. The retinaculum is then reattached to bone over the tendons through drill holes using 3-0 braided polyester suture. If disruption of the peroneus brevis tendon is present, it should be repaired (3). After closure, immobilization for 6 weeks in a weight-bearing cast is recommended. Discussion of the risks of surgery with the dancer is mandatory. Stiffness in the ankle may require 6 months to resolve. Bone block, or periosteal flaps, may permanently stiffen the ankle and are not recommended.

Synovitis of the Ankle

The most common symptom of synovitis is pain at the anterolateral and anteromedial tibiotalar joint line. Motion of the ankle joint at its extremes contributes to the symptoms by the compressive motion of the tibia and talar neck. Pain increases over weeks or months. The diagnosis is made by palpating between the medial malleolus and the tibialis anterior tendon or between the lateral malleolus and the extensor digitorum longus tendons. An effusion is not usually present. Anterolateral pain may be confused with anterior tibiofibular ligament strain (37,38). This differential diagnosis may also be made by injecting 3 ml of 1% lidocaine into the ankle joint. The pain of synovitis disappears, but pain from chronic ligament strain remains. Treatment consists of warm-up periods with slow stretching, use of the foot and ankle exercise board (Fig. 13.9), and NSAIDS along with wrapping of the ankle prior to dance class. If pointe dancing is to be performed, the ankle is plantar-flexed 10° prior to application of the wrap. The wrap consists of an elastic adhesive bandage applied in a figure eight manner about the foot and ankle.

Chronic synovitis may lead to loss of several months of dancing and may even end a career. Steroid injections into the ankle joint in a professional dancer may cause destruction of the articular cartilage. Arthroscopic synovectomy of the ankle is recommended if chronic symptoms do not abate with conservative treatment over several months. Postoperative recovery time is prolonged. Interruption of dance training for periods of up to 1 year has been used as an alternative to arthroscopy but is not recommended. The prognosis for returning to a dance career following chronic synovitis is guarded if dance is interrupted for a year.

Posterior Impingement (Os Trigonum) Syndrome

"Demi Pointe Impingement"

Impingement of the os trigonum is not uncommon. The os trigonum is an accessory bone at the posterior tip of the talus, present in 7.5% of the population. The talar dome and the posterior facet of the talus meet as the dancer stands in *demi pointe*. The posterior border of the tibia presses backward against the posterior talar tuberosity or os trigonum, forcing it against the calcaneus (39). This can become painful and arthritis may develop from the repeated trauma. If osteophytes on the bone grow, the resultant irritation causes pain at the posterior ankle joint. On palpation, tenderness is noted posterolaterally, deep to the peroneal tendons at the joint line. It may also be present posteromedially, confusing the diagnosis with flexor hallucis tendinitis.

The differential diagnosis of this condition includes tendinitis of the flexor hallucis longus, posterior tibial or Achilles tendons, trigger toe, peroneal tendinitis, and synovitis of the ankle. A lateral roentgenogram of the ankle joint may reveal the presence of an os trigonum with or without osteophyte formation. Fragmentation of the bone, a rotated position of the bone (Fig. 13.18), or a prominent posterior talar process may be visible.

Treatment includes warm-ups of the ankle joint and an elastic adhesive dressing to the ankle during class and rehearsals, along with NSAIDS. If symptoms do not abate or progressive fragmentation of the bone or osteophytes develop, steadily decreasing activity in dance may be a necessity. Excision of the bone or posterior talar prominence is then indicated. The 5 cm incision is made in the posteromedial aspect of the ankle behind the medial malleolus. Care is taken to retract the neuro-

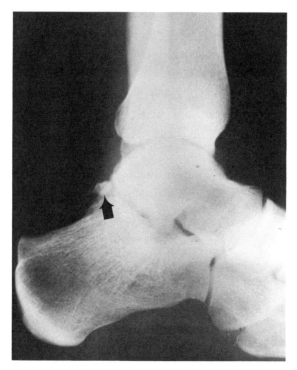

FIG. 13.18. Lateral roentgenogram of a dancer's ankle showing the os trigonum (*arrow*). Relief of symptoms may require surgical excision.

circulatory structures anteriorly. A posterior ankle arthrotomy is performed, and the posterior talar process or os trigonum is excised.

Postoperative healing and rehabilitation may take several months, and the dancer should be counseled accordingly.

Anterior Impingement Syndrome

"Plié Impingement"

During *demi plié*, the anterior distal tibia is pressed against the talar neck. The pressure between these bones and synovial irritation cause pain (40–42). In time, osteophytes form on the talar neck or tibia. The talar neck lesion should not be confused with a dorsal osteophyte, commonly seen in association with tarsal coalition. Pain and asymmetry in performing plié bring the problem to the dancer's attention. Treatment includes a stretching program and non-steroidal, anti-inflammatory medication. If symptoms persist, video arthroscopy of the ankle with excision of the offending osteophytes on either or both bones is indicated. As in all surgery, the dancer is counseled as to the time away from performing dance, which may be 3 months. A rehabilitation program is required postoperatively.

Ligament Injuries

Strains

Inversion injuries resulting from a "bad landing," sickling, or rolling out are accompanied by acute lateral swelling and tenderness, restriction of motion, and lateral pain. If an anterior drawer sign and talar tilt are present, a complete tear of the anterior talofibular and calcaneofibular ligaments may present a serious dance injury. Comparison with the uninjured ankle is necessary, however, as dancers often have lax ligaments without being symptomatic (Fig. 13.19). Roentgenograms may reveal a chip fracture of the fibula adjacent to the talus. In incomplete ligament ruptures, application of a short leg walking cast for 4 weeks is necessary, followed by a rigid ankle orthosis and a program of rehabilitation with water barre for at least 6 weeks. The dancer may not be able to return to dancing *en pointe* for a period of 2 months or more. Complete rupture of both the anterior talofibular ligament and calcaneofibular ligament may require open repair. Chronic lateral instability requires a reconstruction of the ligaments by several methods and up to 1 year for recovery. The younger the dancer, the better the prognosis.

Strain from eversion forces causes injury to the anterior portion of the deltoid ligament and may be associated with injury to the anterior tibiofibular ligament (see previous discussion of synovitis). Rapid turns *sur la pointe* or at $^3/_4$ pointe, as in *fouette*, are a common cause. In modern dance, rising from the floor while pushing

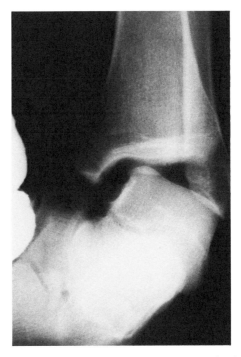

FIG. 13.19. Stress anteroposterior x-ray of ankle showing laxity of calcaneofibular ligament, talar tilt.

off from the medial side of the foot can also cause this injury. Symptoms may also occur from chronic forced dorsiflexion of the ankle. Proper warm-up and multiple rest periods to recover from fatigue are stressed. An elastic anklet gives some support, but strapping the ankle during rehearsal is recommended if vigorous dance steps are to be performed. Elevation of the feet at the end of the day, analgesics and NSAIDS, and an elastic bandage are all helpful.

Pain from ligament strain persists for several months. Most dancers tolerate this. However, occasionally a dancer may require a rehabilitation program including the water barre. If chronic instability requires surgical repair, recovery may be prolonged.

Ankle Fractures

Many factors contribute to the etiology of ankle fractures, including the hardness of the floor and the size, weight, age, and fatigue of the dancer. When a dancer is tired, timing is off and balance is poor. This is when fractures are likely to occur.

TABLE 13.1. *Flexibility program for the foot and ankle non-weight-bearing*

Do each exercise 10 times a day. Increase repetitions of each exercise by 5 each day, up to a total of 30 repetitons.
Do program 3 times daily.
Exercise slowly and do the maximum stretch.

1. Sit on floor with legs straight in front. Place a towel around the ball of the foot. Grasp both ends of the towel with hands and pull foot toward knee. Stretch to the count of 5. Release.

   Same as above except pull more with right hand to bring foot to the right, then pull with left hand to bring foot to the left.
   Repeat with the knee bent about 30°.

2. Sit on the floor with your legs straight out. Flex the foot upward toward your face and curl the toes under at the same time. Now point the foot downward and bring the toes up at the same time. The sequence is: Foot up, toes down, foot down, toes up.

   Sit on the floor with legs straight out in front, putting the foot flat against the wall. With heel and the ball of the foot flat against the wall, pull toes toward your face. Hold to count of 5, relax.

   Do the same exercise with the knee bent 30°.

3. Sit in chair with knee bent and foot flat on floor under knee. Keep heel and ball of foot on floor, raise toes. Keeping toes up, slide foot back a few inches, relax toes. Raise toes again and slide foot back a few more inches. Keep raising the toes and sliding foot back until you can no longer keep the heel on the floor while raising the toes. Bring the foot back out to starting position.

   Repeat from starting position; raise heel, keeping toes flat on the floor, then press down again. Lean upper body forward for increased stretch.

   Same position as above, slide foot forward as far as you can, keeping both the toes and heels in contact with the floor. At this point, keep the heel in place and knee straight. Flex foot up toward the knee, then point the foot and press toes onto the floor. Keep stretching and pointing the foot.

   Repeat from starting position, except keep toes curled as you stretch and point the foot.

4. Sitting with the knees parallel, foot flat on the floor, pull the inside edge of the foot toward you (supinate), keeping the outside edge on the floor. Hold to the count of 5. Flatten the foot, then bring the outside edge of the foot toward you (pronate), keeping the inside edge on the floor, including the big toe. Hold to the count of 5. Do not let the knee move during this exercise.

   Sitting with feet flat on floor, claw the toes and inch foot forward as toes claw, then release. Separate the toes between clawing. Inch out as far as possible, then slide back and start over.

5. Sitting with feet flat on the floor, raise the big toe, then the second, progressing to the little toe. Reverse and go from the little toe to the big toe.

   Sitting with feet flat, slightly lift heel, putting weight on the lateral borders of the feet. Roll from the little toe to the big toe, then back through the heel without letting the heel touch the floor. You are making a complete circle around the ball of the foot. Repeat and reverse.

Weight-bearing

1. Between two chairs, using them for support, stand with one foot 12 inches in front of the other, feet flat on floor. Rock forward onto the front foot, so that the weight is on this foot, leaving the back foot in contact with the floor, toes on the floor, heel lifted. Rock all the way back so that the front foot is on the heel and toes are pulled back. Change position of feet and repeat.

   Between two chairs, stand on the good leg, swing affected leg all the way back, knee flexed, foot pointed, then swing leg forward to an extended leg, foot and toes pulled toward you (dorsiflexed). Keep repeating.

2. With your back to the wall, feet directly under shoulders, weight evenly distributed, slowly bend knees and do not raise heels. Go to the point of maximum stretch and hold 5 counts, then rise up and repeat.

   Standing as above, at the bottom of the knee bend, roll onto the balls of the feet to the maximum arch, then roll down, then straighten legs. Repeat.

3. Standing on a step with feet parallel, heels hanging off the edge so that the calves are maximally stretched, pull all the way up onto the toes, slowly, then lower all the way down to maximum stretch. Repeat up to 10 times. Repeat with feet turned out, then turned in. Progress to using 5 lb to 10 lb ankle weights.

4. Standing with all the weight on one leg, keep the knee straight and raise to a fully arched foot, slowly, then lower down. Repeat up to 20 times.

   Standing with all the weight on one leg, bend knee and keep heel down, then straighten knee and pull up to a full arch. Slowly lower the heel, keeping knee straight. Repeat.

5. Standing, rock back on heels, claw toes; walk on heels and then walk with toes clawed around pencils.

   Walk on heels with 1 lb to 3 lb ankle weights wrapped around forefoot.

6. Standing, raise and lower the inner sides of feet with the toes clawed.

   Standing with feet parallel, on the balls of the feet, weight on the outer borders of the feet, knees about 4 inches apart. Roll the weight from fifth metatarsal to the big toe in a circular motion. The heels stay off the floor. Do this exercise with the feet turned in, then with feet turned out.

Eversion Fracture

"Fouette Fracture"

This fracture is caused by poor balance and fatigue when initiating a turn. It occurs in the "ankle of support."

Fracture of the fibula above the syndesmosis with rupture of the deltoid ligament and diastasis of the syndesmosis is produced by external rotational forces from such steps as *fouette*. Treatment of the fracture is anatomic reduction under general anesthesia: an image intensifier is helpful. If anatomic reduction cannot be achieved by closed methods, open reduction is indicated. Postoperatively, the ankle is placed in a cast in neutral postion for 4 weeks, followed by an orthosis permitting active range of motion and passive stretching. The prognosis is guarded for returning to professional dancing *en pointe*. The female dancer may return to dancing *sur la pointe*, but this may take as long as 2 years.

An epiphyseal fracture of the distal fibula may occur in the dancer who is skeletally immature. Closed reduction in a short leg, non-weight-bearing cast for 6 weeks is the treatment of choice. Because this injury occurs in younger dancers, prognosis is ultimately good, but return to full motion equal to that of the opposite ankle may take 1 year.

Inversion Fractures

"Emboite Fracture"

When the dancer inverts the foot and plantarflexes the ankle from fatigue or poor form, he or she is at risk of incurring an inversion fracture. The abnormal posture of sickling dance steps such as *emboite* or *saut de basque*, for which quick steps are required, predispose the dancer to such an injury. This fracture is more common in males.

Treatment of choice is closed anatomic reduction with plaster immobilization for 6 weeks, followed by a gradual increase in active and passive motion (Table 13.1). Dancing is permitted after 2 months. Prognosis is guarded for recovery of a full range of motion before 6 months. Nonunion of a small fragment may require surgical excision if symptoms warrant.

Fracture of the medial malleolus may also occur. If the dancer is skeletally immature, an epiphyseal fracture may result. Since it occurs in very young dancers, the complete recovery with only a slightly limited range of motion may be expected.

THE FOOT

Orthoses

The use of arch supports in treating dancers is important. The older dancer with the chronic deformities previously noted finds classes painful and fatiguing. A full-insole, semirigid support is recommended, with longitudinal medial arch elevation and metatarsal pad. Appropriate relief is obtained if these arch supports and pads are placed around painful areas such as the metatarsal heads or the hallux. These appliances are not recommended for professional dancers during dress rehearsal or performance. The use of arch supports while dancing stiffens the shoe and compromises foot flexibility, allowing the foot to slide within the shoe itself. In addition, the proprioceptive feedback mechanism in the foot-floor interface is lost, owing to the thickness of the orthosis.

CONCLUSION

While foot and ankle injuries may be devastating to professional dancers, in many cases they can be treated successfully and expeditiously, especially when diagnosed early. Conservative, meticulous therapy is essential, especially in this special group of patients because of the extraordinary demands they place upon their limbs. Fortunately, increased interest and writings about arts medicine have increased the awareness of performance injuries in the dance community. In addition to providing optimal therapy, physicians should make every effort to educate the dancers in their community, as well as company management. Clearly, increased knowledge decreases the likelihood of injury; prevention is still the best form of treatment.

REFERENCES

1. Como W. *Raoul Gelabert's anatomy for the dancer with exercises to improve technique and prevent injuries.* New York: Danad Publishing Co, Inc, 1964;51–57.
2. Frantz C, O'Rahilly R. Congenital skeletal limb deficiencies. *J Bone Joint Surg* 1964;43A:1202.
3. Teitz C, Harrington RM, Wiley H. Pressures on the foot in pointe shoes. *Foot and Ankle* 1985; 5:216–221.
4. Hardy RH, Clapham JC. Observations on hallux valgus. *J Bone Joint Surg* 1951; 33B:376.
5. Sammarco GJ, Miller EH. Forefoot conditions in dancers part I. *Foot and Ankle* 1982;3:85–92.
6. Thomasen E. *Diseases and Injuries of Ballet Dancers.* Denmark: Universitetsforhaget I Arhus Stiftsbogtrykkerie, 1982;29.
7. Ambre T, Nilsson BE. Degenerative changes in the first metatarsophalangeal joint of ballet dancers. *Aeta Orthopaedic Scand* 1978;49:317.
8. Howse AJA. Disorders of the great toe in dancers. *Clin in Sports Medicine* 1983;2(3):499–505.
9. Sammarco GJ, Burstein AH, Frankel VH. Biomechanics of the ankle; kinematic study. *Orthop Clin North Am* 1973;4:75.
10. Nikolic V, Zimmermann F. Functional changes of tarsal bones of ballet dancers. *Rad Med Fak Zagrebu* 1968;16:131.

11. Zimmerman B. Adaptation, function and injuries of the upper and lower foot joint in ballet dancers. *Arh Hig Rada Toksikol* 1970;21.
12. Sammarco GJ. Chapter 9. In: Jahss M, ed. *Disorders of the Foot*. Philadelphia: WB Saunders, 1982.
13. Collis WJM, Jayson MIV. Measurement of pedal pressures. *Ann Rheum Dis* 1972;31:217.
14. Miller EH, Schneider HJ, Bronson JL, McLain D. A new consideration in athletic injuries—the classical ballet dancer. *Clin Orthop* 1975; 111:181.
15. Micheli LS, Sohn RS, Solomon R. Stress fractures of the second metatarsal involving Lisfranc's joint in ballet dancers. *JBJS* 1985;67A:1372–1375.
16. Sammarco GJ. Chapter 42: Dance injuries. In: Nicholas J, Hershman E, eds. *The lower extremity and spine in sports medicine*, St. Louis: C.V. Mosby Co, 1986; 1406–1439.
17. Sammarco GJ, Miller EH. Forefoot conditions in dancers part I. *Foot and Ankle* 1982; 3:93–98.
18. Helal B, Wilson D, Sammarco GJ. The foot and ankle in dancers. In: *Foot surgery*, vol 2. London: Churchill-Livingston, 1988; 1007–1032.
19. Seals J. A study of dance surfaces. *Clin in Sports Medicine*, 1983; 2(3):557–561.
20. Seals J. Dance floors. *Med Probl Perform Art* 1986;1:81–84.
21. Laws K. Physics and the potential for dance injury. *Med Probl Perform Art* 1986; 1:73–79.
22. Liebler AW. Injuries of the foot in dancers. In: Bateman WB, ed. *Foot science*, Philadelphia: Saunders Co, 1976;284–287.
23. Sammarco GJ. Difficult diagnosis in dancers. *Clin Orth Rel Res* 1984;187:176.
24. Jones R. Fractures of the fifth metatarsal bone. *Liverpool Med Surg J* 1902;42:103.
25. Thomasen E. Chapter 9, The Loose Metatarsophalangeal Joint in Dancers. In: Chicago: Pleuribus Press, *Dance medicine: a comprehensive guide*, Ryan, Stephens, eds. Minneapolis: Physician and Sports Medicine, 1987; 135–138.
26. Sammarco GJ, DiRaimondo CV. Chronic peroneus brevis tendon lesions. *Foot and Ankle* 1989; 9:163–170.
27. Novere GD, Webb LX, Gristina AG, Vogel JM. Musculoskeletal injuries in theatrical dance students. *American Journal Sports Medicine* 1983;11:195–198.
28. Quirk R. Ballet injuries: The australian experience. *Clin in Sports Medicine* 1983; 3:509–514.
29. Lindholm A. A new method of operation in the subcutaneous rupture of the Achilles tendon. *Acta Chir Scand* 1959;117:261.
30. Lynn T. Repair of the torn Achilles tendon using the plantaris tendon as a reinforcing membrane. *J Bone Joint Surg* 1966;48A:268.
31. O'Donoghue DH. *Treatment of injuries to athletics*, 3rd ed. Philadelphia: W.B. Saunders Company, 1976;755.
32. Quigley TB, Scheller AD. Surgical repair of the ruptured Achilles tendon. *Am J Sports Med* 1980; 8:244.
33. Garth W. Flexor hallucis tendinitis in a ballet dancer. *JBJS* 1981;63A:1489.
34. Hamilton WG. Stenosing tenosynovitis of the flexor hallucis longus tendon and posterior impingement upon the os trigonum in ballet dancers. *Foot and Ankle* 1982;3:74–80.
35. Hamilton WG. Tendinitis about the ankle joint in classical ballet dancers. *Am J Sports Med* 1977; 5:84.
36. Sammarco GJ, Miller EH. Partial rupture of the flexor hallucis longus tendon in classical ballet dancers. *J Bone Joint Surg* 1979;61A:149.
37. Hamilton WG. Sprained ankles in dancers. *Foot and Ankle* 1982;3:99–102.
38. Hardaker WT Jr, Margello S, Goldner JL. Foot and ankle injuries in theatrical dancers. *Foot and Ankle* 1985;6:59–69.
39. Howse AJG. Posterior block of the ankle joint in dancers. *Foot and Ankle* 1982;3:81–84.
40. Kleiger B. Anterior tibiotalar impingement syndromes in dancers. *Foot and Ankle* 1982;3:69–73.
41. Quirk R. Talar compression syndrome in dancers. *Foot and Ankle* 1982;3:65–68.
42. Stoller SM, Hekmat F, Kleiger B. A comparative study of the frequency of anterior impingement. Exostoses of the ankle in dancers and non-dancers. *Foot and Ankle* 1984; 4:201–203.

Textbook of Performing Arts Medicine, edited
by R. T. Sataloff, A. Brandfonbrener, and
R. Lederman. Raven Press, Ltd.,
New York © 1991.

14

Reproductive Disorders in Female Dancers

Michelle P. Warren

*Department of Obstetrics and Gynecology and Medicine, at
St. Luke's-Roosevelt Hospital and Columbia College of Physicians and Surgeons,
New York, New York 10019*

Dancers who enter national companies as professionals start training at an early age, usually by 8 years or younger, and continue training during adolescence. Only 5% of those enrolled in a prestigious school for the study of ballet will eventually be accepted into a national ballet company. During this critical and stressful time, professional survival depends in part on conformity to the ideal body form needed to project the art (1). This ideal form is thin, ranging from 10% to 20% below ideal body weight (2). For those who have difficulty, particularly during the pubertal period, when weight gain is normal, dieting becomes a way of life. The extensive physical training which accompanies this dieting is associated with physiological changes and medical problems including delayed puberty, delayed menarche, and secondary amenorrhea (3).

The reproductive disorders which affect ballet dancers are similar to the problems which affect female athletes in general. Delayed menarche (age of menarche 14 years or older) occurs in 70% and secondary amenorrhea in 20% to 78% (2,4). Previous study has focused on a critical percent body fat hypothesis which was thought to be the key to puberty onset as well as secondary amenorrhea in this group (5). Although these reproductive disorders are tightly linked to low weight or body fat, causal mechanisms have not been established. The author studied professional ballet dancers with an aim to understanding the contributing environmental and genetic factors and the mechanisms of the hypothalamic dysfunction which occur in this setting. The study's hypothesis was that the reproductive disorders seen in dancers represent an adaptive response in susceptible individuals who maintain body weights below their ideal (6).

DELAYED MENARCHE

Delayed menarche in dancers has been well documented (5,7). The range in age for the first menstrual period is very variable but may be as late as 21 or 22 years, with an average of 15.4 (± 1.9) years (Fig. 14.1) (7). Dancers weigh much less than peers of the same age. Using menarche as a point of reference, dancers achieved a body weight and body fat usually associated with menarche and normal reproductive function well before (4 to 6 months) menarche actually occurred.

Our studies have shown the advancement of pubertal stages occurred during times of rest, suggesting evidence of a training and activity effect (Fig. 14.2). The training and activity effect was all the more impressive because of the rapidity of development during the periods of rest. Normal girls may take an average of 1.9 (± 0.95) years (mean ± SD) to progress from a Tanner breast stage two to stage four (8), whereas in some dancers, during nontraining, an extraordinary progression was noted in as little as 4 months (7). The progression of sexual development and the onset of menarche correlated in ten to fifteen subjects with a decrease in exercise and/or injury, causing forced rest of at least 2 months duration. During this interval, weight gain was minimal or absent, with no significant change in body composi-

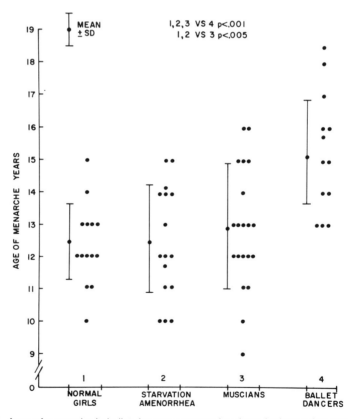

FIG. 14.1. Ages of menarche in ballet dancers compared to those in three other groups (from Warren MP, ref. 7, with permission).

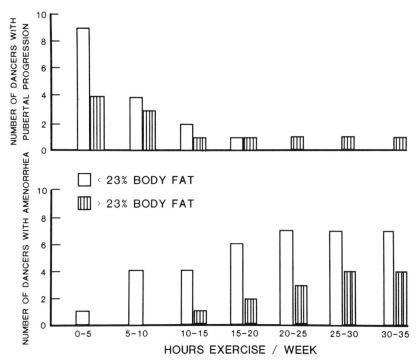

FIG. 14.2. Relationship of exercise to pubertal progression and amenorrhea in ballet dancers (pubertal progression defined as a change in Tanner stage for breast development or achievement of menarche). Cumulative data on 15 dancers over a 3-year period of study were accumulated on a quarterly basis. The exercise level for the preceding 4 months was averaged on a weekly basis. Differences in weight and body fat were calculated for each quarter preceding and during an event (pubertal progression or amenorrhea). Values did not differ significantly. The top part of the figure includes all dancers, including those who developed secondary amenorrhea (from Warren MP, ref. 7, with permission).

tion. The progression of puberty, as manifested by breast development and the onset of menarche, was also more evident in the leaner girls when activity decreased. Thus, ballet training during the adolescent years prolongs the prepubertal state and induces primary amenorrhea in dancers. Rest often leads to a striking "catch-up" in puberty. Although these effects are more notable in women of lower body weight or body fat, it is important to note that these individuals who are training heavily and eating marginally do not generally appear malnourished (7).

The author's study of ballet dancers (7) revealed another interesting abnormality. A remarkable dichotomy is noted in the order of pubertal development: Pubarche, or the development of body hair, is reached at a nearly normal age, but breast development and other estrogen-related factors are suppressed. The fairly normal pubarche and the remarkable delay in thelarche (breast development) in dancers suggests that the mechanism for pubic hair development was either not affected or, was possibly enhanced by the large caloric demands, whereas the mechanism affecting both breast development and menarche is definitely suppressed (7).

Bone age among dancers is delayed, and growth has been noted as late as 18 and 19 years old. Long-term effects of a delay in puberty on growth and development are not known. Skeletal measurements in our dancers suggest that the delay in menarche may influence long bone growth. The dancers were observed to have a decreased upper to lower body ratio and a significantly increased arm span compared to the female members of the family (7). Final heights (2 years post-menarche), however, did not differ. The prolonged hypogonadism (lack of sex hormone secretion) may favor long bone growth, leading to eunuchoidal (long extremities) proportions such as are seen in similar syndromes which are congenital (e.g., sexual immaturity due to lack of pituitary gonadotropic function). Nutritional deprivation may delay epiphyseal closure in the growth centers of the bones as seen in ballet dancers, although a change in skeletal proportions has not been reported on the basis of nutritional factors alone. The altered skeletal proportions may also be due to the fact that the ballet may be attracting girls with these physical characteristics; consequently, these children may represent a select group.

Other authors have suggested that the physical characteristics associated with later maturation in females are more suitable for successful athletic performance (9–12). Another study found that the women, as a group, with later menarche were more successful runners (13). Other studies indicate that gymnasts, runners, and other athletes may have characteristic physiques, suggesting a selective phenomenon (10,11,12); this may apply to ballet dancers as well.

The effects of inheritance on delayed puberty in dancers have also been studied. Since mother and daughter menarcheal age are closely related, Brooks-Gunn, et al. examined a group of dancers as well as a control group and their mothers (14). The dancer's menarcheal age was most influenced by leanness, rather than the mother's menarcheal age. While maternal menarcheal age was the best predictor of menarcheal age in the control sample, body mass (leanness) was the best predictor in dancers. Thus the delay in menarche was not due to genetic factors but rather to leanness, which appeared to be environmental. In examining the causes of leanness in dancers and comparing them to different athletic groups, the groups most apt to have delayed menarche (dancers and figure skaters versus swimmers) scored highest on measures of dieting behavior (15). Thus the leanness which is present in these groups is only partially genetically determined and is contributed to by food restrictions which are an important part of the dancer's behavior to maintain the slim image necessary for professional dance.

SECONDARY AMENORRHEA

Amenorrhea is common in dancers. As many as 78% of adult dancers and 50% of adolescent dancers (2) reported this condition, and the incidence of this problem is influenced by two variables: increased activity and low body weight. The condition can be reversed by reducing the amount of exercise or by a gain in weight.

The impressive temporal relationships between activity, weight, delay in menarche, and amenorrhea are exemplified in Fig. 14.3. The first dancer had her first mensus near her seventeenth birthday during a vacation interval. There was little change in weight or percent of body fat. She developed secondary amenorrhea but menses recurred on two occasions, associated with rest.

A second patient showed the same pattern, with menarche occurring during an interval of forced rest due to an injury at the age of 15. No change in body weight or calculated percent of body fat occurred. With resumption of dancing, however, amenorrhea recurred. Each dancer appears to have her own threshold, and this ties in with the observation that some subjects lose more weight than others before developing abnormalities (7).

A follow-up study of 16 formerly amenorrheic dancers found that resumption of menstruation was associated with a small increase in weight (16). Amenorrhea was again related to dieting and, in particular, the development of eating disorders. In a recent study, one third of a group of 55 dancers reported having had anorexia or bulimia; of the amenorrheic women, 50% acknowledged having had anorexia versus 13% among normally menstruating dancers. Amenorrhea was not related to current activity level or age at which training began, but was significantly related to dieting as measured by the EAT26 scale (Fig. 14.4) (2). The author's studies have also shown that those who do the most dieting are those who may not be genetically programmed to weigh so little, as evidenced by a direct correlation with obesity in the family and a high incidence of eating disorders. Further studies need to be done examining the effects of dieting on athletic amenorrhea, as recent work has suggested it may also be causal in other athletic disciplines.

MECHANISMS

The low gonadotropin secretion and the delay in bone age seen in ballet dancers suggest that the prepubertal state is prolonged. The clinical presentation of dancers differs from the typical constitutional delay of puberty, in that growth is only mildly suppressed, and adrenarche is not delayed (7). The gonadotropin pattern in those patients who developed amenorrhea appears to revert to the premenarcheal pattern, except that the suppression of luteinizing hormone (LH) is more marked than that of follicle-stimulating hormone (FSH) (7). This pattern is also typical of girls who become amenorrheic in the setting of weight loss and in severe nutritional deprivation such as anorexia nervosa (14,17–19). In particular, a reversion to the 24-h prepubertal pattern of gonadotropic secretion has been noted in these patients with weight loss associated amenorrhea or anorexia nervosa (20). The dietary restriction seen in girls who maintain low body weight while exercising heavily may cause a delay in puberty and an amenorrhea which is similar to that seen with dieting and weight loss. The etiology of amenorrhea associated with weight loss is not com-

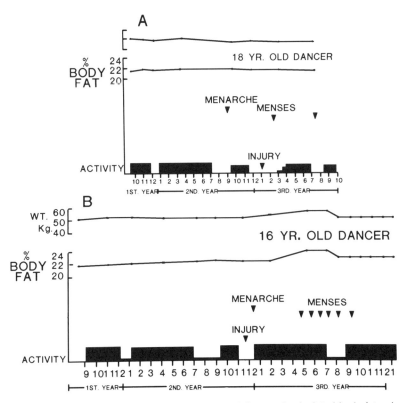

FIG. 14.3. Relationship among menses, exercise, weights, and calculated body fat values in two young ballet dancers (from Warren MP, ref. 7, with permission).

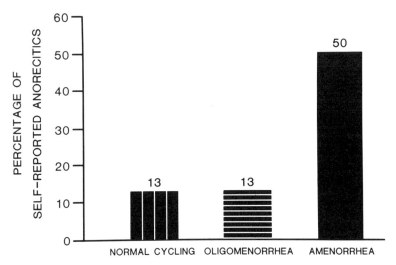

FIG. 14.4. Percentage of dancers with and without menstrual irregularities who reported anorexia nervosa (from Brooks-Gunn J, Warren MP, Hamilton L, ref. 2, with permission).

pletely understood, although diffuse hypothalamic abnormalities (17) have been reported, and a similar mechanism may be operative here (3).

Athletically induced reproductive dysfunctions may be related to eating disorders and dieting (2,21–23). The mechanism may be similar to the problem seen with weight loss. The cause of these dieting-induced menstrual disorders is purely speculative. However, the author and coworkers have hypothesized that a large amount of physical exercise not adequately compensated for by increased caloric intake in lean individuals leads to a form of energy conservation or a metabolic efficiency which is causally related to delayed menarche and secondary amenorrhea. Thus the reproductive disorders are adaptive in nature, similar to those seen with natural environmental stresses. A natural form of this problem occurs in the Kung bushman population, in whom ovulation occurs only at certain times of the year when food is plentiful and hunting activities restricted (24). Other studies have remarked on the small nutritional intake in competitive athletes with amenorrhea (21,22).

The effects of stress have been examined only superficially. Ballet dancers have a higher age of menarche than music students who are exposed to the same stresses of performing professionally (7). In addition, the level of competition is related to eating disorders and therefore amenorrhea, but this is probably due to more rigid standards for thinness in the national versus regional companies (1,4). The influence of stress as a causal factor is difficult to evaluate because of its subjectivity, but it is worthy of further research.

EFFECTS OF REPRODUCTIVE DISORDERS

Delayed menarche and secondary amenorrhea seen in dancers are reversible; their presence would be of no consequence if long-term effects were not present. Recent evidence suggests, however, that intervals of hypoestrogenism, even in young women, may lead to premature bone loss or a lack of bone accretion. The study presented by the author and others reported a high incidence of scoliosis (23%) and stress fractures (46%) in a group of female ballet dancers. Scoliosis was most prevalent in the dancers with delayed menarche. The incidence of stress fractures rose significantly with increasing menarcheal age ($p<0.01$). Scoliosis also rose with increasing menarcheal age ($p<0.05$) (Fig. 14.5) (25).

We have postulated that growth at adolescence may produce a fragile skeleton which is inadequately mineralized without sex hormone secretion. Hypoestrogenism may also delay maturation of osseous centers in the spine, with predisposition to vertebral instability and curvature.

Complications such as collapse of the femoral head resembling osteonecrosis in a 20-year-old dancer who had extreme skeletal delay have also been reported (26). Ongoing studies in dancers indicate that exercise increases bone density only in the presence of normal estrogen secretion, contrary to data reported in postmenopausal women. This may account for the high incidence of stress fractures in young exercising amenorrheic athletes and suggests that a relative osteopenia may exist in this group (27). Deficiency in the exercise-induced increase in bone mass in stressed bones of amenorrheic ballet dancers has also been identified. The lack of bone strengthening which usually occurs in this setting appears to lead to an increase in fracture rate, particularly in women with delayed menarche. This problem is of considerable importance to an exercising female population.

The metatarsal bone, which is especially stressed with exercise, was compared to another weight-bearing bone (spine) and a non-weight-bearing bone (forearm). The findings suggest that the bone most stressed by activity (metatarsal) is the most severely deficient (Table 14.1). The use of the toe shoe in ballet places stress on the metatarsal of the foot; these bones normally have a dramatic increase in cortical thickness. Thus, the bone represents a bioassay for stress-induced exercise effects. The normal dancers studied had a higher metatarsal density than other groups, while the amenorrheic dancers had the lowest. The spine shows similar trends, although the strengthening process was not as marked as in the foot (Fig. 14.3) (3).

Bone density is highly correlated to weight, and the decrease in bone density was significantly lower even when controlling for age for both spine and metatarsal of the foot. As a group, the dancers studied were significantly below their ideal weights. This suggests that the lowered weight itself may be abnormal and contribute to the overall problem.

Hypoestrogenic athletes who practice weight-bearing exercise also appear to be at risk for injury (25,28–32). Normal exercise-induced remodeling is deficient and is

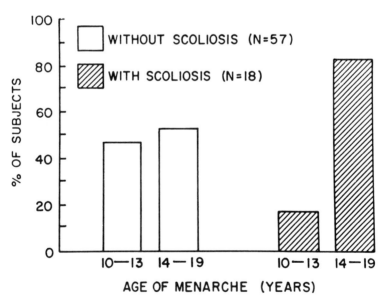

FIG. 14.5. Relation between age at menarche and scoliosis. Most of the subjects with scoliosis were 14 or older at menarche (83% versus 17%; $p < 0.04$) (from Warren MP, Brooks-Gunn J, Hamilton LH, Warren LF, Hamilton WG, ref. 25, with permission).

TABLE 14.1. *Bone mineral density*

	Dancers		Nondancers	
	normal(a)	amenorrheic(b)	normal(c)	amenorrheic(d)
Number	29	22	30	17
Spine[†]				
g/cm^2	1,283 ± .187	1.118 ± .105*	1.266 ± .134	1.154 ± .211*
(wt adjusted)		(*)		
Wrist[†]				
g/cm^2	.658 ± .066	.602 ± .089*	,662 ± .065	.651 ± .077
(wt adjusted)		(NS)		
Foot[†æ]				
g/cm^2	.900 ± .090[††Æ]	.799 ± .080*	.853 ± .111	.842 ± .114
(wt adjusted)	(Æ)	(*)		

Adapted from Warren et al., 1988
[æ]Dancer and amenorrhea interaction p<.04
[Æ]Foot bone mineral density higher than other 3 values
[†]Amenorrheics differ from controls ac vs. bd
[*]differ from their controls a vs. b and/or c vs. d
[††]differ from nondancer normals a vs. c

related to injury in the form of stress fractures, particularly in subjects with delayed menarche (12).

Ballet dancers have multiple reproductive disorders which appear to be due to environmental influence on the hypothalamic-pituitary axis. Secondary effects include changes in the skeleton which predispose the dancer to injury. These endocrine effects are important to the dancer's career and need to be evaluated more extensively. The ability of estrogen replacement to reverse these effects is the subject of ongoing research; the results are not yet known.

REFERENCES

1. Hamilton LH, Brooks-Gunn J, Warren MP. The impact of thinness and dieting on the professional ballet dancers. *The Canadian Association for Health, Physical Education and Recreation* 1986 July/Aug;31–35.
2. Brooks-Gunn J, Warren MP, Hamilton L. The relationship of eating disorders to amenorrhea in ballet dancers. *Med Sci Sports Exerc* 1987;19(1):41–44.
3. Warren MP, Brooks-Gunn J. Abstract. Amenorrhea in young dancers: evidence for a relative osteopenia in weight bearing bones. *Society for Gynecologic Investigation*, 36th Annual Meeting, San Diego, California, March 1989:404.
4. Hamilton LH, Brooks-Gunn J, Warren MP, Hamilton WG. The role of selectivity in the pathogenesis of eating disorders. *Med Sci Sports Exerc* 1988;20(6):560–565.
5. Frisch RE, Wyshak G, Vincent L. Delayed menarche and amenorrhea in ballet dancers. *N Engl J Med* 1980;303:17–19.
6. Warren MP. Reproductive function in the ballet dancer. In: Pirke KM, Wuttke W, Schweiger U, eds. *The menstrual cycle and its disorders. influences of nutrition, exercise, and neurotransmitters.* Springer-Verlag, 1989:161–180.
7. Warren MP. The effects of exercise on pubertal progression and reproductive function in girls. *J Clin Endocrinol Metab* 1980;51:1150–1157.
8. Marshall WA, Tanner JM. Variations in pattern of pubertal changes in girls. *Arch Dis Child* 1969;44:291–303.

9. Wakat DK, Sweeney KA, Rogol AD. Reproductive system function in women cross-country runners. *Med Sci Sports Exerc* 1982;14:263–269.

10. Sinning WE, Lindberg GD. Physical characteristics of college age women gymnasts. *Research Quarterly* 1972;43:226–234.

11. Wilmore JH, Brown CN, Davis JA. Body physique and composition of the female distance runner. *Ann NY Acad Sci* 1977;301:764–776.

12. Malina RM. Menarche in athletes: a synthesis and hypothesis. *Annals of Human Biology* 1983;10:1–24.

13. Feicht CB, Johnson TS, Martin BJ, Sparkes KE, Wagner WW Jr. Secondary amenorrhea in athletes. *Lancet* 1978;2:1145.

14. Brooks-Gunn J, Warren MP. Mother-daughter differences in menarcheal age in adolescent dancers and nondancers. *Annals of Human Biology* 1988;15(1):35–43.

15. Brooks-Gunn J, Burrow C, Warren MP. Attitudes toward eating and body weight in different groups of female athletes. *Int J Eating Disorders* 1988;7(6):749–757.

16. Warren MP. Effects of exercise and physical training on menarche. *Semin Reprod Endocrinol* 1985;3:17–26.

17. Vigersky RA, Anderson AE, Thompson RH, Loriaux DL. Hypothalamic dysfunction in secondary amenorrhea associated with simple weight loss. *N Engl J Med* 1977;297:1141–1145.

18. Warren MP, Jewelewicz R, Dyrenfurth I, Ans R, Khalaf S, Vande Wiele RL. The significance of weight loss in the evaluation of pituitary response to LHRH in women with secondary amenorrhea. *J Clin Endocrinol Metab* 1975;40:601–611.

19. Warren MP, Vande Wiele RL. Clinical and metabolic features of anorexia nervosa. *Amer J Obstet Gynecol* 1973;117:435–449.

20. Boyar RM, Katz J, Finkelstein JW, Kapen S, Weiner H, Weitzman ED, Hellman L. Anorexia nervosa: immaturity of the 24-hour luteinizing hormone secretory pattern. *N Engl J Med* 1972;291:861–865.

21. Deuster PA, Kyle SB, Moser PB, Vigersky RA, Singh A, Schoomaker EB. Nutritional intakes and status of highly trained amenorrheic and eumenorrheic women runners. *Fertility and Sterility* 1986;46:636–643.

22. Nelson ME, Fischer EC, Catsos PD, Meredith CN, Turksoy RN, Evans WJ. Diet and bone status in amenorrheic runners. *Amer J Clin Nutr* 1986;43:910–916.

23. Schwartz B, Cumming D, Riordan E, Seley M, Yen SSC, Rebar W. Exercise-associated amenorrhea: a distinct entity? *Amer J Obstet Gynecol* 1981;141:662–670.

24. Vander Walt LA, Wilmsen EN, Jenkins T. Unusual sex hormone patterns among desert dwelling hunter gatherers. *J Clin Endocrinol Metab* 1978;46:658–663.

25. Warren MP, Brooks-Gunn J, Hamilton LH, Warren LF, Hamilton WG. Scoliosis and fractures in young ballet dancers; relation to delayed menarche and secondary amenorrhea. *N Engl J Med* 1986;314:1348–1353.

26. Warren MP, Shane E, Lee MJ, Lindsay R, Dempster DW, Warren LF, Hamilton WG. Femoral head collapse associated with anorexia nervosa in a twenty-year-old ballet dancer. *Orthopedics and Related Research* 1990;251:171–176.

27. Warren MP, Brooks-Gunn J. Abstract. Menstrual delay in adolescent girls: its relation to premenopausal bone mineral density. 35th Annual Meeting, Society for Gynecol Invest 1988;444.

28. Lindberg JS, Fears WB, Hunt MM, Powell MR, Boll D, Wade CE. Exercise-induced amenorrhea and bone density. *Ann Intern Med* 1984;101:647–648.

29. Marcus R, Cann CE, Madvig P, et al. Menstrual function and bone mass in elite women distance runners. *Ann Intern Med* 1985;102:158–163.

30. Lloyd T, Buchanan JR, Bitzer S, Waldman CJ, Myers C, Ford BG. Interrelationships of diet, athletic activity, menstrual status and bone density in collegiate women. *Am J Clin Nutr* 1987;46:681–684.

31. Lloyd T, Triantafylloy SJ, Baker ER, et al. Women athletes with menstrual irregularity have increased musculoskeletal injuries. *Med Sci Sports Exerc* 1986;18(4):374–379.

32. Barrow GW, Saha S. Menstrual irregularity and stress fractures in collegiate female distance runners. *Am J Sports Med* 1988;16(3):209–216.

Textbook of Performing Arts Medicine, edited
by R. T. Sataloff, A. Brandfonbrener, and
R. Lederman. Raven Press, Ltd.,
New York © 1991.

15

Selected Legal Aspects of Medical Treatment of Performing Artists

Berle M. Schiller

*Partner, Astor, Weiss and Newman, Attorney at Law, Member, Disciplinary Board of the
Supreme Court of Pennsylvania, Philadelphia, Pennsylvania 19102*

Most new areas of medicine are accompanied by interesting legal obligations and questions, as well as by potential legal pitfalls. Arts medicine frequently involves the care of highly talented, publicly acclaimed individuals whose careers have enormous economic impact. The economic consequences of medical care extend far beyond the performer to affect agents, merchandising companies, theater or arena management, recording studios, film companies, and others. In most cases, experienced performers are represented by agents and attorneys and are familiar with their rights and recourse. Consequently, it is important for health care providers to be familiar with their legal obligations and potential problems which may arise from unsatisfactory fulfillment of those obligations.

MALPRACTICE

The phrase "medical malpractice" is a broad description which embraces all liability-producing conduct that ensues from negligently rendered medical care. The spectrum of this liability is vast, ranging from breaches of contracts that seek to guarantee a specific therapeutic result to intentional civil wrongs, accidental civil wrongs, the divulging of confidential information, and defamation. Due to the numerous and distinctive aspects of medical malpractice, it is necessary to dedicate this chapter to addressing only a few selected legal topics as they relate to the liability of the physician of the performing artist.

For the most part, one may describe medical malpractice as fault-based liability. However, the types of fault vary, and each possesses its own unique characteristics. Since a physician/patient relationship may be based on either a contract between the parties (contract basis) or an undertaking to perform (tort basis), medical malpractice liability can arise from a lawsuit based on tort, wrongful breach of contract, or

413

both. Consequently, the foremost question that arises with regard to medical malpractice concerns whether tort or contract law will govern the rights and liabilities of the parties.

Tort Liability

In most cases, a patient sues his or her doctor for failing to perform in accordance with the required standard of care. An example of tortious, medical malpractice may involve the case of a physician's services which are sought by a professional vocal artist who complains of a sore throat. If the doctor mistakenly prescribes an inordinately large dosage of medication and harms the entertainer's vocal cords, he or she may have committed the tort of negligence. In such an instance, regardless of whether or not the physician/patient relationship is in actuality based on a contract, the extent of a physician's malpractice liability is grounded on the extent of departure from the duty of care.

The duty of care is a widespread legal concept reflecting the uniform guideline for behavior, judged by objective criteria, of a *reasonable person* under similar circumstances (Restatement (Second) of Torts 2 §283, American Law Institute 1965 and Appendices 1988). In the medical profession, the standard of care is measured in terms of this fictional reasonable person, except in several respects, where doctors are held to a degree of care exceeding that of a reasonable person. First, doctors are expected to possess and exercise the skill and knowledge of their profession (or specialty) beyond that of a normal individual. Second, a doctor's negligent malpractice must usually be determined by comembers of the profession; that is, through expert testimony.

Contract Liability

A second category of malpractice cases comprises instances where a plaintiff relies on a contractual, rather than a tort, theory of recovery. Instead of charging deviation from due care, in such instances, the plaintiff alleges that the doctor breached an express warranty that he or she would accomplish a specific therapeutic result. For instance, this situation may occur when a doctor promises to the patient, a prominent model, that his radiation treatments will not leave a permanent scar. In the event that they do leave a scar, these statements may not constitute a malpractice action based solely on negligence, since treatment may been have properly performed. Rather, such a malpractice claim, contrary to that of tort, will be grounded on contract principles and the physician's failure to avoid leaving a permanent scar.

Judicial responses to such lawsuits have varied. In some jurisdictions, courts are reluctant to rule in favor of breach of contract medical malpractice claims. Considering the uncertainties which accompany the practice of medicine, those courts conclude that patients can never realistically expect a guaranteed, specific therapeutic result. Moreover, they consider that tort theories of recovery typically afford to most patients complete protection from negligence, so a contract theory of recovery is unnecessary. On the other hand, some jurisdictions do recognize such claims, acknowledging that the threat of liability serves to protect patients who were enticed to accept medical treatment by a doctor's unrealistic guarantee. *Guilmet vs. Campbell* [385 Mich.57,188 N.W.2d 601(1971)] represents a patient-oriented judicial solution. There, the patient recovered $50,000 in damages for breach of contract based on his recollection of his physician's alleged statements that the patient would be out of work for 4 weeks, at the most, that there was nothing at all to the operation, and that the patient could throw the pill box away.

A more restrictive approach is espoused by *Ferlito vs. Cecola* [419 So.2d 102(La.App. 1982)], which held that courts must scrutinize every alleged promise in each case to determine if it qualifies as a guarantee. Specifically, *Ferlito* commented that a dentist's statement that crowns would make his patient's teeth "pretty" neither constituted a guarantee nor negligence.

Yet another solution has been proposed by some state legislatures, which have enacted statutes requiring that contracts guaranteeing specific therapeutic results must be in writing to be enforceable. Since physicians are unlikely to furnish written warranties for treatment, such statutes render virtually obsolete breach of contract medical malpractice lawsuits.

PHYSICIAN–PATIENT RELATIONSHIP

A basic tenet of medical malpractice lawsuits is that no physician may be sued when either an injury occurs after the doctor has completed a procedurally correct surgery or no physician/patient relationship is present. Therefore, a paramount question to address in any medical malpractice lawsuit concerns whether a physician/patient relationship exists.

Usually, the physician/patient relationship and its accompanying rights and duties arise only following a patient's direct employment of a physician. As *Tvedt vs. Haugen* [70 N.D. 338, 294 N.W. 183, 132 A.L.R. 379 (1940)] espouses, "the relation between a physician and a patient is a consensual one wherein the patient knowingly seeks the assistance of the physician and the physician knowingly accepts him as a patient."

However, the physician/patient relationship may arise under alternative circumstances, such as when a doctor renders services for the benefit of the examinee. For instance, if an entertainer's employer hires a physician to physically examine the entertainer, and circumstances exist such that the patient has a right to believe that the information that he is telling the physician is necessary to the diagnosis of an illness and for its treatment, the relation of physician and patient exists. [see also *Rannard vs. Lockheed Aircraft Corporation*, 26 Cal.2d 149, 157 P.2d 1(1945), where the physician/patient relationship *did* arise after the doctor prescribed treatment pursuant to recommendations for a pre-employment physical examination.]

CONFIDENTIALITY

One of a doctor's obligations arising from the physician–patient relationship is the duty of confidentiality. This duty becomes essential for protecting a patient in an instance such as when a performing artist tells his or her physician explicit details of sexual history which the performer wishes to remain private.

The public policy advanced by the privilege of confidentiality aims to encourage patients to fully disclose details of their illnesses without fear of later divulgence by the physician in whom they have trusted and placed their confidence. Often, physician/patient privileges are statutorily defined, with state legislatures recognizing them only if a patient *manifests an intent* to refuse to disclose and prevent the disclosure of confidential communications with the physician.

The protection afforded to confidential communications is broad, and is generally liberally interpreted by the courts. In fact, once the physician/patient relationship is established, there arises a presumption that any information acquired in attending the patient is necessary for his treatment, is in the capacity of a physician/patient relationship, and is protected by the confidentiality privilege.

Nevertheless, a crucial element of confidentiality is the patient's manifested intent, either actual or presumed. Consequently, if a person other than the patient or physician was present at the time of the communication and his presence was not for the purpose of facilitating the physician's diagnosis or treatment, then his presence prevents the confidential privilege from attaching to the communication. The rationale for this rule stems from the logical inconsistency of assuming an intent by the patient to guard communications as privileged when the patient does not object to the presence of a third party.

Medical Evaluations for an Employer

When a physician performs a pre-employment physical examination on behalf of a prospective employer or makes an examination for a life insurance company, a court, or a party adverse to the examinee, the physician/patient relationship does not arise [*Metropolitan Life Insurance Company vs. Evans*, 183 Miss.859,184 So.426(1938)]. Consequently, under such circumstances, liability from the doctor to the performing artist for malpractice and breach of confidentiality may not ensue. Sometimes, an entertainer's personal physician will conduct the pre-employment physical examination. In such a case, the physician/patient relationship and its accompanying rights, duties, and privilege do arise between doctor and entertainer. Nevertheless, regardless of this relationship, the physician still owes certain duties, such as the obligation to disclose, to the entertainer's employer. For example, if a doctor, employed by a musician, discovers during the pre-employment examination that the patient is not physically fit for the job, the duty of confidentiality to the musician does not prevent the physician from disclosing the performer's ailment to the potential employer. Failure to properly disclose the sickness, on the contrary, may constitute a fraudulent misrepresentation, subjecting the doctor to potentially vast liability. This liability may even include damages for breach of the entertainer's employment contract. Therefore a doctor's duty of confidentiality to the patient is not always absolute.

Communications Among Physician's Nurses, Interns and Attendants

Aside from protected communications made by a patient to his physician, the physician/patient privilege also protects the communications spoken by the physician to the patient. That is, the patient can also forbid the disclosure of statements made by the doctor told during the treatment.

Consequently, a communication from physician to patient may pass through the ears of strangers along the way. Thus, most states have adopted a rule to protect such communications. That is, as long as the transmission of the communication stays within the "chain of professional communication" (i.e., among physicians, nurses, interns, attendants, etc.), it retains its privileged character.

Waiver; Relevance in Reports Disclosed Following Waiver

The physician/patient privilege may be waived by the filing of a personal injury action, allowing the disclosure of previously confidential information. However, this waiver affects only information concerning the plaintiff's health and medical history causally relevant to matters that the plaintiff placed in issue by the litigation.

For example, testimony on behalf of a plaintiff-performer in a medical malpractice action against his physician operates as a waiver of the privilege and forbids the performing artist to prevent the physician from testifying. Nevertheless, the physician may disclose information only during procedurally correct and formal discovery proceedings. A physician may not conduct private interviews without his patient's expressed consent.

DIAGNOSIS

There are numerous prongs to diagnosis-related liability. For one, obtaining an appropriate medical history is a crucial requirement to the process of diagnosis. Additionally, failure to ask the patient correct questions and pursue suspicions may constitute an unjustifiable deviation from the standard of care. One must also keep in mind that the information received by a physician while taking a patient history remains privileged and confidential.

Most often, lack of skill or care in diagnosis arises from failure to perform or order appropriate tests. If a doctor fails to conduct a test or perform an examination and there is competent evidence that other skilled doctors in similar circumstances would employ such tests, the doctor has departed from the standard of care and is negligent.

Finally, upon completion of the examination, a physician must provide to the patient an accurate report. Failure to do so constitutes negligence. It is in this area of malpractice law where physicians of performing artists face considerable liability. For instance, a case may occur where a prominent musician approaches a physician, seeking plastic surgery for a scarred neck or a nose operation. A physician who fails to fully inform the patient of the possible side effects that plastic surgery may have on performing ability such as singing or playing the oboe takes the great chance of exposing himself to liability in the event that foreseeable side effects do occur. Similarly, singers who possess voices with distinctive qualities, e.g., raspiness, often complain to their physicians about throat pain. In such cases, each physician must explain any potential adverse effects that a medication or treatment may have on the patient's distinctive voice. If a patient consents to certain treatment but such consent is uninformed because of inadequate disclosure by the physician, the physician may be liable for the tort of negligence.

NEGLIGENT REFERRAL

Barring an emergency, a doctor is expected to consult with a specialist, if available, under the following circumstances: in doubtful or difficult cases, e.g., if the physician knows the treatment is not going well [*Rahn vs. United States*, 222 F.Supp.775(S.D.Ga.1963)], if a patient requests a referral, or if it appears that a referral would improve the quality of the patient's care. Consequently, the inflated ego of a doctor who treats a performing artist and fails to recognize his or her own professional limitations may in the end expose the physician to considerable liability.

A physician is negligent for failing to refer a patient, and also is negligent for referring a patient who is known to be in need of a particular kind of care to a physician who cannot provide it [*Rise vs. United States*, 630 F.2d1068(5th Cir.Ga. 1981).]

However, a prerequisite of negligent referral is that the doctor discovered or should have discovered that the patient's ailment exceeded his ability to treat with a reasonable degree of success. This requirement marks a significant limitation on a doctor's liability for negligent referral; that is, if a doctor is ignorant of a performing artist's ailment because it is a latent, uncommon throat disease, he may escape liability if such ignorance was reasonable.

Finally, if the patient's condition is one which the doctor is competent to treat, his mere failure to reach an early diagnosis, if reasonable, is not negligence. However, if he had contracted with the performer for specific therapeutic results, he may still incur liability for breach of contract.

BEST MEDICAL TREATMENT

In addition to complying with the requisite professional standard of conduct, a doctor must exercise his or her best judgment when he or she knows the prevailing medical practice will have an adverse effect on the patient [*Toth vs. Comm. Hosp. at Glen Cove*, 22 NY.2d 255,263,292 NYS.2d 440,447–8,239 NE.2d 368,373 (1968)], stated:

> If a physician fails to employ his expertise or best judgment . . . he should not automatically be freed from liability because in fact he adhered to acceptable practice . . . (A) physician should use his best judgment and whatever superior knowledge, skill, and intelligence he has.

A controversial situation may arise in the event that a professional vocalist's singing is damaging his or her voice, yet the singer is a highly popular and successful artist. In such a case, should a physician advise the patient to abandon the lucrative profession?

Such a dilemma usually accompanies the best judgment rule, especially in the event that the recognized professional standards to which a practitioner must adhere conflicts with a doctor's best judgment. In such a case, a physician choosing to follow his or her best judgment may be subject to liability for violating the standard of care. Thus, the requirement of best judgment is probably limited to circumstances where either the indicated course of treatment adds no appreciable risk to the patient or the treatment was approved by a reasonable segment of the profession. Therefore, a doctor's best judgment, if reasonable, will not endanger him with malpractice liability.

DAMAGES

Tort Damages

Generally, in tort malpractice actions, a court may hold a physician liable for the following items. In addition to recovering for pecuniary harms such as past and future medical expenses and loss of earning capacity, a patient may recover for pain, suffering, and mental distress. A court can even award punitive damages when a physician's misconduct was sufficiently egregious, as evident from a defendent's evil motive or his reckless indifference to the patient's rights [Restatement of Torts §908(2)].

Contract Damages

When a medical malpractice claim is based on breach of contract, the measure of damages may vary. *Sullivan vs. O'Connor*, [363 Mass.579,296 N.E.2d 183(1973)] a case involving a suit by a performing artist against her physician, identified three alternative measures of damages for breach of contract. The first measure of damages, an expectancy interest, compensates the patient for losing just that—the performance which she expected of the physician. So if an actress expected yet did not receive an attractive nose from plastic surgery, expectation damages will award to her the worth of an attractive nose. This measure of damages however, if often very difficult to calculate, since attractiveness is an extremely subjective term. Therefore, the injured patient usually fails to meet the burden of proving damages with sufficient certainty.

A second theory of recovery is a reliance interest; that is, compensating the patient for costs expended in anticipation of the contract. Finally, a third measure of recovery is restitution interest, which refunds the patient's medical expenses and effectively places the patient into the position in which he or she would be had there existed no contract. So if the surgery cost $4,000, the patient recovers $4,000. Of course, a performing artist will endeavor to recover the highest measure of damages which can be proven with reasonable certainty.

One final limitation on contract recovery is that of mitigation. A patient-performer must attempt to avoid any costs that are within his or her control. The performer cannot recover for speculative harm. A patient-entertainer must prove the calculation of lost value with sufficient evidence (probably with testimony provided by experts such as producers and management specialists), and the performer may not recover for injuries which were preventable by actions that reason dictates a plaintiff to take. The rule of mitigation is not a defense to the existence of a tort or contract cause of action. It applies only to the diminution of damages, denying recovery to a plaintiff for the portion of her loss that could be avoided by her reasonable efforts. Therefore, if a doctor injures a performing artist, causing loss of a job, the damages for loss of employment are limited to the present value of the money that would have been earned under the original contract, less that which he or she has earned and can reasonably be expected to earn during the unexpired term of the contract.

CONCLUSION

Medical treatment of performing artists can be a legal minefield for the treating physician. Breaching confidentiality by talking about a famous performer who has just sought medical care is a particularly common error. In some cases, prescribing rest and abstinence from performance seems conservative, but if not really necessary, such prescription may cause substantial monetary loss and liability to the physician. It is generally advisable for doctors to initiate and maintain early contact with their attorneys whenever a questionable situation arises.

Subject Index

Gender differences, *see* Sex differences
Genius, *See* Prodigies
Giant cell arteritis, 135
Glare, 291–292
Glossodynia, 134–135
Glossopharyngeal neuralgia, 133
Glottal efficiency, 251–252
Glottal impedance, 253
Gonadotropins, 409
Graffman, Gary, 40
Grand plié, 370,373
Guillain-Barré syndrome, 183
Guilmet vs. Campbell, 415
Guitar picks, 49
Guitarists, 48–49
Gum chewing, 158–159

H

Herpes viruses
  brass players, 55
  voice effects, 235
Hi-Notes, 13
High radial nerve compression, 210
  High school musicians, 26
Hoarseness, 234
Homosexuality, 333–334
Hormones, voice problems, 241–242
Hot-wire anemometer, 253
Hyperabduction position, 187
Hyperextensible joints, 63–64
Hyperkinetic dysarthria, 260
Hypermobility, 63,85–93
  biochemical defects, 90
  follow-up, 92
  medical needs, 62–64,92–93
  point system, 87–90
  prevalence, 85–86
  temporomandibular joint, 118,132
  treatment, 92–93
Hyperopia, 287–289
Hypnosis, 358
Hypoestrogenism, 409–411
Hypogonadism, dancers, 406–411
Hypopharyngeal dilatation, 53
Hypothyroidism, 241

I

Idiopathic condylolysis, 131
Idiopathic epilepsy, 176
Idiopathic facial paralysis, 181

Idiopathic toothache, 134
"Idiot savant," 173
Imaging methods, 122–124
Immobilization therapy, 161,208
Impingement syndrome, 81–82
Implant arthroplasty, 222
Incidence, 16
Inderal, 10,180,325,356
Index Medicus, 4
Indirect laryngoscopy, 6
Inhalers, 268
Inner ear, 302,305–306
Instrument choice, 327–328
Instrumentalist, 7
Intelligence, 339–340
Interdigital neuroma, 380
Internal locus of control, 361
International Arts Medicine Association,
  14
International Conference of Symphony
    and Opera Musicians, 13
  survey of 15,26–27,31,156,320
International Musician, 13
International Trumpet Guild Newsletter,
  9
Interphalangeal joints
  dancers, 385–386
  osteoarthritis, 97
  triggering point, 216
Intraoral appliances, 160–161
Intraoral pressure, 148
Intratracheal pressure, 253
Inverse pressure theory, 232
Inversion fractures, 400

J

Jazz musicians, 17
Jazz pianists, 40–41
Joint laxity, 62–64; *see also*
    Hypermobility
*Journal of the American Medical
    Association*, 10
Journal of Voice, 6,16
Juvenile rheumatoid arthritis,
    101–103,131

K

Keyboard instruments
  choice of, personality, 327–328
  injury etiology, 37–41

Warm-up exercises (*contd.*)
  evidence for value, 66
  and musculoskeletal injury, 73–74
Weight change, 239–240
Wind instrumentalists
  cardiovascular aspects, 52–54
  dental problems, 5,136–157
  injury etiology, 52–58
  pulmonary aspects, 52–54
  temporomandibular joint, 127,136–157
Wind instruments, mouthpiece, 139–140
"Wobble board," 378
Woodwind players
  injury etiology, 56–58
  pulmonary function, 52–53
  temporomandibular joint, 57,127,
      136–157

Woodwinds, mouthpiece, 139–140
Worker's compensation, 314–315
Wrist position, pianists, 39
Writer's cramp, 193

X
Xanax, 180,325
Xomed injection, 273

Y
Yergason's sign, 82–83

Z
Zyderm Collagen injection, 273